# *Understanding*
# NURSING RESEARCH:

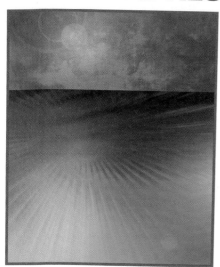

## Reading and
## Using Research
## in Practice

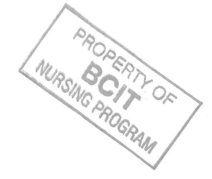

# *Understanding*
# NURSING RESEARCH:

## Reading and Using Research in Practice

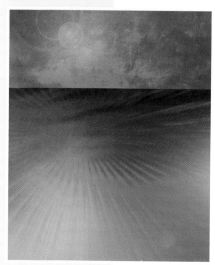

## CAROL L. MACNEE, RN, PHD
**Director of Research and Professor**
East Tennessee State University College of Nursing
Johnson City, Tennessee

LIPPINCOTT WILLIAMS & WILKINS
A **Wolters Kluwer** Company

Philadelphia • Baltimore • New York • London
Buenos Aires • Hong Kong • Sydney • Tokyo

*Acquisitions Editor:* Margaret Zuccarini
*Managing Editor:* Joseph Morita
*Editorial Assistant:* Carol DeVault
*Production Editor:* Danielle Litka
*Senior Production Manager:* Helen Ewan
*Art Director:* Doug Smock
*Manufacturing Manager:* William Alberti
*Indexer:* Ellen Brennan
*Compositor:* Peirce Graphic Services
*Printer:* R.R. Donnelley-Crawfordsville

9  8  7  6  5  4  3  2  1

*Library of Congress Cataloging-in-Publication Data*

Macnee, Carol L. (Carol Leslie)
  Understanding nursing research : reading & using research in practice / Carol L. Macnee.
    p. ; cm.
  Includes bibliographical references and index.
  ISBN 0-7817-4271-4 (alk. paper)
  1. Nursing—Research. I. Title.
  [DNLM: 1. Nursing Research. WY 20.5 M169u 2003]
  RT81.5.M235 2003

                                                          2003047626

# Preface

I have always loved research and the research process. Nonetheless I earned a B in my first formal research course, and was somewhat discouraged at the conclusion of that undergraduate class. Since then I have completed many research courses, conducted a number of research studies, and taught research to students at the undergraduate and graduate levels. I still love research, but as I have taught the subject I have frequently been frustrated in my seeming inability to effectively communicate that enthusiasm to my students, particularly undergraduates.

As I have considered what it was about undergraduate research courses that left students disinterested and even phobic about research, I have concluded that the problem lies in our tendency to teach as if students were going to implement research, rather than use research in their practice. This has led to my shifting my perspective from what knowledge is needed to implement research, to what a nurse needs to know to use research in practice. That in turn led to the idea for this book.

This book differs from existing undergraduate research textbooks in a number of ways. The premise of this book is that nursing students need to understand the language of research and the underlying concepts in the research process, but not necessarily be prepared to conduct a research study. The second premise is that nursing students and practicing baccalaureate-prepared nurses are motivated to read and use research only as it relates to their practice. Given these two premises, it becomes logical that many nursing students and nurses read only the abstract and the conclusion sections of research reports. Those two sections usually contain the least amount of technical language of research and will most directly address the clinical meaning of a research study, and so they are viewed as both understandable and useful for practice. Therefore, this book is organized around the sections of a research report rather than the steps of the research process, and it starts at the end of the report—the conclusions—and moves forward to the beginning to help the student recognize the relevance of each section of the research report for understanding and using research in practice. Five questions that a nurse might ask when reading research are used to organize the text, and throughout the chapters the emphasis is on reading, understanding, and using research. In keeping with this emphasis on using research in practice, each chapter of the book begins with a clinical vignette that ends with the nurse seeking information about a clinical question from the research literature. One or two published research articles that directly relate to the vignette are identified and are used throughout the chapter for specific examples of the concepts addressed in that chapter. The published research articles are all provided in the appendices, and on our Connection Web site.

It is a challenge to represent the breadth and depth of nursing practice and nursing research in a single textbook. A real effort has been made to include vignettes that reflect nursing practice in a variety of settings ranging from acute care to public health, and across a range of specialties. In addition, articles used as exemplars in the chapters were selected to reflect the common quantitative and qualitative research methods used in nursing research. This text differs from other undergraduate research texts in yet another way because it addresses both qualitative and quantitative research in almost every chapter. As nursing evolves as a science, we have recognized the need for use of methods from both the positivist and naturalist views to develop knowledge that reflects our holistic perspective. Both qualitative and quantitative methods are used to build knowledge in nursing, and rather than artificially separate the discussion of these two approaches, this book contrasts the approaches while identifying the broader conceptual base that is common to both. However, recognizing that combining quantitative and qualitative methods in each chapter may at times be confusing, content specific to each method has been clearly identified using icons that clearly identify the method being described within a paragraph.

Lastly, recognizing that learners learn best by doing, each chapter of this book ends with a specific learning activity that prepares students for the concepts addressed in the following chapter. The learning activities are discussed in the following chapter and are directly related to the examples and the vignette in the chapter. To provide an opportunity for students to be active learners, an in-class questionnaire that can be used as a mini-research study is included in the appendices, and a fictional article that could have been based on results from the in-class questionnaire also is provided. This fictional article intentionally contains flaws that are slightly more glaring than one is likely to find in any published peer-reviewed research report. This fictional article is used throughout the text as an example along with the real published research reports.

The goal of this text is that students finish it feeling able to read and intelligently understand published research to use it in practice. Associated with this goal is the hope that students will develop and maintain a real interest in research rather than a desire to avoid it at all costs. The text is designed to be friendly, taking a somewhat casual tone in order to minimize the already intimidating nature of the language and concepts of research. To increase the usefulness of the text, the glossary at the back of the book is printed leaving space for students to add their own notes about different research terms, and each term is indexed within the glossary itself for easy reference. The mark of a really good textbook is that it is one that students decide to keep so they can use it in the future, rather than sell it after they complete their course. I hope this will be one of those textbooks.

I believe that learning to understand and use published research can be fun and interesting for students if they can see the direct relevance to their practice. The organization of this book is unconventional and the tone conversational to address the subject of research from the perspective of a reader and user rather than a creator of research. Students tell me this is a helpful perspective that they enjoy. As a nurse researcher, it is always my greatest hope to foster an appreciation and enthusiasm for the process that I find so challenging and meaningful. I hope this text contributes to accomplishing that goal.

# *How to Use* UNDERSTANDING NURSING RESEARCH:

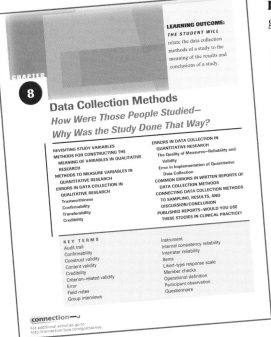

**LEARNING OUTCOMES** let students know what they're going to learn in each and every chapter.

**KEY TERMS** are listed at the beginning of every chapter and bolded in the text; this helps students stay focused on important topics.

**CLINICAL CASES** at the beginning of each chapter help the student think about a specific situation where research can be used in practice.

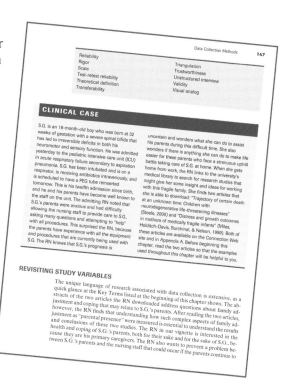

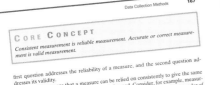

Data Collection Methods     **167**

CORE CONCEPT

*Consistent measurement is reliable measurement. Accurate or correct measurement is valid measurement.*

first question addresses the reliability of a measure, and the second question addresses its validity.

**Reliability** means that a measure can be relied on consistently to give the same result if the aspect being measured has not changed. Consider, for example, measuring the gender of a sample: if three independent observers each record the gender of 1000 adults as they individually walk into a room, there will be a quite high level of consistency in the final count of the numbers of men and women in the sample. However, if even five or six of the sample are androgynous in their appearance, there may be some small differences in the final counts provided by the three observers. We have already said that this leads to some small error in the measure. If we changed our sample to 1000 diapered infants all dressed in white, we would expect much more inconsistency in the final totals, because gender identification of infants by observation is much more difficult to do consistently. If, instead, three laboratories conducted genetic testing of each of the 1000 infants, there should be no differences in the final totals for boy and girls (assuming no laboratory error). Thus, the data collection on gender (particularly for infants) using the method of observation is less reliable than the data collection on gender using the method of genetic testing.

The reliability of a measure becomes more difficult to ensure as the measurement process becomes more complicated, because complexity allows for more opportunities for error through inconsistency. Several approaches are taken to ensure or examine the reliability of measurement in quantitative research, depending on the type of measurement being used. When data are being collected by observation, a researcher often trains the observers and then tests them with different cases, until all the observers agree on their observations the majority of the time.

The maternal distress study provides a good example of this when it describes the use of the HOME scale. The authors tell us that the "HOME was administered by three observers who were trained by an experienced HOME tester until they had a minimum interrater reliability of 95%" (Miles et al., 1999, p. 132).

In other words, the observers practiced making the observations needed to obtain a score on the HOME scale until they each reached the same score at least 95% of the time. The authors also tell us that "the interrater reliabilities for the data collectors averaged 97%" (Miles et al., 1999, p. 132). **Interrater reliability** is present when two or more independent data collectors agree in the results of their data collection process. In the case of the HOME scale when the three independent observers collected data from the families in the study, they agreed an average of 97% of the time. By providing this information, the authors help the RN in our vignette to know that this complicated procedure to get a measurement of parental competence was used consistently across the different families. That consistency in use decreases the chances that any differences between families were due to inconsistent

---

**CORE CONCEPTS** highlight essential information for the student.

---

**QUALITATIVE AND QUANTITATIVE ICONS** help students differentiate between these two important, but sometimes confusing, concepts.

---

be perceived as interfering with S.G.'s nursing care. She knows that these parents have dealt with S.G.'s being so ill in the past, so she believes that the current problem is not a lack of understanding or unfamiliarity with the ICU, but rather what this most recent health crisis means to these parents. With a desire to work with S.G. and his parents in mind, the RN begins to read about the data collection in the two studies she has found.

To examine the measurement approaches taken, the RN first has to identify the variables in each study. We discussed variables in Chapters 4 and 5, defining them as some aspect of interest that differs in different groups or situations. Both qualitative and quantitative studies have variables, but only quantitative studies use the categories of independent and dependent variables. Independent variables are those factors in the study that are used to explain or predict the outcome of interest and also are sometimes called predictor variables, because they are used to predict the dependent variable. In the article the RN found about maternal distress, the authors write of predictor variables rather than independent variables. Dependent variables are the variables that depend on other variables in a study or are the outcome variables of interest. The maternal distress article refers to the dependent variables as outcome variables.

The variables studied in both articles on family adjustment to severely ill children are listed in Table 8–1. The article about trajectory of certain death describes a qualitative study that has three variables: (1) families' perceptions and experiences living with a child who has a neurodegenerative life-threatening illness (NLTI), (2) impact on family of living with a child with an NLTI, and (3) factors that influence family care of a child with an NLTI. The study reported in the maternal distress article addressed distress and growth as the two outcomes of interest and examined maternal attitudes, maternal role attainment, child-illness characteristics, and maternal illness-related distress as predictor variables.

QUALITATIVE

Before we continue, let's look at how we determine the variables in a study. Although it is logical that variables differ across groups or situations, many research reports will not explicitly identify the study variables. For example, the trajectory of certain death article never specifically lists the variables studied, as is done in Table 8–1. The variables for a study obviously should reflect the topic of interest, which, in turn, should be described in the purpose, background, and research questions for a study. Because a qualitative study usually begins with one or more broad questions and uses open-ended approaches to collecting data, the variables of interest often are identified within the research questions. The study variables are not mentioned in the data collection and analysis section of the trajectory of certain death article, only the methods used for that study. The RN in our vignette, therefore, had to read the previous section of the report that described the specific aims of the study to identify clearly the variables under study.

QUANTITATIVE

In contrast, reports of quantitative studies should clearly describe the variables included in the study, even if they are not explicitly labeled as such, because the data collection methods in quantitative research are specifically aimed at measuring the variables in the study as objectively as possible.

of certain death article, the RN is comfortable that the experiences described in that article are credible and transferable to S.G.'s parents' experiences. The researcher developed a trusting relationship with the families, used several methods to triangulate the data, used member checks to ensure credibility, and systematically analyzed the data to generate the dimensions described in the findings of the study, thus ensuring confirmability. The RN is comfortable that the results of this study will help her understand the crisis S.G.'s parents are probably facing falling off their plateau with S.G. However, the RN is not sure why the researcher chose to use a method called grounded theory for collection of the data or why children with NLTI were specifically targeted for data collection. To answer these questions she must read the section of the report that describes the research design.

After reading about the data collection methods used in the maternal distress study, the RN was sure that great effort went into measuring several abstract and complex variables. She was sure that each variable has been carefully defined, both theoretically and operationally, and that the reliability of the different measures is discussed. Validity of the measures is not discussed as completely as reliability was, and the study itself is complex because of both many measures and many points of measurement. The RN wonders why so many variables were included in this study and why the study was carried out over so many time points. She believes that the findings have given her some insight into how she might take a more active role in working with S.G.'s parents, as well as S.G. himself. However, she would like to understand better the design of this study and what this type of design may mean for the applicability of the results to practice.

**OUT-OF-CLASS EXERCISE:**

**Free Write**

The next chapter continues to address the question of why a study included the people it did and why the study was done the way it was by talking about research designs. Before reading that chapter, consider the question of whether being in nursing school affects the students' well-being. If you were going to conduct a study to address this question, how would you go about it? What do you think would be the best way to conduct a study to answer this question, and what do you think would be the most realistic approach? Are they the same or different, and why? Think about this, then write, in as much detail as possible, your ideas about how to conduct a study to determine if and how being a nursing student affects the manner on which you have decided. Wherever you can, write your rationale for conducting the study in the manner on which you have decided. After you have completed this assignment, you will be ready to move on to read about research designs in Chapter 9.

**References**

Bliss, D. Z., Johnson, S., Savik, K., Clabots, C. R., & Gerding, D. N. (2000). Fecal incontinence in hospitalized patients who are acutely ill. *Nursing Research, 49*(2), 101–108.

Denzin, N. K. (1989). *Interpretive interactionism.* Newbury Park, CA: Sage Publications.

**OUT-OF-CLASS EXERCISES** at the end of every chapter give the students a way to put their knowledge to use.

**REFERENCES** are provided for students and faculty who seek more information.

**RESEARCH ARTICLES** are provided in the appendices and discussed at length in the chapters, so students are dealing with actual research.

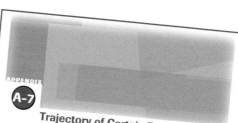

APPENDIX

**A-7**

## Trajectory of Certain Death at an Unknown Time: Children With Neurodegenerative Life-Threatening Illnesses

Rose G. Steel

Children with neurodegenerative life-threatening illnesses (NLTIs) account for a significant proportion of children requiring palliative care. Most of their care is provided at home by their families over many years, yet there is a paucity of research examining families' experiences when a child with an NLTI is dying at home. In this grounded theory study, data were collected from 8 families through observations and audiotaped interviews. Families moved through a process of navigating uncharted territory as they lived with their dying child. The illness trajectory of certain death at an unknown time was not a steady decline. Instead, families lived much of their lives on plateaus of relative stability where they often felt alone and isolated from health-care professionals. Inevitably, periods of instability originated in subsequent precipitating events in the process that led to families dropping off the plateau on the way to the child's inevitable death. Implications for research and practice are discussed.

The numbers of children with a prolonged terminal illness are low when compared with adults. At any one time, there are over 200 children in the province of British Columbia living with progressive life-threatening illnesses (PLTIs) (Davies, 1992). One estimate from the United Kingdom is that 1:1000 children may be affected by PLTIs (Goldman, 1996). Although the numbers are relatively small, these children pose substantial management problems (Caring Institute of the Foundation for Hospice and Home Care, 1987). Additionally, the numbers are projected to increase as the incidence of life-threatening diseases rises and advances in technology and medicine reduce mortality rates (Broome, 1998; Davies & Howell, 1998). Care for these children is typically provided at home by their families over an extended period of time, often years (Burne, Dominica, & Baum, 1984; Goldman, 1998; Stevens, 1998), yet there is little available research to guide professionals in assisting such families.

Children in pediatric palliative care suffer from a wide variety of diseases and syndromes. About 20% of these children have cancer. Many have progressive neuromuscular or neurodegenerative conditions (NLTIs) that will eventually cause their death (Ashby, Kosky, Laver, & Sims, 1991; Davies & Howell, 1998; Goldman, 1996). There is a lack of knowledge about the experiences of their families. Health

*Canadian Journal of Nursing Research, 2000, Vol. 32, No. 3, 49–67*

## ACKNOWLEDGMENTS

I would first like to acknowledge and thank the many students I have taught at East Tennessee State University who have patiently but stubbornly insisted that they were in nursing to practice, not to be researchers, and in so doing have pushed me to make my case for the relevancy of nursing research to their practice. I also want to acknowledge my colleagues who, like me, recognize that if we fail to instill a valuing of research in the baccalaureate student, we do a great disservice to our profession and its growth as a science. I want to thank the three most important mentors in my career: Jean Goeppinger, Lauren Aaronson, and Carol Loveland-Cherry. Each has shared with me her excitement and love of knowledge development, along with many practical opportunities to learn the research process. I hope this book passes some of that enthusiasm and knowledge on. Finally I want to thank Margaret Zuccarini of Lippincott Williams & Wilkins for taking a risk with a new author and a new idea, Production Editor Danielle Litka for all of her work, and Managing Editor Joe Morita for guiding me on this journey into the world of publishing.

# Contents

**CHAPTER**

## The Research Process   232

### How Is the Research Process Related to a Published Research Report?

**CHAPTER**

## The Role of Research in Nursing   253

**CHAPTER**

**1**

# Using Nursing Research in Practice

**KEY TERMS:**

Abstract

Electronic databases

Evidence-based practice

Internet

Key words

Knowledge

Printed indexes

Quality assurance

Systematic

Systematic reviews

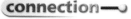

**connection**

For additional activities go to
http://connection.lww.com/go/macnee.

## CLINICAL CASE

M.K. is a 16-year-old female patient who was admitted to the intensive-care unit (ICU) 24 hours ago after a motor vehicle accident (MVA) in which she sustained a moderate concussion, lacerations, and a second-degree burn to her right leg. She was acutely hypoglycemic at admission. M.K. was diagnosed with type I diabetes when she was 5 years old. She has recently started using an insulin pump, which she loads every 2 days. When on a date with her boyfriend at a local pizza parlor, she gave herself a bolus injection of insulin to cover the pizza that they had just started eating when she and her boyfriend got into an argument. M.K. angrily left after eating only a few bites of the pizza and drove home. The MVA occurred approximately two blocks from her home when she lost control of the car and hit a tree. She was wearing her seatbelt but struck her head on the side window. The cigarette she was smoking at the time fell onto her lap and burned through her skirt, causing the second-degree burn. M.K. had a random blood sugar reading of 35 mg/dL at admission; her Hb A$_1$ was 9%, and her total cholesterol was 199 mg/dL. M.K. has demonstrated excellent knowledge of her diabetes self-care, both testing her sugar and loading her pump, since shortly after her admission. She acknowledges that it was a dangerous mistake to forget that she had self-administered a bolus injection with insulin but also says that she has "to be able to live her life" without diabetes controlling it. The RN who cared for M.K. during the first 12 hours of her admission, and who will be assigned to her tomorrow when she will likely be discharged, realizes that some level of teaching related to M.K.'s glycemic control and health is needed. Because a review of basic diabetic self-care is not needed, the RN conducts a short literature search for information about diabetes and risk factors using her home computer and locates an online abstract of a study titled "Risk factors for cardiovascular disease in children with Type I diabetes" (Lipman et al., 2000).

## INTRODUCTION

This book discusses using nursing research in nursing practice. The goal of this book is to teach you, a practicing nurse, to find answers to clinical questions you may have by using nursing research. Another way to phrase this goal is that this book is about practice based on research evidence, or evidence-based practice. To base your practice on research evidence, however, you must be able to understand both the research language and the research process.

Because answering clinical questions is important for a practicing nurse, this book begins at the end of the research process—the conclusions—and moves forward through the process. Research study conclusions often lead to further questions. You may wonder, for example, why the author(s) reached these conclusions. That question may lead to the results section of the study where specific numbers and measurements are described. You also may wonder to what types of patients these research results apply. That question may lead to the description of the study sample. If you wonder why this type of patient was studied, or how the author(s) measured some aspect studied (eg, pain), you must read and understand the methods section of the research study. Finally, the methods section may direct you to review what has been done before and what nursing theory and other theories may suggest about this clinical question. That information is in the beginning or background section of the research report.

Therefore, this book begins at the end of and moves forward through a research report to understand both the research language in a report and the research process underlying it. The five general questions that are described in the previous paragraph are used to organize the end-to-beginning approach utilized in this book. Each chapter in this book discusses a different component of the research report and how that component can help to answer the five general questions. These questions also can be used to organize your own reading and understanding of research. They are:

- What is the answer to my practice question—what did the study conclude?
- Why did the author(s) reach these conclusions—what did they actually find?
- To what types of patients do these research conclusions apply—who was in the study?
- How were those people studied—why was the study performed that way?
- Why ask that question—what do we already know?

This book focuses on reading and understanding research reports to use them intelligently to guide clinical practice. Therefore, each chapter begins with a vignette that results in a clinical question that might be addressed in nursing research. A published research report that is related to the clinical vignette is part of the required reading for the chapter, and each chapter focuses on what can be decided about practice based on an understanding of the article. To help bring the language and process of research to a practical level, you and your classmates also may participate in a small practice "study" that will be used in the text as a concrete example of different aspects of the research process.

When you finish reading this book, you will be prepared to read nursing research critically and use it intelligently. Critically reading research means reading it with a questioning mind: knowing what information should be presented in a report, understanding what is reported, and critically asking yourself whether the research is good enough for you to accept and use in your practice. You will not be prepared to be a researcher yourself, but you will understand some of the processes of nursing research and how that research can help you in your practice.

## QUESTIONS FOR PATIENT CARE

In the vignette at the beginning of this chapter, the nurse faces a clinical question. M.K., the patient, is physiologically safe and has demonstrated a clear understanding of the basics of care for her chronic disease. Despite this, the nurse knows that M.K. is still at risk for future diabetes crises and for major long-term health problems related to her poor glycemic control. The nurse has many options about what to include in discharge teaching: a review of signs and symptoms of hypoglycemia, a review of the potential complications of diabetes, a discussion of the risks of smoking, or a discussion of the risks of high cholesterol. The nurse wonders which issue to focus on or whether there might be a way to combine several different issues without giving M.K. a lecture or list of "don'ts."

This nurse's question is just one example of the kinds of questions nurses face each day in clinical practice. Any nursing student knows that not all nurses do everything the same way. Therefore, the question arises: which is the best way to flush a percutaneous endogastric (PEG) tube, maintain an indwelling urinary catheter, or prepare a patient for surgery? And then there are questions about the differences in patients. Why do male patients have a quicker postoperative recovery from coronary artery bypass grafts than do female patients? Why do some patients quit smoking when they are pregnant and others do not? Why do some patients with AIDS keep recovering from infections, when others seem to weaken and die as soon as the first severe complications occur? Which is more helpful to a patient with major depression, to urge them to get up and moving each day or to urge them to listen to themselves and follow their own natural schedules? Although nursing knowledge has grown steadily and we know a great deal about providing optimal health care, there are still more questions than there are answers about how to promote health.

## Finding Answers to Patient Care Questions

How do you, as a nurse, find answers to clinical questions such as those listed in the previous section? Although there are several approaches one can take, four commonly used approaches include:

1. Consulting an authority to answer the question.
2. Using intuition and subjective judgement to answer the question.
3. Turning to experience to answer the question.
4. Reading nursing research to find an answer to the question.

The first approach, using an authority to answer the question, might include asking someone who knows more than you do or looking for the answer in the texts, practice journals, and reference books that may be available. You also might directly ask the patient or someone who has had similar health problems, recognizing that he or she has direct knowledge of the question. As a nursing student, you will often use authorities to answer your patient care questions. Graduate nurses also regularly seek answers to questions from such authorities as reference books, practice journals, other members of the health care team (such as the pharmacist), or the patients.

A second approach to answering clinical questions is to use your own intuition or subjective judgment. Nursing is both a science and an art, and intuition or subjective judgment can be an important way of knowing what to do in clinical situations. Intuition is knowledge that is not explicit and articulated. Intuition differs from common sense or arbitrary choice because it is knowledge, but knowledge that we cannot explicate in detail. Intuition may tell you that a particular day is not the day to push a depressed patient to get out of bed. Intuition may tell you that one patient with AIDS has given up and will not survive a hospitalization, whereas another who is equally ill is determined to live. Such intuition will guide your care for each of these patients, perhaps leading to a focus on social support and spiritual care for the first patient and a focus on independence for the second patient.

A third approach to answering questions about nursing care is to depend on one's own experience. Experiences may indicate that patients who had their indwelling urinary catheters changed every 72 hours had fewer urinary tract infections (UTIs) than did those who had theirs changed every 48 hours. Experiences may also indicate that depressed patients who were strongly encouraged to get out of bed and follow a daily morning routine were discharged sooner than those who were not encouraged. Personal experience with a health problem may also provide answers to clinical questions: you may know what worked for you or your family, so that is what you will offer or do for your patient.

Each of these ways of answering clinical questions can be helpful and appropriate. However, sometimes you cannot get the answer from an authority and have no intuitive or experiential basis on which to answer the question. Sometimes the answers from these different approaches may differ. Take the clinical question about what type of teaching to plan for M.K. for example. The nurse in the vignette talked to the charge nurse about M.K. and was told that reviewing the rationale for blood sugar control was the most appropriate plan. The nurse also checked the standardized care plan for patients with type I diabetes and found that a review of the signs and symptoms of hypoglycemia and hyperglycemia was recommended. The nurse's experience with her 15-year-old daughter tells her that "lecturing" about anything will not be helpful in this case but that sharing concerns and ideas may work. Given these possible scenarios, the question of how to address discharge teaching with this patient remains.

The fourth approach to answering clinical questions, nursing research, may provide this nurse with an answer to her question that avoids the subjectivity of the other approaches. Often it is exactly the types of questions that are not answered in textbooks and that everyone has a different idea about or experience with, that are the questions studied in nursing research.

## Finding Answers Through Research

Reading and using research is not necessarily the easiest possible approach to seeking answers for clinical questions. To look for answers in research you must: (1) identify research in the area of interest, (2) access the research report(s), (3) read and understand the research report(s), (4) decide whether the research is relevant and useful in answering your question, and (5) decide whether to accept and use what you find in the research. Rather than completing all these steps, it is easier to ask someone whom you consider an expert or an authority, hoping that, perhaps, he or she has read the research. However, it is not uncommon for the answer to a question to be "I do not know" or for the answer to differ between sources. As a professional nurse, you will shortly *be* the authority from whom others will be seeking answers. Part of your role as a professional nurse is to use nursing research intelligently in your patient care.

Using research in clinical practice can broadly be called evidence-based practice. That is, a nursing practice that is based on evidence from research. **Evidence-based practice** is broadly defined as the conscious and intentful use of research- and theory-based information to make decisions about patient care delivery. Research is not the only evidence that nurses use as a basis for their practice. As described, there are other sources of knowledge or evidence on which nurses base their practice, including authority, intuition, patient feedback, and textbooks. However, currently there is an emphasis in nursing on the use of systematic reviews of research as evidence for practice. **Systematic reviews** are the product of a process that includes asking clinical questions, performing a structured and organized search for theory-based information and research related to the question, reviewing and synthesizing the results from that search, and reaching conclusions about the implications for practice. This is similar to how an individual nurse might obtain answers to clinical questions, but it involves a more structured process. Systematic reviews, such as reports of individual research studies, use research language and are based on the research process. The quality of systematic reviews differs, just as the quality of individual research studies vary. Therefore, intelligently reading these reviews is another part of finding answers to practice questions.

Another way that nurses regularly use research in their practice is in developing and implementing quality assurance. **Quality assurance** includes a range of activities, such as licensing, and maintenance of regulatory and credentialing procedures. One important aspect of quality assurance is the development and implementation of standards for quality of health care. Standards of care may take numerous forms, including clinical pathways, identification of clinical indicators, or descriptions of clinical outcomes. In all cases, these standards of care reflect the expected processes and outcomes of care and are often based on research findings.

For example, a standard of care in an ICU unit may be that each patient is asked to rate his or her pain level on a 10-point scale once during each shift. This standard is likely based on research findings about patients' perceptions and experiences of pain and the best approaches to pain management. Despite quality assurance standards being based on research, research also is often used to revise standards of care or to evaluate whether selected standards are effective.

As a practicing professional nurse, then, your practice should be based, in part, on research, but it will also often formally be evaluated by research-based standards. This book attempts to give you the skills needed to use research intelligently in your practice, whether for answering direct clinical care questions based on systematic reviews or individual research reports or for developing and evaluating quality of care standards. However, to read and understand research, you first must know what research is.

### Identifying Applicable Research Reports

Finding research reports is the first step in using research in clinical practice. Identifying research has become easier with the ever-increasing use of the Internet and the increasing numbers of journals that are published electronically. In the clinical vignette for this chapter, the nurse used a home computer to search for research concerning the needs of adolescents with type I diabetes. However, to find research reports, it is important to know for what you are looking. Not all articles about a health condition are research. In fact, most information one can access through journals, texts, and the World Wide Web is not research. So what is nursing research?

The definition of nursing research includes two key ideas. First, for a written report or a Web site to describe research, it must describe the systematic gathering of information to answer some question. **Systematic** means that a set of actions was planned and organized. The information-gathering actions may include interviews,

> C ORE  C ONCEPT
>
> *Nursing research is the systematic gathering of information to gain, expand, or validate knowledge about health and responses to health problems.*

observations, questionnaires, or laboratory tests, but they must have been guided by a plan and administered methodically or systematically.

Second, the information must have been gathered to answer a question that addresses a gap in our knowledge about nursing. **Knowledge** is what is understood and recognized about a subject. Information can be gathered for many other purposes, including evaluation, reporting, or accounting for resources. Research seeks to gather information so that we can understand or know something about which we do not yet have an answer. Research begins with a question, an unknown, and develops new knowledge. In contrast, evaluation, reporting, and accounting usually describe or validate something that is known or already occurring.

An article found by the nurse caring for M.K. describing known factors that increase the risks of long-term complications among adolescents who have diabetes, for example, would not be a research report. Even if the article provided statistics or numbers about these risks, such as the percentage of U.S. adolescents who smoke or the average cholesterol level of adolescents with type I diabetes according to the Centers for Disease Control and Prevention (CDC), it still would not be a report of research. An article about the risks of complications in type I diabetes that was a research report would describe a question about those complications and then describe the process and results of a systematic effort to answer that question. Therefore, facts and numbers alone do not make a source of information a report of research. A research report provides a description of systematic gathering of information to gain, expand, or validate knowledge.

Not only is it important to differentiate research reports from those that are not research, but also it is important to identify and find primary sources of research. A primary source is a report of the research written by the original author(s). Professional newsletters and journals often include summaries of research that have been presented at a conference or published elsewhere. Although these summaries are a quick source of information, they do not allow you to understand fully and evaluate the actual research because they are another individual's summary of that research. These types of summaries are helpful, however, for identifying research studies that may be potentially interesting and important in your practice. To use research intelligently you must find and read the original research.

As you read more research, the difference between reports of research and other scholarly and informative work becomes clearer. In fact, many of the computer sources used to find research reports have an option that allows you to select only reports that are research, eliminating the need to even decide if an article is a research report. But it is important to understand that what you find when you read a research report is not just a description of facts, ideas, theories, or procedures, but also a question and a systematic effort to gain information to address that question.

*Accessing Research Reports*

Once you know what you are looking for, the next step in finding research reports is knowing where to look. As nursing students, you are probably already aware of numerous nursing research reports. One of the obvious sources is a journal that includes the words "nursing research" in its title (ie, *Research in Nursing and Health* or *Nursing Research*). Most professional nursing journals, even those whose primary purpose is not publishing research, do include research articles, often specifically labeled as research in the table of contents. However, simply picking up and scanning journals at the library or at a hospital is a somewhat hit-or-miss approach if you are interested in a specific clinical question. Three primary sources that allow you to search for research on a specific question or topic are (1) printed indexes, (2) the Internet, and (3) electronic databases. Table 1–1 lists examples of these three primary sources.

*Printed Indexes*    **Printed indexes** are written lists of professional articles organized and categorized by topic and author, and they cover from 1956 to today. They usually can only be found in formal academic libraries and are used more infrequently, given the development of computerized electronic databases. Printed indexes are, however, the only source that lists and categorizes research that was done *before* 1982. Because indexes are tedious to use, are not as available as other sources for finding research, and provide a catalog of studies that are older and, so, not current, they should be considered a last resort for acquiring research. However, indexes can be helpful in providing ideas for key words to use in a computer search on a topic, as well as indicating the kinds of research that have generally been done in your area of interest.

*The Internet*    The **Internet** is the worldwide network that connects computers throughout the world. Several programs, called search engines, are used to search the Internet; they are often already loaded on the hard drive of a personal computer. Because the Internet is a source of information from computers throughout the world, a tremendous and potentially overwhelming amount of information can be found using it. However, because almost anyone can put information on the Internet, the accuracy, completeness, and even honesty of information found there must be considered carefully.

When you use the Internet to search for research, it may help to use the word "research" in the search, in addition to words that describe your question. Initially, you will probably get thousands of results, or "hits." These vary from connections to large databases, connections to specific journals or newsletters, and connections to organizations to connections to individuals' Web pages. You then narrow the search to specific links that will give you research reports. Examples of sites that may provide links that could be helpful in answering clinical questions are the CDC (http://www.cdc.gov) and the National Institute for Nursing Research (NINR) (http://www.nih.gov/ninr). Links to large and well-established health-related organizations such as these can assure you high-quality information, and many of these sites provide selected research reports. Links to little known organizations or sites, however, should be used cautiously because the information found may be incorrect or incomplete. When the RN in our vignette used the Internet to search for ideas about discharge teaching for M.K., her search led to a link with the American Diabetes

| TABLE  1–1   Sources to Search for Nursing Research About a Specific Clinical Topic | |
|---|---|
| **Type of Source** | **Specific Examples** |
| **Print**<br>Indexes: provide lists of articles that are organized by topic and author from a range of journals; include all types of articles, including research articles published as early as 1956 | Printed *CINAHL* (*Cumulative Index to Nursing and Allied Health Literature*), also known as Red books<br>*Index Medicus*<br>*International Nursing Index* |
| Card catalogs: list all materials held by the library, including books, audiovisuals, theses, and dissertations organized by topic and by author | |
| Abstract reviews: summaries of research studies and prepared bibliographies | *Dissertation Abstracts International*<br>*Psychological Abstracts*<br>*Sociological Abstracts* |
| **Electronic**<br>World Wide Web (WWW): an information service that provides access to the Internet using numerous programs called search engines | Popular search engines include:<br>  http://www.yahoo.com<br>  http://www.infoseek.com<br>  http://www altavista.com<br>  http://www dogpile.com<br>  http://www.google.com<br>Relevant nursing-related Web sites include:<br>  http://www.ana.org–American Association of Nursing<br>  http://www.nih.gov/ninr–National Institute of Nursing Research<br>  http://www.cdc.gov–Centers for Disease Control and Prevention<br>  http://www.dhhs.gov–Department of Health and Human Services<br>  http://www.nursingsociety.org–Sigma Theta Tau International Nursing Honor Society<br>  http://www.cna-nurses.ca/–Canadian Nurses Association |
| Electronic databases: categorized lists of articles from a range of journals, organized by topic, author, and source | CINAHL–includes articles from 1982 to the present<br>MEDLINE (Medical Literature analysis and retrieval system)<br>PsycInfo (psychology information)<br>PUBMED (database provided by the National Library of Medicine) |

Association (http://www.diabetes.org). This link includes a site for health professionals, and the health professionals site includes a link to selected new diabetes research. There the RN seeking information about discharge planning with M.K. might have found the article about risk factors for cardiovascular disease.

*Electronic Databases*    Besides using search engines on the Internet, you also can use the Internet to make a connection with an academic library through most university Web sites. Once you make that connection, you can usually access the large electronic databases available at these libraries. **Electronic databases**, the most commonly used source to find research reports, provide categorized lists and complete bibliographic citations of sources of information in a broad field of knowledge. Examples of computer databases include the Cumulative Index to Nursing and Allied Health Literature (CINAHL), which categorizes information that relates to the practice of nursing and allied health professions, and PUBMED, which is a database provided by the National Library of Medicine and provides access to more than 11 million health-related and medicine-related citations. Electronic databases can be found in CD-ROM format as well as online. Most are organized similarly so that you can initiate a search for information using **key words**, terms that describe the information for which you are interested in getting information. In the case of the clinical question about M.K., some of the key words used to search might have included "diabetes," "type I," "discharge teaching," "complications," and "risks." Sometimes the most difficult part of using an electronic database is determining which key words to use. As mentioned, a quick look at printed indexes may help identify appropriate key words.

Electronic databases also allow you to search for information written by a specific author or for a specific article using its title. Searches can be limited by date of publication or type of information sought, such as research only. The results of an electronic search include a list of references with bibliographic citations and, usually, an abstract or summary of the article. Again, remember that not all articles found in a search will be research articles unless you have specified that you only want research articles. Although occasionally the title of an article alone may clearly tell you that it is relevant to the question you are asking, you may also need to read the abstract to decide whether it is relevant. Abstracts are discussed in detail later in this chapter.

After finding a citation for a possibly relevant research report, the next challenge may be actually to acquire a copy of it. Copies of research reports may be acquired in several ways. One way is to subscribe to those journals that usually print the types of research articles that are of interest to you. This allows the article you are interested in reading to be available in your own home. A second way is to join one or more professional organizations that provide subscriptions to their journals as a membership benefit. For example, membership in Sigma Theta Tau International includes a subscription to *Image: Journal of Nursing Scholarship,* which includes many research reports. Another option for acquiring research reports is obtaining them from your place of practice, because most health care organizations subscribe to several professional journals.

Because numerous journals are now published online as well as in print format, a third way to acquire a research report is to get it online. Although most online journals only provide full-text articles to subscribers, many academic libraries have subscriptions to both print journals and online journals, so, as a nursing student, you may be able to get articles online. You also may be able to request an interlibrary loan of an article from a journal to which your library does not subscribe. If you do so, be sure to find out whether there is a charge for the article. Finally, you can acquire articles by visiting the closest academic library that subscribes to the journal you need.

### Reading and Understanding Research Abstracts

The nurse in our vignette will read the published online abstract to decide whether to take the time and trouble to acquire the entire text of the research article. However, reading and understanding the abstract to decide whether the report is potentially useful may be a challenge. Because the abstract for a research report is frequently available when a nurse uses one of the different sources to find research, let us examine what usually is included in an abstract of a research report.

An **abstract** is a summary or condensed version of the research report. Although one meaning of "abstract" is to summarize, another is to "take away." Because an abstract is a condensed summary, it does "take away" from the total picture or information about a research study and gives only limited information about the study itself. Therefore, the abstract should not be depended upon for understanding a research study or making decisions about clinical care. However, if you are trying to decide whether to acquire the full report of a research study, the abstract can certainly be useful. Abstracts vary from journal to journal in format and length. They also vary depending on the type of research performed. Abstracts may be organized by headings, such as Background, Problem, or Results, or they may be written as a single paragraph. However they are organized, almost every abstract identifies the general problem or research question and the general approach taken to implement that research. Most abstracts also briefly describe the people included in the study (called the subjects or participants) and one or two of the most important findings. Abstracts vary in length from 100 to 500 or more words; those that are more limited in the number of words obviously provide less information. Even longer abstracts, however, provide only a "skeleton" of the key ideas from the research report.

Despite the abstracts' limitations, they still can be useful in determining whether the research study reported is one that you want to acquire and read. The abstract usually provides a clear idea about two important factors: (1) whether the research addressed the clinical question of interest and (2) whether it studied patients or situations that are similar to your clinical case so that the research is relevant.

Often you can determine from reading an abstract whether the study addressed the topic you are interested in exploring. For example, a search of the CINAHL database using the key words "diabetes" and "risk factors" might return a citation for an article titled "Risks for increased lipids and heart disease among diabetics," a fictional title simply used as an example. This title suggests that the research might be relevant to discharge planning for M.K. The abstract for this article, however, might indicate that the purpose of the study was "to describe the incidence of increased blood lipid values in patients taking sulfonylureas to see how these medications contribute to risks of cardiovascular disease." Because M.K. is a type I diabetic and is not taking any sulfonylureas, a review of the abstract would allow you to conclude that this article is not worth acquiring at this time. It is also possible that although the purpose of this study does not fit with the clinical question about M.K., the RN may choose to acquire this research report anyway because of its general clinical interest. Besides giving you information about the purpose of a study, most abstracts include information about who was included in the study. Regarding the question about discharge teaching for M.K., if an abstract tells you that the people (subjects) in the study were all adults who were vegetarians, you may decide that this study will probably not be helpful for your specific purpose. Be careful, searching for research on a topic of interest can be a bit like eating peanuts—each one leads to yet another. That is to say that it is easy to become distracted from the clinical question of interest by related studies. Because we often have limited time and resources, it may be important to have as clear an idea as possible regarding the clinical question of interest before you begin searching and reading abstracts of research reports.

## PUBLISHED ABSTRACT: WHAT WOULD YOU CONCLUDE?

To better understand the usefulness of reading and understanding research report abstracts, read the abstract of the article found by the nurse in our vignette, "Risk factors for cardiovascular disease in children with Type I diabetes" (Lipman et al., 2000). You can find this article on the Internet at the Connection Web site for this textbook and in Appendix A. Remember that the nurse in the vignette is trying to decide what should be the focus of her discharge teaching with M.K. the next day, and consider the following questions as you read the abstract:

1.  What do you understand or not understand in the abstract?
2.  Do you believe reading the entire report will be helpful in deciding what to teach M.K.? Why or why not?
3.  Based on the abstract alone and what you know about M.K., can you make a decision about what to teach M.K.? Why or why not?

It is likely that you did not understand all the language in the abstract; do not be discouraged. The goal of this book is to help you learn to understand that language, so the next chapter directly addresses the research language. It also is likely, however, that you *did* understand some of the abstract, and that even reading this limited information about the research has added to your knowledge about risks for adolescents with diabetes.

The abstract is organized by six major headings that can be helpful to your understanding. The abstract indicates that atherosclerotic cardiovascular disease is a major problem for children with type I diabetes. It tells you that the study examined 140 children with insulin-dependent diabetes mellitus (IDDM). The results indicate that "diabetes control and physical activity were correlated with TC (total cholesterol) in the risk sample of children at highest risk" (Lipman et al., 2000, p. 160). Because M.K. has type I (or insulin-dependent) diabetes and has an increased TC, even if you did not understand the entire abstract, this research report is relevant to discharge planning for M.K.

Clinical practice-related decisions cannot be based on information gleaned from the abstract of a research report alone. Specifically, the research abstract does not have enough information to: (1) understand all the results of the study, (2) identify

> ### CORE CONCEPT
>
> *Abstracts from research reports can be helpful in narrowing, or focusing on the appropriate research to acquire and read. They cannot, and should not, be depended upon to provide a level of understanding of the research that would support clinical decision-making.*

who was in the study, (3) recognize how the results fit or do not fit with existing knowledge, or (4) decide intelligently whether the study was performed in a way that makes the results realistic for clinical practice. For example, the abstract from the Lipman et al. article (2000) does not tell you that many of the children included in the study had fairly good Hb $A_1$ values. This result is reported only in the main report of the study, and the authors indicate that this result made it difficult for the researchers to answer questions about the role of Hb $A_1$ in blood lipid levels. The abstract also does not tell you what was meant by "physical activity." Because the RN in the vignette is interested in health risks in general, it is important to determine whether "physical activity" in this research means a structured therapeutic program that might not be appropriate for M.K. or common daily exercise activities that M.K. could implement. The RN must read the research report to find the description of physical activity and to decide if the study's findings can be helpful to M.K.

## SYSTEMATIC REVIEWS IN EVIDENCE-BASED PRACTICE

This book treats evidence-based practice in the broadest sense by including all types of research, as well as other sources of knowledge, as evidence. Currently, however, there is a particular emphasis in nursing on a *process* of evidence-based practice that addresses clinical questions by searching the literature, evaluating evidence, and choosing an intervention. The product of this process is a systematic review of the research regarding a particular clinical question. Thus there is a process that is often referred to as implementing a systematic review as a basis for evidence-based practice, and there is a product that also is often referred to as a systematic review. Although it might be easier to refer to the process of implementing a systematic review as the process of evidence-based practice, doing so significantly limits the breadth of evidence that may be used in nursing. Therefore, throughout this text whenever the word systematic review is used, the specific usage of the word will be made explicit to avoid confusion. An example of a systematic review titled "Exercise in heart failure: A synthesis of the current research" (Adams & Bennett, 2000) can be found at the Connection Web site listed and in Appendix A. Like individual research reports, a synthesis review includes an abstract and a statement of the problem. However, rather than developing a systematic plan to directly gather information from patients about that question, a synthesis review systematically gathers reports of research studies that have already been completed that address the problem. The review summarizes these studies, considering aspects of the research process (such as designs and samples), and then draws conclusions about what is known about the clinical question based on the entire group of studies. Here, as with abstracts on individual studies, a nurse can review the abstract to decide whether the review is directly related to the question of interest. Here again, even reviewing the abstract requires a basic understanding of the research language.

This chapter starts you on the way to critically reading, understanding, and intelligently using research in practice by: (1) defining research, (2) describing sources of research reports, and (3) discussing the use of abstracts to select research to read. The next chapter discusses the language of nursing research, as well as the components of published research reports and how they can guide your understanding and decisions about using the research in clinical practice.

## OUT-OF-CLASS EXERCISE:

### Get Ready for the Next Chapter

To prepare for the next chapter and to give you a concrete example of the components of a research report, read the fictional research report titled "Demographic characteristics as predictors of nursing students' choice of type of clinical practice" on the Connection Web site for this text and in Appendix B. This report describes a fictional study similar to one in which you may participate during your first class period. As you read this report, make two lists, one containing important words or ideas that you understand in the report and one listing important words or ideas that you do not understand. Once you have read the report, you are ready to read the next chapter.

## References

Adams, C. D., & Bennett, S. (2000). Exercise in heart failure: A synthesis of current research. *The Online Journal of Knowledge Synthesis for Nursing, 7*(5).

Agan, R. D. (1987). Intuitive knowing as a dimension of nursing. *Advanced Nursing Science, 10*(1), 63–70.

American Nursing Association (ANA). (1989). *Education for participation in nursing research.* Kansas City, MO: American Nursing Association.

Carper, B. A. (1978). Fundamental patterns of knowing in nursing. *Advances in Nursing Science, 1*(1), 13–23.

Cronin-Stubbs, D. (1992). Publishing research for staff nurses' use. *Applied Nursing Research, 5*(4), 157.

Heath, H. (1998). Reflection and patterns of knowing in nursing. *Journal of Advanced Nursing, 27,* 1054–1059.

Huycke, L. I. (2001). Evidence-based nursing practice. *Southern Connections, 15*(2), 2.

Lipman, T. H., Hayman, L. L., Favian, C. V., DiFazio, D. A., Hale, P. M., Goldsmith, B. M., et al. (2000). Risk factors for cardiovascular disease in children with Type I Diabetes. *Nursing Research, 49*(3), 160–166.

Nahas, V. L., Chang, A., & Molassiotis, A. (2001). Evidence-based practice: Guidelines for managing peripheral intravascular access devices. *Journal of Nursing Administration, 31*(4), 164–165.

Stevens, K. R., & Long, J. D. (1998). Incorporating systematic reviews into nursing education. *The Online Journal of Knowledge Synthesis for Nursing* [On-line serial], *5*(7). Available: http://www.nursingsociety.org/library.

Thompson, C., McCaughan, D., Cullum, N., Sheldon, T. A., Mulhall, A., & Thompson, D. R. (2001). Research information in nurses' clinical decision-making: What is useful? *Journal of Advanced Nursing, 36*(3), 376–388.

## Resources

Burns, N., & Groves, S. K. (1999). *Understanding nursing research* (2nd ed.). Philadelphia: W.B. Saunders Company.

LoBiondo-Wood, G., Haber, J., & Krainovich-Miller, B. (1998). Overview of the research process. In G. LoBiondo-Wood & J. Haber (Eds.), *Nursing research: Methods, critical appraisal, and utilization* (4th ed.). St. Louis: Mosby.

Polit, D. F., & Hungler, B. P. (2002). *Nursing research: Principles and methods* (7th ed.). Philadelphia: Lippincott Williams & Wilkins.

**LEARNING OUTCOME:**

*THE STUDENT WILL* differentiate the components of and associated terminology in research reports.

CHAPTER

**2**

# Components and Language of Research Reports

**KEY TERMS:**

Conclusions
Data
Data analysis
Descriptive results
Hypothesis
Limitations
Literature review
Measures
Meta-analysis
Methods
Multivariate

Problem
Procedures
*P* values
Qualitative methods
Quantitative methods
Results
Sample
Significance
Themes
Theory

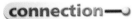

## CLINICAL CASE

J.K. is a 68-year-old man who has Parkinson's disease. He has had two admissions in the past year to the medical intensive care unit (ICU), one for acute dehydration and electrolyte imbalance, and the other for a head injury resulting from a fall. On each occasion, he developed complications that required a stay of more than 1 week. During these hospitalizations he became incontinent of stools, and this led to significant skin irritation and breakdown on his buttocks, which required home health care after his discharge. J.K. is being admitted to the unit again, with a primary diagnosis of bacterial pneumonia. The admitting RN has come to know J.K. and his wife from his last two hospitalizations and realizes that, given his history, he is at high risk for developing fecal incontinence. Although the RN is knowledgeable about skin care and treatments once fecal incontinence occurs, she wonders what factors put J.K. at greatest risk for this problem and how to anticipate and prevent it from developing during this admission. The RN visits the hospital library after her shift and quickly performs a search on CINAHL, using the key words "fecal incontinence" and specifying research articles only. One result is a citation for an article titled "Fecal incontinence in hospitalized patients who are acutely ill" (Bliss, Johnson, Savik, Clabots, & Gerding, 2000). The article is from a journal that is available in the library, so the RN photocopies the article and takes it home to see if it contains any suggestions that might be included in her plan of care for J.K. the next day. This article is available in Appendix A and on the Connection Web site. Read through it quickly to make the best use of the examples that are provided in this chapter. Do not worry about fully understanding the article, but do keep a list of words or ideas that you do not understand.

A t the end of Chapter 1, you were asked to read the fictional article about nursing students' choices of practice and to list the important words that you understood and those that you did not understand. This chapter provides an overview of the major components or sections in most research reports and some of the unique research language that identifies these different sections. As you probably discovered when reading the fictional article, not understanding certain terms in a research report is frustrating and creates barriers to use of the research intelligently in practice. This chapter discusses the meanings of some of the language of research. The remaining chapters examine the individual sections of a research report and the definition of terms used in those sections in more detail. Viewing the entire report first allows you to see the whole "picture" and will help you to understand where each section fits when we begin to review each specific part. Recognizing and understanding some of the nursing research language will make it easier for you to start reading and comprehending the research and to use it in your practice.

The language and style of research reports are unique and, therefore, difficult to read. Research reports are generally written in a scientific writing style, the goals of which are to be clear, precise, and succinct. Like the health care language, the research language is formal, technical, and terse, with many ideas compounded into each sentence. This makes research reports reliable methods of communication for anyone immersed in the language of science, but it also makes them inscrutable to the novice who is just beginning to read research.

Learning to read research reports is similar to learning to read a patient's chart. The first time that you read a sentence such as "The patient is a 64 yo w m, presenting c̄ RUQ abd pain, post a MVA yesterday a.m.; denies LOC or pain at time of accident," it probably made little, if any, sense to you. Now, however, you know that this sentence refers to a patient being a 64-year-old white male who has come to seek health care because he has pain in the upper half and right side of his belly. He was in a motor vehicle accident yesterday morning but says that he did not lose consciousness or have pain at the time of the accident. Notice that it took two sentences and many more words to say the same thing in everyday prose. The language of research is much like the language of health care—it too is packed with meaning in every sentence and uses unique terms that communicate clearly to anyone familiar with it. Just as you have mastered or are mastering the language of health care, you will master the basics of the language of research.

## COMPONENTS OF PUBLISHED RESEARCH REPORTS

In addition to an abstract, almost every research report has at least four major sections: (1) Introduction or **Problem**, (2) **Methods**, (3) **Results**, and (4) **Conclusions** or discussion. Table 2–1 describes each of these sections and lists some of the research terms associated with each section. Because this book discusses research by beginning at the end of the process and moving backward, we look at each of the sections of a research report, starting with the end.

### Conclusions

The word "conclusions" is used in research reports much as it is generally used outside of the research setting: conclusions complete a report and identify an outcome. The **conclusions** in a research report specifically describe or discuss the researcher's final decisions or determinations regarding the research problem.

In nursing research reports, conclusions also usually include a description of implications for nursing practice. That is why practicing nurses often start with the conclusions of a report—here, the meaning of the research for practice is specifically addressed. What distinguishes conclusions in a research report from those in other reports is the expectation that they contain either new knowledge or confirmation of previous knowledge. The goal of the research process is to generate knowledge that can be used in practice: in the conclusions section of a research report, the findings or results of a study are directly translated into that new knowledge. That is, the conclusions go beyond simply saying what was found in a study; they present the implications or meaning of those findings for future practice. As such, the conclusions of research reports are powerful. They are used as the basis for decisions about direct patient care, whether one-on-one care, such as that provided by the RN to J.K., or developing clinical standards or pathways that direct patient care for large groups of patients.

Because of the power and importance attached to them, the determinations or decisions described in the conclusions of a research report are carefully worded and list any relevant cautions or limitations. This cautious presentation may, however,

| TABLE 2–1 | The Sections of a Research Report and Associated Terms |
|---|---|

| Research report section | Associated terms |
|---|---|
| *Problem or Introduction:* describes the gap in knowledge that will be addressed in the research study | ■ Literature review<br>■ Theory<br>■ Research question<br>■ Hypothesis |
| *Methods:* describes the process of implementing the research study | ■ Qualitative<br>■ Quantitative<br>■ Measures<br>■ Sample<br>■ Procedures |
| *Results:* summarizes the specific information gathered in the research study | ■ Data<br>■ Data analysis<br>■ Themes<br>■ Descriptive<br>■ Significant<br>■ Multivariate |
| *Conclusions:* describes the decisions or determinations that can be made about the research problem | ■ Limitations<br>■ Implications for practice |

make the conclusions weak or not helpful to the nurse who is looking for answers to clinical questions.

For example, the RN who is looking for ways to prevent fecal incontinence in J.K. finds the conclusions of the report described in a section labeled "Discussion." From reading this section, she learns that fecal incontinence is a common problem and that the length of hospitalization does not make a difference in the development of fecal incontinence. Exposure to antibiotics or sorbitol-containing medications also was not connected to fecal incontinence. Although it is useful to know that the antibiotics that J.K. is taking for his pneumonia will not contribute to his development of fecal incontinence, this does not help the RN identify what *is* a contributor or how to prevent incontinence. The discussion in this article goes on to state: "therapies that make stool consistency less loose or liquid *may* be useful in managing fecal incontinence" (Bliss et al., 2000, p. 106 [emphasis added by author]), and that "increased severity of illness and older age" (p. 107) also are risk factors for developing fecal incontinence. The authors clearly express their conclusions cautiously and may be do so for several reasons. Chapter 3 examines in more detail why conclusions often are constrained or hesitant.

The conclusion section of a research report usually has fewer unique research terms than does the rest of the report. This is probably another reason why the conclusion section is sometimes the first part read by many nurses. One term that regularly appears in the conclusions section is limitations. **Limitations** are the aspects of a study that create uncertainty concerning the meaning that can be derived from the study, as well as the decisions that can be based on it. The description of a study's limitations often addresses the beginning sections of the report, such as the study's methods and sample.

Just as the cautious language used in the conclusions section can be frustrating when you are looking for answers to clinical questions, the limitations described may make you wonder whether you can use the information or conclusions in your practice. That is why the limitations are included in the conclusions: to remind the reader that there are constraints or limits to the knowledge being reported. Limitations do not mean that the results of a study are flawed or meaningless. They do, however, indicate the boundaries of or constraints to the knowledge generated by the research. One might view the research study limitations as the fence that surrounds and "limits" the new knowledge contained in the report. To decide whether to use the knowledge described in a research report and how you will use it, you must understand not only the knowledge itself but also the "fence" around it (*see* Figure 2–1), which requires you to understand the aspects of the research process, such as sampling or methods, that may constrain the new knowledge.

Finally, the conclusion section of a research report usually contains recommendations for future research regarding the problem of interest. These recommendations often directly address the limitations that have been described and suggest additional studies that are needed to further build on the new knowledge generated from the study described in the report.

**FIGURE 2–1** **Limitations of the research process constrain knowledge acquired.**

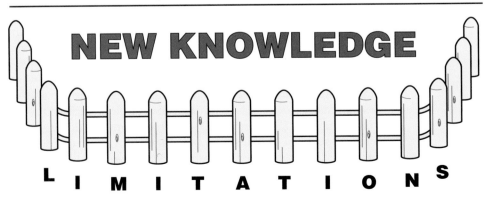

## Results

The **results** section of a research report summarizes the specific findings from the study. Almost no research report can give all of the information that was actually gathered during a research study, so the results section contains a summary or condensed version of what the authors believe are the most important findings. **Data** are the information collected in a study. Organizing and compiling data is called data analysis. **Data analysis** pulls elements or information together to present a clear picture of all of the information collected, but it does not interpret or describe the implications for practice of that picture of the information.

The data analysis methods used to summarize the information collected in a research study create some of the unique language found in this section of a report. Results or findings of a study may be reported in the form of numbers, words, or both. Which form is used depends on the type of information or data that was collected. If the study collected information about people's beliefs and experiences, the results section summarizes the words collected using terms such as themes or categories and concepts. **Themes** are abstractions that reflect phrases, words, or ideas that appear repeatedly when a researcher analyzes what people have said about a particular experience, feeling, or situation. A theme summarizes and synthesizes discrete ideas or phrases to create a picture from the words that were collected in the research study. For example, in the fictional research report about nursing students' choices of type of clinical practice, the results section mentions "three distinct themes that represent the meaning of life experiences related to choice of field of nursing." The author does not list the answers given by 30 different nursing students; rather, she has looked for recurring ideas or words in those answers and categorized them into three themes: personal life experience, experience with nursing role models, and experiences with fictional media.

In contrast, the research study on fecal incontinence collected information in the form of numbers, such as age, scores for severity of illness, and proportion of stools with unformed or liquid consistency. Again, the authors do not list all the scores or ages for 152 patients; rather, they summarize the numbers in several different forms, such as percentages, proportions, and averages. The language that describes data analysis of information in numbers is called statistics, and the language of statistics is often some of the most intimidating language to readers of research. We do not have to be statistical experts to develop a greater understanding of that language, and we focus on the language of statistics in Chapter 4. However, a few key terms are worth highlighting.

Almost any research report, even those that are mostly reporting results of interviews in the form of words, includes descriptive results. **Descriptive results** sum-

## Core Concept

*The difference between results and conclusions is that results are a summary of the actual findings or information collected in the research study, whereas conclusions summarize the potential meaning, decisions, or determinations that can be made based on the information collected.*

marize information without comparing it to other information. For example, descriptive results may state how many people were in a study, the average age of those studied, or the percentage of male subjects studied. In the fecal incontinence article, the first two paragraphs of the results section are descriptive (*see* Box 2–1). Here, the authors describe the patients in terms of how many were tube fed, their diagnoses, the units the patients were on, and types of tube feeding the patients received. The authors do not compare these findings to any other group; they simply describe what they found using language that summarizes the information such as percentages or averages.

The authors of the fecal incontinence article also provide average scores and ages in Table 1 of the report, but they do more then just describe the findings because they divide the patients into two groups, those with and those without fecal incontinence, and compare the groups' scores. The comparison of these scores requires a consideration of two important statistical concepts: significance and *P* values. Table 1 in the article indicates that there is a significant difference between those with and those without incontinence by providing *P* values at the bottom of the table. **Significance** is a statistical term indicating a low likelihood that any differences or relationships found in a study happened by chance. In research, we often try to make decisions about clinical care for a large group of patients based on what we have found in a small group of patients. Statistical significance is important because of the need to be sure that what was found in the small group of patients studied is not something that happened by chance rather than because of some factor we are studying.

***P* values** indicate what percentage of the time the results reported would have happened by chance alone. For example, a *P* value of .05 means that in only 5 out of 100 times would one expect to get the results by chance alone. If it is unlikely that

---

**BOX 2–1    Descriptive Results From Fecal Incontinence Study**

"The study consisted of 152 patients (150 men and 2 women): 76 were tube fed and 85 were not tube fed. The primary diagnoses of the patients were categorized as follows: peripheral vascular disease ($n = 36$), head or neck cancer ($n = 34$), neurologic disorders ($n = 19$), pulmonary disorders ($n = 18$), gastrointestinal disorders ($n = 10$), cardiac disorders ($n = 10$), abdominal aortic aneurysms ($n = 9$), genitourinary or renal disorders ($n = 6$), and miscellaneous (eg, leukemia, hip fracture) ($n = 10$). None of the patients had a primary or comorbid diagnosis of dementia at admission. A history of fecal incontinence was not documented in the medical record of any study patient on admission to the MAMC. The patients were located on the following units: surgical ($n = 73$), medical ($n = 27$), mixed neurologic and neurosurgical ($n = 12$), surgical intensive/transitional care ($n = 29$), medical intensive/transitional care ($n = 9$), and coronary care ($n = 2$).

Of the 67 tube-fed patients, 66 started tube feeding using continuous administration and 1 used intermittent administration. During the study, 29 patients changed the tube feeding administration method. The following formulas were used when patients started tube feeding: Osmolite . . . At the time of the study, all nasoduodenal and nasojejunal feeding tubes were inserted using fluoroscopy. During the study, 14 patients changed types of feeding tubes." *Bliss, et al., 2000, pp. 103–104.*

the results happened by chance, then we can summarize the findings by saying that the results are statistically significant. In the fecal incontinence study, the patients' ages, severity of illness scores, nursing care scores, proportion of stools with unformed or liquid consistency, and proportion of surveillance days with diarrhea, for example, were all significantly different between the patients who did and did not have fecal incontinence. What that difference means and how it affects our clinical decision making are not discussed until the conclusions section of the report. However, summarizing and reporting the finding of a difference that is not likely to happen by chance alone is important so that the reader knows why the researchers reached their conclusion.

Another term that is often found in the results section of a research report is multivariate. **Multivariate** indicates that the study reports findings for three or more factors and includes the relationships among those different factors. Both the fecal incontinence article and the fictional article report multivariate results, because they look at relationships and differences between more than two factors. The fecal incontinence article uses the word "multivariate" in the section where the authors describe a regression analysis looking at the relationships among four factors: presence of fecal incontinence, unformed and loose or liquid stool, age, and severity-of-illness index. In contrast, the fictional article does not use the word multivariate, but it does describe results of a logistic regression with age, rating of health, and choice of field of nursing. Now that you know what the word means, you can count the number of factors analyzed and identify that this study is, indeed, multivariate. "Regression analysis" and "logistic regression" are both statistical procedures that allow us to look at relationships between more than two factors and test whether those relationships are likely to occur by chance. Statistical language such as this is discussed further in Chapters 4 and 5.

The information summarized in the results section of a report depends on who was studied, how the study was conducted, what the research question asked, and how the researcher(s) analyzed the information. To understand more completely what was implemented in a study and who was studied, we must look at the methods section of the research report.

## Methods

The methods section of a research report describes the overall process of implementing the research study, including who was included in the study, how information was collected, and what interventions, if any, were tested. Remember from Chapter 1 that one of the things that distinguishes research from other ways of answering questions is its systematic collection of information. The methods section of a research report should describe those systematic procedures used to collect information to the reader. Chapter 8 examines, in detail, the variety of research methods, along with the many names used for them. For now, remember that research methods can be broadly categorized under two major headings: qualitative and quantitative methods. Because qualitative and quantitative methods are used both separately and together in nursing research, both methods are discussed throughout this text. To assist you in understanding the differences between the two methods and how the differences may affect your use of the research in practice, icons, such as those used in the following two paragraphs, are included in most of the chapters to identify selected key ideas regarding either qualitative or quantitative methods.

QUALITATIVE

**Qualitative methods** focus on understanding the complexity of humans within the context of their lives and on building a whole or complete picture of a phenomenon of interest. Therefore, qualitative methods involve the collection of information as it is expressed naturally by people within the normal context of their lives.

QUANTITATIVE

**Quantitative methods** focus on understanding and breaking down the different parts of a phenomenon or picture to see how they do or do not connect. Therefore, quantitative methods involve collecting information that is specific and limited to the particular parts of events or phenomena being studied.

Throughout the book, we will talk a great deal more about both qualitative and quantitative research and highlight important distinctions between the two methods using the icons in the preceding paragraphs. However, beginning to use these words now is important because the methods sections of qualitative and quantitative studies look different.

Figure 2–2 illustrates the differences between knowledge building using qualitative vs. quantitative methods: qualitative research assembles the pieces of a puzzle into a whole picture, whereas quantitative research selects pieces of a completed puzzle and breaks them down into their component parts.

Methods sections of research reports, whether they use qualitative or quantitative methods, usually include information about three aspects of the research method: (1) the sample, (2) the data collection procedures, and (3) the data analysis methods.

### Sample

A **sample** is the smaller group, or subset of the group, of interest that is studied in a research study. In the fecal incontinence study, the researchers were interested in gaining knowledge that can help any patient at risk of fecal incontinence, but they only had the time and resources to study a group of 152 such patients.

Therefore, one thing the RN who wants to try to prevent fecal incontinence in J.K. must consider is whether the 152 patients described in the research report are similar to patients such as J.K. so that what was found in that study is likely to reflect what will happen in J.K.'s case. The effort to assure that the subgroup or sample and

---

## CORE CONCEPT

*Most research attempts to gather information systematically about a subset, or smaller group of patients or people, to gain knowledge about other similar patients or people. Many of the methods in research are aimed at assuring that what happens in the subgroup or sample studied is as similar as possible to what would happen in other larger groups of patients or people.*

**FIGURE 2-2**   **The differences between qualitative and quantitative methods.**

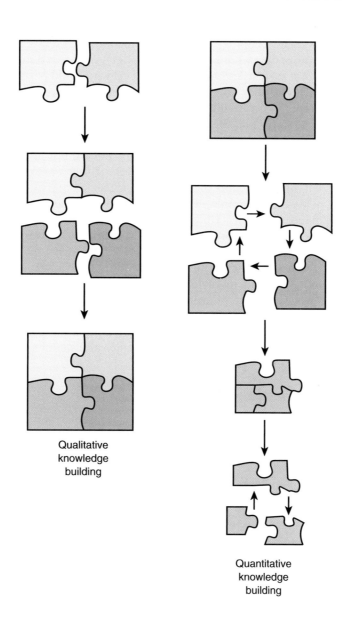

Qualitative
knowledge
building

Quantitative
knowledge
building

what happens to them is similar to the other patients or people about whom we hope to gain knowledge is emphasized in quantitative research methods. However, describing the sample, that is, who was studied, is important for understanding the results of a qualitative study as well as those of a quantitative study.

The sampling subsection in the methods section of a research report describes how people were chosen for the study, what was done to find them, and what, if any, limits or restrictions were placed on who could participate in the study. It also usually describes how many patients or people declined to be in the study, withdrew from it, or were not included in it for specific reasons. For example, the fictional article states that the sample was one of convenience, meaning that no special efforts were made to get a particular type of student to participate. The students chose whether to participate in the study and did not provide identifying information on the questionnaire. Therefore, no restrictions were placed on who would participate: all the researchers did was approach a class of students and ask them to volunteer. This is an example of a simple sampling procedure. In contrast, the fecal incontinence article describes a method in which "secondary data analysis of data [was] collected during a prospective cohort investigation" (Bliss et al., 2000, p. 102), and says that the original sample included 92 tube-fed and 92 non–tube-fed patients from acute and critical care units at a veterans hospital. This is a more complicated sampling method, involving the analysis of information from a previous study that used two groups, or cohorts as researchers sometimes call them, of patients and followed them prospectively, that is, moving forward in time. Understanding samples and sampling is an important part of making intelligent decisions about the use of research in practice; therefore, samples and sampling are discussed in more detail in Chapters 6 and 7.

### *Procedures*

In addition to information about samples, the methods section usually includes information about procedures used in the study. Nurses are familiar with procedures within the context of health care. Research **procedures** are similar because they are the specific actions taken by researchers to gather information about the problem or phenomena being studied.

QUALITATIVE

Because the systematic collection of information in a qualitative study involves looking at as much as possible of the whole phenomena being studied, qualitative studies' procedures are systematically planned activities—such as observations or open and unstructured interviews of people in their natural life situations—to see and hear as much as possible of the complexity of those situations. A qualitative researcher may videotape or audiotape interviews with individuals so that every word, expression, and pause can be carefully considered and studied. In addition, qualitative researchers keep detailed notes of their own observations of the environment where the information is collected and of the expressions and actions of individuals when the information is being collected. This is not a haphazard process but an organized, systematic, and intensive process to collect and then analyze the complexity of experiences.

QUANTITATIVE

In contrast, because the methods used in a quantitative study involve identifying specific aspects of a problem, the procedures involve actions to isolate and examine those particular aspects or pieces. The focus of a quantitative study is on clearly defining and examining selected aspects that are believed potentially to be relevant to the problem being studied. Therefore, procedures may involve carefully defined repeated observations at set time intervals, such as taking a blood pressure reading immediately before and after a patient is suctioned. Another example of a procedure in a quantitative study may be a specific protocol for teaching, in exactly the same manner, each patient to use visualization to relax before surgery.

In summary, quantitative and qualitative methods lead to different approaches and procedures. Timing and actions are carefully planned and controlled in detail for a quantitative study, whereas timing and actions as they naturally occur are what is being studied in a qualitative study.

Often, the procedures in a quantitative study involve taking measurements, sometimes directly, such as taking a blood pressure reading, but often indirectly, such as in a written questionnaire. **Measures** are the specific method(s) used to assign a number or numbers to an aspect or factor being studied. For example, in the article about fecal incontinence, stool consistency is categorized at four levels, ranging from hard and formed to liquid. The authors report that when a description of stool consistency was not recorded on the stool record, the "investigator checked the nurses' notes in the patient's chart or spoke with the nurses responsible for recording the patient's bowel movements" (Bliss et al., 2000, p. 102). The final number given to describe stool consistency is the proportion of stools that were either unformed or liquid, calculated by dividing the number of stools that were described as unformed or liquid by the total number of stools. Thus, the measure of stool consistency included defining four levels, collecting information about the consistency of each stool, and converting that information into a number for each patient. Box 2–2 summarizes this process.

Another example of measures is found in the fictional article that describes a study that is looking at factors that cannot be directly observed in the way that stool consistency can be observed. The fictional article has a section labeled "Measures,"

---

**BOX 2–2 Logarithm for Measuring Stool Consistency in Fecal Incontinence Study**

Stool consistency defined as: (1) hard and firm, (2) soft but formed, (3) unformed and loose, or (4) liquid
↓
Information about consistency of each stool retrieved from stool record or nurses notes
↓
Total number of stools calculated, total number of stools that were level 3 or 4 calculated (unformed or liquid)
↓
Number of unformed/liquid stools divided by total number of stools

which describes a three-part written questionnaire. This questionnaire was used to assign numbers to aspects that were studied, such as previous education or choice of field of study.

Based on the previous discussion of qualitative and quantitative studies, it is probably clear that the fecal incontinence study used a quantitative method, because its goal was to break down and define the different pieces of the puzzle that lead to fecal incontinence. It carefully defined the factors to be studied and established set points in time to record information to create consistency in data for the patients in the study. Similarly, the fictional article describes measures used to translate the factors that were studied into numbers, indicating a quantitative approach, but also includes what the author calls a "qualitative question." By using the word "qualitative," the author indicates that this part of the research attempted to look broadly or holistically at the students' experiences, without selecting specific pieces and asking focused questions. Therefore, the fictional article describes the use of both qualitative and quantitative procedures in its methods section.

An important point to understand is that although this book describes and defines many of the terms used in the research process and found in research reports, the terms have various meanings and can, at different times, be used broadly or more specifically. This can be frustrating or discouraging, because the words or ideas are new and you are just beginning to understand them. However, the more experience you gain from reading and learning about research, the easier understanding it will be. You will find the same situation with many of the words used in the health care field. For example, "normal" body temperature is defined as 98.8°F. Fever is clearly present when a patient has a temperature of 100°F or higher, but a temperature between 99°F and 100°F is not considered either febrile or "normal" and a patient can feel "feverish" with a "normal" temperature. With practice, nurses learn to recognize these variations in the meaning of the words "fever" and "feverish." Similarly, with practice, you will learn to recognize and be comfortable with the variations in meanings or use of research terms. In the case of the fictional article, although we have said that quantitative and qualitative methods usually look different, which suggests that an individual research study will use only one of the two broad approaches, at times, researchers use a combination of the two methods to address the same research problem.

### Data Analysis Plan

In addition to describing the sample and the procedures used in a study, the methods section often includes a description of the data analysis. Remember that data are the information collected in a study and data analysis is a description of what was done with that data to obtain a clearer picture of what the information tells us. Although the results section summarizes the outcome of data analysis, the meth-

---

## CORE CONCEPT

*Many of the terms used in research have a range of meanings rather than a single discrete, locked-in meaning.*

ods section often describes in detail how the researchers worked with or analyzed the data. In the article about fecal incontinence, the authors describe in some detail the computation of scores and statistics for the various values they found from measurements in the clinical setting. The report's subsection is labeled "statistical analysis," because it describes the statistical procedures that were carried out to provide a meaningful summary of the collected information. The fictional article has a much shorter "Analysis" subsection. In the analysis subsection, the author informs the reader that a specific computer program was used to analyze the data that were numbers and then describes the analysis procedures for the data that were words. Again, the approaches to analyzing quantitative and qualitative data are different and are discussed further in Chapter 4.

## Problem

So far, we have reviewed the conclusions, results, and methods sections of research reports: conclusions discuss the outcomes, decisions, or potential meanings of the study; the results summarize what was found; and the methods describe how the study was implemented. This brings us to the beginning of a research report, a section often labeled "Problem" or "Introduction". Just as the word suggests, the **problem** section of a research report describes the gap in knowledge that is addressed by the research study. In this section of the report, the researcher explains why the research study was needed, why the study was carried out in the manner that it was, and, often, what the researcher is specifically asking or predicting.

The introduction or problem section of a research report usually includes a background, or **literature review** subsection, which is a focused summary of what has already been published regarding the question or problem for which there is a gap in knowledge. The literature review gives us a picture of what is already known or has already been studied in relation to the problem and identifies where the gaps in knowledge may be. It may report, for example, that studies have only been done with selected types of patients, such as with children but not with adults. Or it may report that no one has ever tried to ask a particular question before: perhaps studies have examined how to treat diarrhea and fecal incontinence caused by a specific bacterium such as *Clostridium difficile* but not examined general causes of fecal incontinence.

The literature review does not necessarily only include published research studies. It also may include published reports about issues related to practice or a description of a theory. A **theory** is a written description of how several factors may relate to and affect each other. The factors described in a theory are usually abstract; that is, they are ideas or concepts, such as illness, stress, pain, or fatigue, that cannot be readily observed and immediately defined and recognized by everyone. Nursing theories such as Roy's (1984) Theory of Adaptation, Neuman's (1982) System Model, and Watson's (1985) Theory of Human Caring are examples of written descriptions of how the four major components of nursing (persons, health, environment, and nursing) may interrelate.

Lazarus's (1993) Theory of Stress and Coping is another example of a theory that most nurses know and that is somewhat simpler than most nursing theories. It proposes relationships among four abstract factors: life events, perceptions of threat, perceptions of ability to manage a threat, and stress. The relationships proposed in

**FIGURE 2-3**    **Proposed relationships among the four factors in Lazarus's Theory of Stress and Coping (1993).**

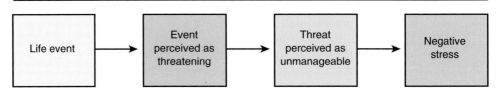

the theory are: if a life event occurs that is perceived as threatening, and there are no perceived approaches to manage or mitigate that threat, then stress results. Figure 2–3 illustrates the proposed relationships among these four factors.

When a research report discusses a theory in its introduction or problem section, the study usually tests or further explains the relationships proposed in that theory. Therefore, if a study report discussed Lazarus's Theory of Stress and Coping (1993) in the introduction, we expect that the study will be based on, that is, examine, some aspect of how life events and perceptions affect stress as described in that theory. If a research study is based on an existing theory, then the researcher often already has an idea of what relationships are expected to be found. These ideas are stated in the form of a **hypothesis**, a prediction regarding the relationships or effects of selected factors on other factors. For a study to include a hypothesis, there must be some knowledge about a problem of interest, so that we can propose or predict that certain relationships or effects will occur. Neither the fecal incontinence article nor the fictional article explicitly includes either a theory or a hypothesis. Both studies do describe several factors that may influence the problem of interest, but the problem statements in both studies suggest that the knowledge gap results from not knowing the effects or relationships among these factors. As a result, both studies present purposes or research questions but do not include hypotheses that make predictions. Research questions, purposes, and hypotheses are discussed in Chapter 10.

## RESEARCH REPORTS AND THE RESEARCH PROCESS

So far, we have discussed mainly the elements of a published research report. However, in doing so, we have had to at least touch on what a researcher does to conduct a research study. Although this book is not intended to teach you how to be a researcher, it is impossible to use research intelligently if you do not understand the basics of the research process. Fortunately, the research report is written in a manner that closely mirrors the actual research process, so, as we focus on understanding and intelligently using research, we also can learn the basics of the research process. We overview the steps in that process now and then discuss the different steps further in the following chapters.

### Steps in the Research Process

Figure 2–4 illustrates the five steps in the research process and the relationship between them and the sections of a research report. The first step is to define and describe a knowledge gap or problem. Frequently, this first step begins with a clinical

**FIGURE 2-4**    **The relationship between the research process and the sections of a research report.**

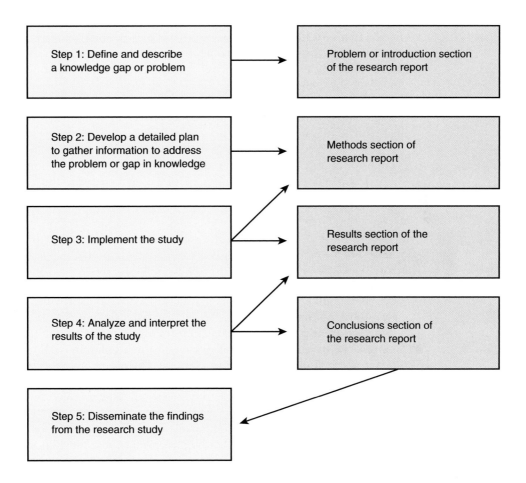

question, such as the one raised by the RN in the vignette, who wants to prevent the complication of fecal incontinence and the associated skin breakdown in her patient, J.K. A researcher interested in this type of clinical question then performs a literature review to determine what is already known about the problem. Performing a literature review requires using databases, as discussed in Chapter 1, except that the researcher attempts to find and read as many as possible of the pertinent published articles on the topic. As part of defining and describing the knowledge gap, the researcher also investigates whether anyone has ever implemented a study addressing the clinical question, as well as how other people have studied or described aspects of the problem. Although this process may help the researcher to gain a clearer picture of how to construct a study to address the clinical question, it also may make the problem more complicated and confusing. Often, a researcher's question changes as he or she learns about what has already been studied or described. Therefore, the focus of the first step in the research process is to narrow and identify the specific focus for the research study and its culmination is a statement of a problem or purpose for the study. The problem section of a research report partially reflects this first step in the research process by providing a description of the relevant literature, possibly a theory, and one or more of the following: a research problem, question, or hypothesis. However, the neatly written problem or introduction section of a research report certainly will not reflect all of the thinking, sorting, and comparing involved in the first step of the research process.

The second step in the research process is to develop a detailed plan for gathering information to address the identified knowledge gap. Planning the research study depends on the problem or question being asked, and the designs of qualitative and quantitative studies differ, partly because of the type of questions asked and partly because of the researcher's beliefs about how best to gain meaningful knowledge.

**QUALITATIVE**

Knowledge gaps that lend themselves to studies using qualitative methods are usually related to the experiences, beliefs, feelings, or perceptions of individuals, and, often, little is known about the area in question. Because little is known or understood about the problem, qualitative methods provide a broad picture by describing the whole of the experience from the patient's viewpoint. In addition, a researcher may approach knowledge gaps using qualitative methods, because he or she believes that we can best learn and understand the phenomena of interest by examining the whole of a phenomena in its usual context.

**QUANTITATIVE**

In contrast, knowledge gaps that involve a concrete response or action, such as fecal incontinence, lend themselves to a quantitative approach, in which each factor that might contribute to a disorder is identified, defined, and measured. A researcher who uses a quantitative approach believes that knowledge can best be generated by breaking down a phenomenon into its different pieces and objectively measuring and examining each piece and its relationship to the other pieces.

In the second step of the research process, the specific methods that will be used to study the problem are planned, including who will participate in the study, what will be done to collect information, and how that information will be analyzed. This step requires understanding the various approaches that can be taken to systematically gather information, considering what has been done in the past and what kinds of problems have occurred, and planning carefully to maximize the knowledge that will be the product of the study. The methods section of the research report, like the problem section, summarizes the decisions that were made in this step of the research process by specifically describing the sample, procedures, and data analysis used in the study. For example, in the fictional article about nursing students' preferences for first clinical jobs, the report tells us that the study included junior-year undergraduate nursing students and that, in this program, traditional 4-year, RN-to-BSN and LPN-to-BSN students were included in the study. The report also tells us that a written questionnaire was used to collect the data. The researcher in this study could have decided to study graduating seniors rather than juniors or to conduct in-depth interviews with selected students rather than using a questionnaire. The researcher had reasons for using juniors and having them complete a questionnaire, such as time constraints, student availability, and the researcher's view on meaningful ways to gather knowledge. What we read in the research report usually only reflects the final decisions of this step of the research process, and the researcher will likely only provide a limited explanation of the methods used.

Because research is a process, a study may not occur as it was designed and planned; therefore, the methods section also may describe any changes made to the study plan as it was implemented. In the fecal incontinence study, for example, the authors tell us in the methods section that 32 of the 184 subjects in the original study were disqualified for several reasons. This change meant that the researchers no longer had two groups of patients (tube-fed and non–tube-fed) who were matched so that they had the same balance of risk factors for *C. difficile*. When subjects withdrew, the groups were not matched, that is, the same, on the presence or absence of *C. difficile*. Therefore, the researchers had to analyze the entire sample as one group and include the risk factors for *C. difficile* as one aspect that they studied.

The third step in the research process is to implement the study by gathering and analyzing the information in the systematic manner planned in the second step. As mentioned in the discussion of procedures, this may involve numerous different actions, such as tape-recording interviews, performing carefully controlled clinical experiments, or mailing and compiling responses to a questionnaire. In addition to gathering the information, this step involves managing, organizing, and analyzing the information to address the problem being studied. The outcome of this step is reported in the results section of the research report, which is why that section describes the sample and summarizes the answers or outcomes for each measure. Those results may not directly answer the research question, but they do allow the reader to understand better what happened during the study. For example, it is likely the researchers in the fecal incontinence study did not seek to have mostly men in their study. However, it may be that the only site that they could access for their study was a veterans' medical center. As we learn in the results section, this led to a sample that included 150 men and only 2 women. It is important to remember this when reviewing the conclusions, because they can only be applied to men.

The fourth step in the research process is the detailed analysis and interpretation of the results. In qualitative research methods, this fourth step of the process is woven closely with the third step, with analysis often guiding additional data collection. In quantitative methods, some preliminary analysis and summary of the data usually occur during the implementation step of the research process. However, additional analysis and careful interpretation of the meaning of the findings occurs only after all the information from the study is gathered. The researchers will analyze the data, compare their findings to those from previous studies, and decide what they can conclude from the study. At this point, the researcher hopes to answer the question posed, confirm or not confirm the prediction made, or create a meaningful understanding of the phenomena of interest. The actual findings from the study are summarized in the results section of the research report, whereas the implications, or potential meaning of those findings, are included in the conclusions section of the report. As with all the other sections of a research report, what is actually included in the report does not reflect everything that the researchers did during this step: they will distill their analysis into a few paragraphs to provide the reader with a succinct summary of what they found and what it may mean for clinical care.

The fifth and final step of the research process is the sharing or dissemination of the findings. Gathering information to gain new knowledge is not a particularly useful activity if no one ever learns about the new knowledge, so an important obligation and commitment of the researcher is to share that research through publications, presentations, posters, and teaching. Research reports, such as the one on fecal incontinence, are obviously a major method for disseminating research. However, research reports do not accomplish the goal of disseminating research if the people who need the knowledge cannot understand them. This brings us back to the importance of understanding and intelligently reading and using research in nursing practice.

### The Language of Research

So far, this chapter has presented several terms that are unique to research. Although each of these terms has been defined in this chapter, do not be discouraged if you are not completely clear about all of them. They are also included and defined in the glossary, and we will revisit them as we discuss the different sections of a research report in more detail in the following chapters. The learning outcome for this chapter is that you differentiate the different sections or components of a research report and the language associated with each of those sections, not that you understand in-depth each of the terms. Table 2–1 provides a summary of the sections of a research report and the associated language of those sections.

You were asked at the end of Chapter 1 to read the fictional article and compile a list of terms you did and did not understand. Hopefully, this chapter has touched on some of the terms that were not clear to you and, perhaps, added to your understanding of terms that you believed you already understood. Again, you can think of reading research as being similar to reading a patient's chart. The first time you read a patient's hospital chart, a great deal of the information in it did not make sense to you and you may not have even known which section to look in for different types of information. With time, however, you learned the unique language of the health care field and found your way around a chart with ease. The same thing will happen with research reports. Just as you learned where to look for physicians' orders and the unique language used in those orders, you will learn where to look for specific information about a research study and to understand the unique research language used. For example, you have already learned where to look for information about procedures in a research study and some of the unique language used to describe those procedures, so you have a good start at reading and better understanding research reports. As you read the different research reports used in this book, keep adding to your list of words or ideas that you do not understand, then periodically review it and cross out those words you believe you understand. You can use this list to guide your own reading and can share the list with your fellow students and your faculty to assure clarification of the words to facilitate your own and fellow students' learning.

## Meta-Analysis and Systematic Reviews as Evidence for Practice

The two examples we have been using in this chapter are both reports of a single research study. Other research reports, however, report studies of a group of single research studies or meta-analysis. **Meta-analysis**, a quantitative approach to knowledge development, applies statistics to numeric results from different studies that addressed the same research problem to look for combined results that would not happen by chance alone. Meta-analysis is similar to systematic reviews for evidence-based practice, the form of research that summarizes multiple research studies, along with other evidence. However, systematic reviews do not generally apply statistical procedures to the information collected from individual studies.

The sections of reports of meta-analyses and systematic reviews resemble those of single studies but may differ in some important ways. Table 2–2 summarizes what you might expect to find in the different sections of reports of a systematic review and of a meta-analysis. Both a systematic review and a meta-analysis begin with a section that identifies the problem of interest. In a meta-analysis, the problem identified may be anything that has been addressed in several individual research studies. For example, a recent report of a meta-analysis addressed studies of fall prevention in the elderly (Hill-Westmoreland, Soeken, & Spellbring, 2002), and another meta-analysis study addressed diabetes patient education research (Brown, 1992). In contrast, a systematic review addresses a specific patient care or clinical practice question, because the intent of the review is to provide evidence for practice.

A systematic review has defined procedures, but they are not always described in the report under a heading titled "Methods." The procedures in a systematic review involve searching and identifying all primary studies that examine or are related to a particular clinical care problem. The researcher has to define the problem and which studies are related and not related to that problem. The researcher also describes the procedures used to search the literature after describing the problem, or perhaps at the end of the report, under a heading such as "search strategies."

In contrast, a meta-analysis report usually has a clearly identified methods section in which the search strategies used, the inclusion and exclusion criteria used for the sample of studies, and the statistical analyses applied are all described. Notice that a meta-analysis examines a sample of research studies rather than a sample of patients.

The results sections of meta-analyses and systematic reviews differ because the meta-analysis specifically describes the numeric values from findings of the different studies and the statistical tests used to test those numbers, whereas the systematic review does not. Therefore, a report of systematic review primarily uses words to summarize the available studies that address a clinical care question, although it may report individual numbers from some of those studies. A meta-analysis may summarize the nature of the studies used, but the core of the findings is numeric. Both systematic reviews and meta-analyses usually provide a table identifying the basic characteristics of the individual research studies that were included, which allows the reader to view the individual studies as needed.

**TABLE 2–2**    **Components of Reports for Individual Research Studies, Meta-Analyses, Systematic Reviews, and Quality Assurance Reports**

| Components of Reports | Traditional Research Study | Meta-Analysis | Systematic Review | Quality Improvement Study |
|---|---|---|---|---|
| Problem or Introduction | Review of the literature; theory; statement of a knowledge gap; predictions or hypotheses | Identification of a problem that has been addressed in several studies with inconsistent results | Statement of a practice problem, including a broad overview of the relevant clinical questions related to that problem | Statement of a standard for patient care that is measurable and specific, usually including a summary of the basis research and clinical basis for the standard |
| Methods | Description of quantitative or qualitative procedures; sampling methods; data analysis methods | Description of the procedures used to find and select the individual research studies; description of procedures used to code and analyze results from the individual studies; table of studies usually included here | Description of search strategies used and criteria used for including a study in the review | Description of the procedures used to identify selected patient care situations and the methods used to collect information about the care in those situations |
| Results | Description of findings; summary of themes or concepts or results of statistical procedures | Summary of the results of statistical tests on groups of results from individual studies | Summary of the research findings categorized and synthesized under clinically meaningful topics; usually includes a table of studies here | Summary of the patient care practices that were identified |

| TABLE 2–2 | Components of Reports for Individual Research Studies, Meta-Analyses, Systematic Reviews, and Quality Assurance Reports (Continued) | | | |
|---|---|---|---|---|
| **Components of Reports** | **Traditional Research Study** | **Meta-Analysis** | **Systematic Review** | **Quality Improvement Study** |
| Discussion or Conclusions | Summary of key findings; comparison of results to previous studies; speculation about meaning of results in relation to theory; description of limitations; recommendations for additional research and final conclusions | Summary of key findings and identification of how these differ from what may be generally accepted understanding; identification of needs for additional research and of limitations in existing studies | Specific identification of practice implications derived for the synthesis of the literature; identification of needs for additional research | Summary of key findings; comparison of findings to established standards; speculation about reasons for differences found; recommendations for changes to remedy any deficits found |

Finally, both meta-analyses and systematic reviews have a conclusions section in which the potential meaning of the findings are described. As with single research reports, a meta-analysis and a systematic review may identify limits to what has been reported and usually recommend areas for future research. A systematic review always addresses implications for clinical practice.

Another important type of written report that describes research is a quality improvement study report. A quality improvement study report resembles a report of a traditional research study, but there are some differences between the two. The problem addressed in a quality improvement study usually concerns whether certain expected clinical care was completed, so the question involves discovering what is being done or what has happened, rather than trying to understand a phenomenon. As with traditional research, a quality improvement study usually examines only a subset of all the occasions when a specified type of care was given. Methods to collect data for a quality improvement study include questionnaires, direct observation, and chart reviews. The report of a quality improvement study describes how information was collected concerning the clinical care and a summary of what was found. This is similar to the methods and results sections of a research report. The conclusions of a quality improvement report include recommendations for improving the quality of care, based on what was found regarding the care currently given. The recommendations are similar to the conclusions that are drawn from a research study.

(See Table 2–2 for a summary of the sections of quality improvement reports compared to individual research reports, meta-analyses, and systematic reviews.)

## PUBLISHED REPORT—WHAT DID YOU CONCLUDE?

We have discussed briefly all of the sections in the published research study about fecal incontinence in patients who are acutely ill. The authors in that study report directly that stool consistency, severity of illness, and older age are risk factors for fecal incontinence and that "Treatments that result in a more formed stool may be beneficial in managing fecal incontinence and warrant further investigation" (Bliss et al., 2000, p. 107). If you were the RN in the vignette, would you now know what you would do tomorrow to decrease J.K.'s risk of fecal incontinence? Why or why not?

One reason it may be difficult to decide what to do for J.K. based on the research report is that the nurse may still have questions about the research. What kinds of questions do you think the RN may have about how to approach her care of J.K.? One question might be whether she can believe the results of this study or whether the results are "strong" enough that she is willing to try a different approach with J.K. A second question might be why only three factors were considered; what about diagnosis, infection, or mobility, for example? A third question might be: what is meant by "severity of illness" and how can the RN assess this in her setting? You can probably think of other questions. With a further understanding of the research language and the research process, it is possible to answer most of the questions posed by reading the published report in more detail. In the next chapter, we look more closely at the conclusions of research reports and what they can tell us about patient care questions.

## OUT-OF-CLASS EXERCISE:

### Differing Conclusions From the Class Study

The fictional article in Appendix B represents the kind of report that might be written based on the questionnaire you may have completed in class. In that article, the author suggests that older students may be interested in nonacute settings, because they have had more experiences with health care in several settings. In preparation for the next chapter, write a paragraph that ends the fictional article by taking the position that nursing programs must focus on recruiting older students so that more nurses can be obtained for general care and nursing home settings. Then write a paragraph taking the opposite position that age should not be considered because it is not clear whether it contributes to choice of nursing practice after graduation. *Base your arguments on the findings reported in the fictional article*—not solely on your opinions or ideas. Once you complete this exercise, you are ready to read Chapter 3.

## References

Bliss, D. Z., Johnson, S., Savik, K., Clabots, C. R., & Gerding, D. N. (2000). Fecal incontinence in hospitalized patients who are acutely ill. *Nursing Research, 49*(2), 101–108.

Brown, S. A. (1992). Meta-analysis of diabetes patient education research: Variations in intervention effects across subjects. *Research in Nursing and Health, 15,* 409–419.

Hill-Westmoreland, E. E., Soeken, K., & Spellbring, A. M. (2202). A meta-analysis of fall prevention for the elderly: How effective are they? *Nursing Research, 51*(1), 1–8.

Lazarus, R. S. (1993). Coping, theory and research: Past, present and future. *Psychosomatic Medicine, 55,* 234–247.

Neuman, B. (1982). The Neuman system model: Application to nursing education and practice. East Norwalk, CT: Appleton-Century-Crofts.

Roy, C. (1984). Introduction to nursing: An adaptation model (2nd ed.). Englewood Cliffs, NJ: Prentice-Hall.

Watson, J. (1985). *Human science and human caring: A theory of nursing.* Norwalk, CT: Appleton-Century-Crofts.

## Resource

Locke, L. F., Silverman, S. J., & Spirduso, W. W. (1998). *Reading and understanding research.* Thousand Oaks, CA: Sage Publications.

LEARNING OUTCOME:

*THE STUDENT WILL* interpret the conclusions of research reports for their potential meaning for clinical practice.

CHAPTER

**3**

# Discussions and Conclusions

## *What Is the Answer to My Question?*
## *What Did the Study Conclude?*

**KEY TERMS:**

Conceptualization
Confirmation
Discussion
Generalization

Replication
Speculation
Study design

**connection**—◡

## CLINICAL CASE

C.R. is a 32-year-old woman who is homeless and is a frequent patient in the emergency room, where she has been treated for numerous infections, including several sexually transmitted diseases. Now she is concerned that she might be pregnant. C.R. currently lives at a shelter for homeless women and states that she does not want to be pregnant because a shelter is no place to raise a child. The RN has seen C.R. on several of her visits, as well as several other homeless women who have come to the emergency room for pregnancy tests or concerns about having contracted a sexually transmitted disease. The RN recognizes a need for health promotion with these women to decrease their risks for contracting HIV and for unwanted pregnancy, and the director of the women's shelter has suggested that she offer a program on HIV risk reduction at the shelter. The RN asks C.R. what she thinks about the idea of a program at the shelter to discuss risks for HIV and unwanted pregnancy. C.R. replies: "It all depends on how you decide to talk to us—if you treat us like real people or not." When the

RN thinks about C.R.'s words, she realizes that the people in the homeless shelter may have special needs that should be considered when planning for their health care and wonders what might be the most effective way to provide health care, particularly HIV education, to this unique population. A search in the hospital library on PUBMED during the weekend yields numerous hits regarding health care for the homeless, and two appear useful. The RN finds both of them that day. The first is "Homeless patients' experience of satisfaction with care" (McCabe, Macnee, & Anderson, 2001), and the second is "Evaluating the impact of peer, nurse case-managed, and standard HIV risk-reduction programs on psychosocial and health-promoting behavioral outcomes among homeless women" (Nyamathi, Flaskerud, Leake & Dixon, 2001). Both of these articles are available in Appendix A of this book and on the Connection Web site. Reading the conclusions or discussion sections of these two articles will help you to understand the examples discussed in this chapter.

## THE END OF A RESEARCH REPORT—DISCUSSIONS AND CONCLUSIONS

In this chapter, we address the first of the five questions that are used to organize this book: **What is the answer to my question—What did the study conclude?** Because, as mentioned earlier in Chapter 1, the major reason a practicing nurse wants to read and understand research is to answer clinical questions, nurses, such as the one in the vignette, often go directly to the last section of a research report. That section is sometimes labeled "Discussion," "Conclusions," or both, but its content usually includes both a discussion and conclusions as described here.

When the RN who is interested in HIV prevention for homeless women reads the discussion section of the report on patient satisfaction, she learns that five themes representing dimensions of satisfaction for the homeless population were identified in this study. She also reads that these five satisfaction themes were supported by other themes regarding health and homelessness and that there were positive aspects to homelessness imbedded in some of the themes. The RN then reads the "Discussion and Conclusion" section of the report about evaluating HIV programs with

homeless women, where she learns that all three programs that were tested led to significant improvements in behavioral, cognitive, and psychological risk factors. She
also learns that self-esteem was not improved across any of the three groups studied.
The RN's likely response to reading the discussions and conclusions sections of these
two reports is: "that is all interesting, but I still do not know how to most effectively
teach HIV prevention to the homeless women at the shelter."

The discussion and conclusions section of research reports initially may not be
helpful in clinical questions for several reasons, including:

- the study may not address the question you are asking,
- the researchers may have had problems implementing the study, resulting
  in an unclear answer, or
- the results of the study may have been unexpected and increase, rather than
  decrease, the complexity of possible answers to the question.

Later chapters address why research questions may not directly address clinical
questions and the many problems that can occur when carrying out a research study.
Although this chapter discusses briefly how unexpected results can affect clinical usefulness, understanding results and the results sections of research reports are discussed more completely in Chapter 4. This chapter focuses on a fourth reason that
the conclusion of a report may not answer a clinical question: inappropriate or unclear expectations about what information can be found in the conclusion of a research report. Just what should we expect to find from the discussion and conclusions
sections of research reports?

## DISCUSSIONS

This book treats discussions and conclusions as two separate sections, but remember that you often find them combined in published reports. Table 3–1 summarizes
the major components of most discussion and conclusions sections. The **discussion**
section of a research report summarizes, compares, and speculates about the results
of the study.

### Summary

The first part of the discussion section in a research report usually includes a summary of the study's key results. This summary usually addresses the results that directly relate to the major research question posed by the researcher(s). It also
includes the unexpected results or the results that stood out as particularly meaningful. However, this summary usually is brief, because it follows a detailed description of the results. It is also likely, unless the study had few findings, that it will
not include all of the results from the study. What this brief summary does include
are the results from the study that the researcher believes are particularly important
and meaningful.

For example, the discussion section in the qualitative satisfaction study tells us
that five themes were found that capture the dimensions of satisfaction with health
care for a homeless population. It also states that themes capturing the experiences
of homelessness and of health were identified. The authors specifically identify some

| TABLE 3–1 | General Components of the Discussion and Conclusion Sections of Research Reports |
|---|---|
| **Section of Report** | **Major Components of the Section** |
| Discussion | ■ Summary of key findings<br>■ Comparison of results to those of previous studies<br>■ Description of whether findings confirm results of similar studies or predictions based on theory<br>■ Speculation regarding possible interpretations of results |
| Conclusion | ■ Description of the new knowledge that can be accepted based on the study<br>■ A conceptualization of the meaning of the results or a generalization of the findings<br>■ A description of study limitations |

of the themes, including "self-knowing," "resourcefulness," "respectful engagement," and "committed care," but they do not tell us all the themes or explain the meaning of the themes in this section of the report. Similarly, the discussion section of the report of the HIV program evaluation study tells us that all three HIV risk-reduction programs led to significant improvements in all studied areas, except self-esteem. It does not describe the specific psychological, behavioral, and cognitive improvements that occurred, although there are references to select cognitive aspects, such as hostility. The section also does not explain what constituted and differentiated the three programs that were tested.

## Comparison

After a brief summary of key or important results, the discussion section of a research report debates the possible meanings of the study results. Questions addressed in research studies are rarely simple or readily answered completely by only one study; therefore, the results of a study provide information that can be explained or understood in several different ways. Hence, the pros and cons of different

## CORE CONCEPT

*The summary of findings in the discussion section of a research report only contains selected results from the study. It does not give the reader a complete picture of the results found in the study but does give information about some key or important results.*

explanations for the results may be described, forming a written debate. Further, the meaning of the findings usually must be interpreted within the context of existing knowledge, so the discussion section frequently compares the results of the study to those of previous studies. The match or lack of match of the results of a study to results from previous studies support the different explanations offered about the results. Another important reason for comparing is to provide confirmation of previous findings. **Confirmation** is the verification of results from other studies. Rarely are we comfortable deciding that we are completely certain of the answer to a clinical question based on the findings of only one study. One goal of research is to build knowledge, with each individual research study adding a new piece to our understanding. However, as with the parts of any building that is going to be stable and strong, the pieces of knowledge must overlap and unite to make a cohesive whole. A study that is a duplication of an earlier study is called a **replication** study, and its major purpose is confirmation. Usually, however, a research study differs from past studies in some ways by, for example, using a different patient group in the study or using different procedures on the subjects. Whether a study is a replication or a variation on previous studies, the discussion section of the research report describes how the findings from the study do or do not overlap with previous knowledge.

In addition to discussing how the results of a study do or do not confirm those of previous studies, the authors may compare their findings to the predicted results that were based on existing theory. Theory might be considered to be the plans for the knowledge being built about a clinical question: like a building plan, a theory provides the description of how all the parts of a phenomenon should fit together. Not all research studies are based on a theory or test a prediction from a theory, because not enough may be known about a clinical question. However, if the study tested a prediction or hypothesis that was based on a theory and the results of a study show the pieces fitting together as the theory predicted, then the results are considered to confirm that theory. We discuss how theory directs and is built by research in Chapter 10.

Neither of the studies on homeless patients that the RN found specifically tested theory, but both compare their results to the results of previous studies. For example, the discussion in the article on homeless patients' satisfaction with care states that previous studies found seven dimensions of satisfaction that differ from the themes identified in the present study. The discussion in the HIV program evaluation article states that although pretest and posttest counseling was not successful in previous studies, it was successful in their sample of homeless women. It is not uncommon for results from an individual study to differ from previous studies: that is why we usually need multiple studies to make clinical decisions. Results that differ from findings in previous studies require that the author(s) suggest reasons for those differences, which leads us to the third component of most discussions.

## Speculation

In addition to comparison, the discussion section of a research report speculates regarding the reasons for the results of the study. **Speculation** is the process of reflecting on the results of a study and offering some explanation of them. The debate,

> # CORE CONCEPT
>
> *The discussion section of a research report contains a debate about how the results of the study fit with existing knowledge and what those results may mean.*

or speculation, in a discussion generally considers several alternative explanations for the results of the study and provides a rationale for the author's judgments about which is the best explanation.

As a core concept from Chapter 2 stated, the results section provides the findings of the specific study, whereas the discussion and conclusions sections of a report interpret those findings in light of existing knowledge and theory. This interpretation is appropriately called a discussion, because it is open to debate. It reflects not fact, but thoughtful informed speculation. Although such speculation is thoughtful and informed and considers alternative possibilities, it is based on the particular author's knowledge of and selection of previous research or theory. Another author might know or select a different theory or body of research to use in his or her discussion.

Why are the meanings of results from almost any study open to debate? The answer lies, in part, in the nature of research. We learned in Chapter 2 that research usually examines a question using a subgroup or sample of people. Although great pains often are taken to include diversity in the people, samples cannot possibly reflect all of the variation that exists in humans. What works with or happens to a few subjects is unlikely to be exactly what happens with many patients or with everyone.

QUALITATIVE

In fact, qualitative methods assume that experiences are unique and that, although we can increase our understanding regarding a particular question, we will never be able to answer it definitely. Returning to our analogy of building knowledge piece by piece, the qualitative research perspective is that the picture of the phenomenon, which is the product in knowledge building, is constantly evolving because our world and our individual experiences are always changing.

**Conceptualization** is a process of creating a picture of an abstract idea; in the case of nursing research, it is a picture of some aspect of health. Discussions and conclusions of qualitative studies conceptualize some phenomenon related to health as opposed to those of quantitative studies that objectify and isolate parts of the phenomenon. If theory is the plan for a building, we can view a qualitative study as providing results that are an artist's rendition of a building, rather than a detailed blueprint of that building, which would reflect quantitative results. The picture provides a clear sense of how a building might look or even feel and smell, whereas the blueprint of a building gives us a sense of how it is put together but not of how we will actually experience the building once it is complete. Figure 3–1 illustrates this concept.

From a qualitative perspective, knowledge is built by creating a "picture album" filled with different "pictures" of a particular aspect of health. Each study result, or "picture," gives a sense of the aspect of health at a unique moment in time. As we look at more and more "pictures," we get a greater sense of the whole phenomenon. For example, the final sentences of the satisfaction study convey the

**FIGURE 3-1**

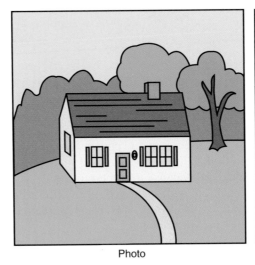 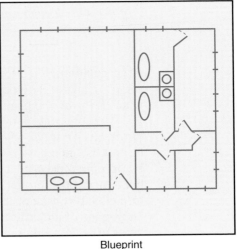

Photo                                                  Blueprint

Product of qualitative research is like        Product of quantitative research is like a
an artist's rendition.                                blueprint, showing details and
                                                            how parts go together.

conceptual conclusions drawn by the authors. The authors state that a model of care for homeless should include "process activities facilitating respectful engagement, and the presence of committed, inclusionary care practices" (McCabe et al., 2001, p. 84). The words create a picture of care, but they do not suggest specific practices.

QUANTITATIVE

Quantitative methods do not assume that knowledge is always changing and evolving; they assume that there are answers to questions and that we can find those answers by objectifying and quantifying the components of a phenomenon to understand the relationships among the components. Quantitative methods assume that we get closer and closer to "knowing" the "real" answer to questions the more often we get the same results in different studies with different groups.

Returning to the analogy of a picture album vs. a blueprint, the qualitative researcher expects each study to be a unique "picture" that adds to our overall understanding. The quantitative researcher, however, does not expect that each study will be a different blueprint but that each study will add more details to the same blueprint.

The goal of quantitative research is to generalize a study's results. **Generalization** is the ability to apply a particular study's findings to the broader population represented by the sample. The authors of the evaluation of HIV programs study, for example, conclude that standard care approaches can be effective with homeless women in general. They also describe in their discussion a breakdown of the different aspects of the standard approach, including the provision of access to care and the presence of a caring health care professional. They then generalize that the specific aspects of their standard HIV program that were effective in their study are likely to be important factors for all homeless women.

### Implications for Practice

The discussion in a nursing research report often includes a debate about the meaning of the study results for nursing practice. For example, the satisfaction article suggests that because several of the themes identified in the study reflected that there are positive facets to being homeless, such as a sense of pride in survival, nurses can use these positive facets as a basis for building additional strengths to promote health. Another less positive clinical interpretation that the authors might draw is that positive facets, such as pride, are not strengths but defenses that separate homeless patients from others and make it difficult to work with them. The authors have not chosen that interpretation in their discussion of the study results, possibly because it does not fit with their philosophy of nursing and health care. However, it is important to realize that choices are made concerning the best clinical interpretation of results, just as choices are made about how the results add to existing knowledge in general.

The RN who reads the discussions in the two articles about homeless patients is reading the different authors' interpretations of what they believe to be their key findings. In the satisfaction study, the authors clearly state that an important finding was the difference in what constituted satisfaction for their homeless sample compared with what constituted satisfaction in other populations, such as middle-class workers who had health insurance. The authors interpret their findings to mean that homeless clients have unique needs that should be considered when providing care to them. In contrast, the authors of the evaluation of HIV programs study interpret their results of no differences among the three different programs to mean that standard programs that are productive for people who are not homeless will work adequately for homeless patients. Neither study is right or wrong. Both studies speculate about the meaning of their results, considering previous research. However, the RN in the vignette now has two different possible answers to her question about unique needs for the homeless women she plans to educate. The RN must read previous sections of the reports to decide how to combine the findings of the different studies. We return to the RN's dilemma later in this chapter.

## CONCLUSIONS

The conclusions of a research report describe the knowledge that the researcher believes can be gained from the study, given its "fit" with other studies and theories. As stated in Chapter 2 in the discussion of sections of a research report, conclusions from a research study can be powerful because they are used to guide practice. Conclusions move beyond debate or speculation about the results to a statement of what is now "known" about a question or problem. As a result, they generally are worded carefully and cautiously. Conclusions also may be statements about what we do not know, particularly if the study results do not fit with theory or replicate previous studies. Therefore, it is possible for a conclusion to state that we now know we cannot get the answer for our question using the methods or measures or sample that was used in the study being reported. More often, conclusions include recommendations for building knowledge about a clinical question or health aspect. In either case, the conclusion section almost always describes the limits that must be placed on the knowledge that has been gained from the study.

Neither the satisfaction study nor the evaluation of the HIV programs study provides absolute concrete answers to the questions they addressed. We have identified that one reason for this is that when questions are complex, the research results are open to debate and interpretation. Another reason that study results are open to speculation or debate is that almost every study has limitations. Remember from Chapter 2 that limitations are the aspects of a study that create uncertainty about the meaning or decisions that can be derived from it. We suggested that limitations can be viewed as a fence around the results of a research study that confine or limit what we can conclude.

Several aspects of a study may be viewed as limitations, and Figure 3–2 illustrates some of these. We have already alluded to one factor that often limits a study: the sampling—who was included in the study. Although the satisfaction study included homeless men and women from several different locations, most were identified as White. This aspect of the sample leaves us with uncertainty about the meaning of the results for homeless individuals who are Black, Latino, or Native American. Because the satisfaction study was qualitative, it did not aim to have a representative sample so that results can be generalized to a similar population. The satisfaction study aims to produce findings that can be used in various settings, so the limit on the sample indicates that the picture provided by the study results is a picture of only homeless people who are White and from southern Appalachia.

**FIGURE 3-2**    **Some limitations of the research process, represented by the fence posts.**

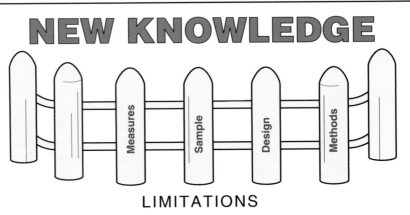

Unlike the satisfaction study, the evaluation of the HIV programs study aims to generalize its findings to all homeless women. However, the authors include in their description of limitations: "the West Coast perspective of this sample may limit generalizability of findings to other samples" (Nyamathi et al., 2001, p. 420). By doing so, the authors recognize that attitudes and beliefs that are pervasive on the West Coast may not be held by homeless women in other parts of the country. These attitudes and beliefs may have contributed to the effectiveness of the standard HIV program's effectiveness; therefore, it might not be effective with homeless women in the Midwest or the South. As we see in Chapters 6 and 7, many other sampling-related aspects can create limits to a research study.

A second factor that may be a limitation is the **study design**, the overall plan or organization of a study. Some study designs create more uncertainty than others do. For example, if the RN in the vignette read a study that described only the cognitive, behavioral, and psychological levels of homeless women at one time point after participating in an HIV education program, she would be uncertain about whether those levels were present before the intervention. A study that uses a pretest and posttest design, in which measures are taken before and after an intervention, such as the HIV program evaluation research, removes some of the uncertainty about the results, because we know that actual outcome changes occurred between the beginning and the end of the study. Many factors affect a researcher's decision about a study design, including the type of question being asked, the level of existing knowledge, and the availability of resources. Chapter 9 discusses research designs in more detail.

A third factor that may be a limitation involves the measures used in the study. Several problems can occur with the study measures. For example, a study's measures may be inconsistent. If a study measures blood sugars using a glucometer that loses calibration halfway through the study, the resulting blood sugar measures will be inconsistent. Sometimes paper-and-pencil questionnaires are unclear or confusing, causing people to be inconsistent in their understanding of and, therefore, answers to the questions. A second possible problem is that measures may be inaccurate or incomplete. Returning to the study using a glucometer for measuring blood sugars, if the glucometer had gone out of calibration before the study began, the resulting measures would be consistent but inaccurate throughout the study. That is, the measures will consistently be inaccurate. Accuracy and consistency of measures are referred to as validity, rigor, and reliability in research. The examples given in this paragraph are all reflective of quantitative research, although accuracy and consistency are also a problem in qualitative research. These ideas are the focus of Chapter 8.

Finding accurate measures of concepts in quantitative research is a problem in nursing, because it is difficult to find ways to quantify some concepts that are important to nurses, such as anger, quality of life, pain, or self-confidence. If measures do not exist, the researcher will either have to make one or not include that factor in the study. Excluding an important factor limits the conclusions that can be drawn. For example, in the conclusion of the evaluation of the HIV programs study, one limitation that was identified was that the authors did not measure or examine the effect of referrals on psychological, behavioral, and cognitive outcomes. The authors do not mention if they did not measure the effect of referrals because there was no established way to do so or because they did not anticipate the need for that measurement. The lack of that measurement presents the possibility that the standard program was effective because the women received referrals, rather than because the program led to different behaviors. It may be less obvious, but if a measure of an important factor is new and has never been tested to show that it works, we must wonder how accurate and consistent it may be, which also can be a limitation.

The methods used in a study are a fourth factor that also may limit the conclusions. Not only does a measurement need to be consistent and accurate, but it also must be used consistently and accurately. An appropriately calibrated glucometer will still provide results that are inconclusive regarding a person's blood sugar if it is used at different times during the day and with different techniques to acquire the blood samples. Similarly, a measure of knowledge about HIV will not be conclusive if one group answered it immediately after a program and the other group answered it a week after their program. Therefore, the methods used to conduct the study also may lead to limitations in the conclusions.

For example some participants declined to provide urine specimens, which created a limit to the study of the HIV programs. Because one of the measured outcomes was drug use, the methods would have been better if they had assured that all the women study participants provided urine specimens for drug assays. That some of the women refused to provide the specimen that was needed to confirm what they reported about their drug use casts some doubt about the conclusions from the study.

The discussion and conclusions section of a research report, then, includes a summary of key results, a comparison of those results to findings from other studies or to existing theory, speculation and debate about the possible explanations for the results and how they fit with current knowledge, and, finally, some carefully worded decisions about new knowledge gained in the study. The discussion and conclusions section includes debate, speculation, and cautious language because research questions are complex, each study contributes only one new piece to the puzzle or one more picture to the phenomenon, and almost every study has some limitations.

## Can Conclusions Differ?

At the end of Chapter 2, you were asked to write two concluding paragraphs for the fictional article, taking two different positions regarding who should be recruited for nursing programs based on the results reported in the fictional article. Reviewing the results reported in that study, we find that age, type of program, and rating of health affected choice of nursing field. We assume that the goal is to focus recruitment of students on increasing the number of graduates that enter fields that are not considered acute, a goal with which you may not personally agree. One way to interpret the results is to focus on the finding that age was an important factor in choice of field and conclude that older students should be recruited. Therefore, the new knowledge gleaned from the study would be that recruiting older students will increase the numbers of new graduates entering nonacute nursing fields.

However, the finding that health rating was important could mean that the relevant factor is not age and experience as the author suggests. Rather, the relevant factor may instead be level of health, with students who perceive themselves as less healthy selecting fields of practice that are generally considered less physically strenuous. If this is true, then age is not the relevant factor. Rather, schools of nursing must recruit students who want less physically strenuous positions. This second conclusion would probably be considered relatively implausible, but it illustrates that conclusions can differ based on the interpretation of the results. Because the conclusions drawn from study results can differ, as you read discussions and conclusions of research reports, you should carefully consider whether the interpretation provided makes sense to you in terms of your own knowledge and practice.

### Do We Change Practice?

We have emphasized that the conclusions of research reports can be powerful because they are used to change practice. We also have pointed out some of the uncertainty that is reflected in most conclusions. Most importantly, we have said that the purpose for you to intelligently understand research is for you to use it in practice. Recognizing the limitations of each individual research study and the complexity of building new knowledge does not imply that research cannot and should not be used in practice. However, it does mean that it is essential to have some understanding of more than just the study conclusions. We must understand why and how much the limitations, such as sampling, measures, methods, or design, make the results uncertain, and we must look intelligently at the study findings and if the author's interpretation is logical.

Each individual research study reflects only one piece or picture in the process of knowledge building, which is why nurses and other health professionals emphasize the use of systematic reviews. Systematic reviews include the results from many studies as evidence for practice. Systematic reviews compile the results of multiple studies regarding the same clinical question and organize the findings around key aspects related to practice. A systematic review also addresses differences in research studies, such as design, sample, and methods. The end of a systematic review is usually titled "practice implications" and summarizes the practice-related points that are most strongly supported by different research studies.

As with individual studies, however, systematic reviews are open to interpretation because the findings of particular studies can be given more or less attention. For example, the author of a systematic review may place less emphasis on negative findings about a procedure and interpret the positive findings to warrant a change in clinical practice. An author may also believe that any negative finding about a procedure questions its use and interpret any negative research to indicate that a procedure should not be adopted in practice. As in individual studies, the conclusions of systematic reviews include some hesitancy or caution and almost always include recommendations for further research. Systematic reviews as evidence for practice can be helpful, but the nurse still must read the review carefully and intelligently to decide how the findings should be used in practice.

## COMMON ERRORS IN RESEARCH REPORTS

To be read and used intelligently in practice, the research report must clearly and completely give the reader the information he or she needs. Many nurses assume that if they are not comfortable in their understanding of a research study, it is be-cause they lack knowledge. This may be the case, but it is also possible that part of the problem lies in the research report. Therefore, we discuss common errors that may be found in research reports in each chapter to help you recognize that some-times the problem lies not with your knowledge but with the information provided to you.

One error may be a failure to include one or more of the major aspects of a dis-cussion and conclusion in a report. The authors of a research report should provide the information discussed throughout this chapter in the discussion and conclusions section. As a research reader, you should expect to find there a summary of key find-ings, a comparison of the findings to previous research, and an interpretation of the meaning of the findings within the context of current knowledge. Also, you should find some discussion of the study limitations. The fictional article provides an ex-ample of a report that does not include important aspects, because it neither com-pares its results to previous studies nor includes any discussion of study limitations.

A second common error is presenting a confusing summary of key findings or presenting new results. The summary of key findings should use language that is con-sistent with both the common use of terms and how the terms were used through-out the report. The summary should not include key findings that were not already described in more detail in the results section. Because we are starting at the end of a report, we might not know that information in the discussion was not addressed in the results, but we can quickly find this out if we read the results section. The sum-mary of key findings is a brief, succinct summation. If a result is only provided at the end of a report in this manner, we will likely not have enough information about it to judge intelligently the usefulness of that finding for practice.

A third common error in research reports is overinterpreting the results. Like nurses in practice, researchers want answers to the questions they study. Therefore, it is tempting to overinterpret results by reading into them, generalizing the results of a study beyond what was actually found, or discounting the limitations of the study. It is expected that a researcher will understate or be conservative when in-terpreting study results. However, occasionally a report presents an interpretation that makes suggestions that are more than what can reasonably be concluded based on the results of the study. For example, if the authors of the satisfaction article had concluded that perceptions of trust were the most important theme for homeless pa-tients, they would have drawn a conclusion that interpreted their results beyond what they indicated—they did not ask the homeless study participants what was most important to them; rather, they asked what satisfaction meant to them. Trust was one of the themes identified, but no grounds exist for claiming that it was the most important theme.

Similarly, occasionally a research report draws conclusions that are not directly related to the question under study. Suppose, for example, that the authors of the HIV programs article had stated in their conclusions that having an ongoing inti-mate partner made homeless women more likely to decrease risky behaviors. Yet, the HIV program study compared the effectiveness of three different programs, not the role of personal relationships on behaviors, so such a conclusion would not fit with what was studied. In fact, the authors of the HIV program evaluation article clearly state in their conclusion that they did not compare women with or without intimate partners because the researchers did not have a specific group that did not have intimate partners.

## PUBLISHED REPORTS—WHAT WOULD YOU CONCLUDE?

The discussion and conclusions of the two reports found by the RN in the clinical vignette tell us several different things. They tell us that dimensions of satisfaction with care for homeless clients differ from those identified in earlier studies with people who were not homeless. This confirms the RN's impression that homeless individuals may have different needs or views based on C.R.'s comment about treating them as real people. The conclusion also suggests that homeless individuals have strengths as well as deficits. The discussion did not tell the RN what the themes for satisfaction were; she will have to read the results section to answer that question. The evaluation of the HIV programs study tells the RN that a standard program that works with nonhomeless people also worked as well as other HIV programs with homeless women. The authors of that study describe why a standard program may meet the special needs of homeless women.

The conclusions from these two reports may contradict one another. However, it is possible to fit the conclusions of these studies together in a meaningful way. For example, the RN might decide from the satisfaction article that she must recognize and look for some of the strengths in the homeless women whom she has cared for and consider how she might use those strengths in an HIV prevention program. At the same time, the RN might plan to use already-prepared HIV prevention materials developed for general community presentations, recognizing that they will likely be effective with this population if they are presented thoughtfully and reflect the unique needs of homeless women.

The discussion and conclusions section of a research report provides useful information for using research in practice, including a summary of key findings from the study, a comparison of the findings to previous research and theory, and an interpretation of the meaning of the findings. However, although the conclusions begin to answer the RN's clinical question, she will probably want to know more about the themes for satisfaction among the homeless and to know more about how the different HIV programs affected the outcomes studied. This means that she must read the proceeding section of the research report—the results section.

## OUT-OF-CLASS EXERCISE:

### How Do We Organize a Large Amount of Information to Make Sense of It?

The next two chapters discuss the results section of research reports. As we mentioned in Chapter 2, the results sections of research reports often include some of the most complex and confusing language for readers who are not advanced researchers themselves. We look at some of the key terms in results sections that can readily be understood without having an advanced degree in statistics, and discuss how to determine what you need to really understand and intelligently use nursing research in practice.

To prepare for Chapter 4, summarize some of the data from your in-class study exercise in a way that makes it easier to understand or that makes sense of it. When doing this, think about why the organization you are using helps make it easier to understand. If you did not have an in-class study, your faculty may provide you with some data to use for this out-of-class exercise. Once you have completed this exercise, you are ready to read Chapter 4.

## References

American Psychological Association. (2001). *Publication manual of the American Psychological Association* (5th ed., pp 26–27). Washington, DC: American Psychological Association.

Locke, L. F., Silverman, S. J., & Spirduso, W. W. (1998). *Reading and understanding research.* Thousand Oaks, CA: Sage Publications.

McCabe, S., Macnee, C. L., & Anderson, M. K. (2001). Homeless patients' experience of satisfaction with care. *Archives of Psychiatric Nursing, 15*(2), 78–85.

Nyamathi, A., Flaskerud, J. H., Leake, B., Dixon, E. L., & Lu, A. (2001). Evaluating the impact of peer, nurse case-managed, and standard HIV risk-reduction programs on psychosocial and health-promoting behavioral outcomes among homeless women. *Research in Nursing & Health, 24,* 410–422.

## Resource

Polit, D. F., & Hungler, B. P. (1999). *Nursing research: Principles and methods* (6th ed.). Philadelphia: Lippincott.

**CHAPTER**

**4**

# Descriptive Results

## *Why Did the Authors Reach Their Conclusion—What Did They Actually Find?*

DIFFERENTIATING DESCRIPTION FROM
  INFERENCE
UNDERSTANDING THE LANGUAGE OF THE
  RESULTS SECTION
  Language Describing Results From
    Quantitative Studies
  Language Describing Results From
    Qualitative Studies

CONNECTING RESULTS THAT DESCRIBE TO
  CONCLUSIONS
COMMON ERRORS IN THE REPORTS OF
  DESCRIPTIVE RESULTS
PUBLISHED REPORT—WHAT WOULD YOU
  CONCLUDE?

**KEY TERMS:**

Bivariate
Categorization scheme
Coding
Content analysis
Data reduction
Data saturation
Demographics
Dependent variable
Distribution
Frequency distribution
Independent variables
Inference

Mean
Measures of central tendency
Median
Mode
Normal curve
Predictor variables
Skew
Standard deviation
Theme
Univariate
Variable
Variance

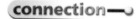

connection—⊃

For additional activities go to
http://connection.lww.com/go/macnee.

## CLINICAL CASE

During the past 5 years, the RN at the county Public Health Department has noticed a steady increase in the number of patients who are Mexican American, as well as migrant workers from Mexico. This increase was confirmed at a recent staff meeting, when it was revealed that the Women, Infants & Children (WIC) program, the well-baby program, and the infectious disease surveillance program had all documented major increases in the past year in the number of patients who are Mexican American and Mexican migrant workers. The staff decided that revising or developing programs to meet the needs of this increasing population would be their goal for the coming year. To begin planning for this goal, each RN was asked to bring with them to the next staff meeting a summary of at least one study examining the health and health practices of Mexican Americans or migrant workers. The RN has worked with the tuberculosis (TB) program for a while and has noticed that family support plays an important role in the screening and treatment of tuberculosis. Last week, he worked with the

Hernandezes, a young family in which the father recently had a skin test that was confirmed as active TB by a chest radiograph. He wondered how a low-income family dealing with the stress of living in a new country copes with an infectious illness that requires long-term treatment. A search of CINAHL using the key words "tuberculosis," "Mexican," and "family" yielded no results. When he limited the search to "Mexican" and "tuberculosis," several articles were identified, and when he used only "Mexican" and "family," several other articles were listed. The RN selected one article from each search to read before the next staff meeting: "Factors associated with participation by Mexican migrant farmworkers in a Tuberculosis screening program" (Poss, 2000) and "Mexican American family survival, continuity, and growth: The parental perspective" (Niska, 2001). Both of these articles are available in Appendix A and on the Connection Web site. Reading these articles, particularly the results and discussion sections, will help you to understand the examples in this chapter and in Chapter 5.

## DIFFERENTIATING DESCRIPTION FROM INFERENCE

At the end of Chapter 3, we concluded that to base clinical decisions on the conclusions of a research report, we need to understand better the study results. The results of a study are the specific findings of that study, which can provide an answer to the second question we are using to organize this book: *Why did the authors reach their conclusion—What did they actually find?* This chapter and Chapter 5 address this question.

The results sections of reports summarize findings with two broad goals: (1) to describe or explain the phenomenon of interest and (2) to predict aspects related to the phenomenon of interest. Because qualitative studies approach knowledge development with an expectation of increasing understanding to inform practice, their results use data analysis methods to provide description and explanation. In contrast, quantitative studies may predict, in addition to describe and explain, because the assumption behind them is that results can be generalized to other groups. Quantitative data analysis aims to not only describe and explain but also to allow us to infer what would happen with other similar groups based on what was found in the present study. **Inference** is the process of concluding something based on evidence. The statistical procedures used in most quantitative studies, therefore, are called inferential statistics.

It is important to differentiate between results that merely describe and results that are intended to allow inference, because it directly affects what we can conclude from a study. The knowledge we gain from description can be used to understand better a situation or phenomenon, and that understanding can help us in our clinical practice. For example, the results in the article about Mexican family survival that the RN found include four characteristics that all of the families interviewed viewed as essential to family growth: (1) having shared communication, (2) growing in togetherness, (3) planning ahead, and (4) helping the children become part of the family (Niska, 2001). The RN can use this description of what these families considered essential as he works with the Hernandez family. What he cannot do, however, is predict that if he intervenes to improve the family's communication, the family will survive, because description does not allow us to predict the future nor to understand what causes the phenomena that we have described. To understand cause and make predictions, we must know not only what is present at a given point in time but also the order of factors or events and the timing of such events or factors. When we describe the presence of two or more factors, we know they are present concurrently, but we do not know if one came before the other, if one caused the other, or if both were caused by some other outside event.

Only results that allow us to infer provide information that is useful to predict future responses or situations if the same set of circumstances applies. Results that allow us to infer include information about the order of events or factors and the timing of those events or factors. Therefore, results that are intended to allow inference may be used in clinical practice to predict future health-related outcomes under similar circumstances. The second article uses inferential statistics in the results section and found that perceptions of susceptibility to TB and the intention to get a purified protein derivative (PPD) to screen for TB contributed significantly to whether individuals in the study actually had a PPD. These results can be used in clinical practice to predict that clients who plan to have a PPD and believe that they are susceptible to TB will most likely participate in a screening program. Not all inferential statistics lead to an understanding of causation, but they are all used to infer that what was found in the specific results tested is also likely to be found in other similar cases. Understanding some of the language that is used in the description of results and in inferential statistics is the first step in understanding what results mean for clinical practice. The RN in the vignette found both a qualitative and a quantitative article. In this chapter, we use both of these articles to gain a better understanding of the language in results sections of research reports that reflects descriptive data analysis; we then look at the language of

## CORE CONCEPT

*Research results that only describe or explain cannot be used to predict future outcomes or to directly identify the cause of the findings.*

inferential statistics in Chapter 5. We will continue to use the fictional article as an example in this chapter.

## UNDERSTANDING THE LANGUAGE OF RESULTS SECTIONS

Most research reports' results sections begin by providing information summaries about individual study variables. A **variable** is an aspect of the phenomenon of interest or research problem that differs among people or situations. Therefore, a variable is something that varies: it is not the same for everyone in every situation. Research aims to understand, explain, or predict those differences or variations. A variable may be some attribute of a person, such as age, health, or beliefs. A variable may be a test score, such as a score for anxiety level, or a physiological parameter, such as body temperature. A variable may be an environmental aspect, such as community resources, family support, or employment rates. In all of these examples of variables, we know there will be differences among people or situations.

Research attempts to gain new knowledge about variables that have been identified as important. In the research article for Chapter 1, the variables studied were total cholesterol (TC), diabetes control, and risk factors, such as blood pressure, smoking, and physical activity (Lipman et al., 2000). The goal of the study was to understand better what makes TC and diabetes control vary, so that we can encourage that they vary in the healthiest direction. In the fecal incontinence study (*see* Chapter 2), the variable that the study hoped to explain was fecal incontinence, and other variables, such as stool consistency, tube feeding, and illness severity, were examined to see if their occurrence and extent explained the presence of fecal incontinence (Bliss, Johnson, Savik, Clabots, & Gerding, 2000). The variables for the two studies found by the RN in the vignette for this chapter are identified in Table 4–1.

QUANTITATIVE

In quantitative research, there are two types of variables: independent (or predictor) and dependent. Because the purpose of quantitative research is to explain or predict a particular variable, we call that variable the dependent variable. The **dependent variable** is the variable that is determined by, that is, depends upon, other variables in the study or is the outcome variable of interest. In the fictional article about nursing students' preferences for practice (*see* Appendix B), the outcome that the research is trying to explain or predict is choice of field of nursing practice, so it is the dependent variable. The other types of variables that we discuss in quantitative research are independent variables. **Independent variables** are those variables in the study that are used to explain or predict the outcome of interest, that is, the dependent variable. In the fictional article, the independent variables included age, perceived well-being, race, and marital status. These were factors that differed among students and may explain or predict their choice of field, the dependent variable. Independent variables also are called **predictor variables**, because they are used to predict the dependent variable.

Notice that Table 4–1 classifies the variables from the TB study as independent or dependent but does not classify the variables from the family survival article. The TB study is quantitative and attempts to explain or predict the use of TB-screening pro-

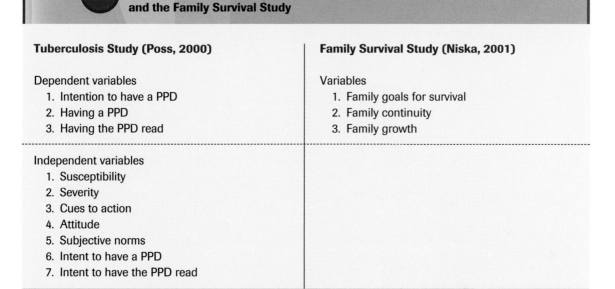

| TABLE 4–1 | Identification of the Specific Variables in the Tuberculosis-Screening Study and the Family Survival Study |
|---|---|
| **Tuberculosis Study (Poss, 2000)** | **Family Survival Study (Niska, 2001)** |
| Dependent variables<br>  1. Intention to have a PPD<br>  2. Having a PPD<br>  3. Having the PPD read | Variables<br>  1. Family goals for survival<br>  2. Family continuity<br>  3. Family growth |
| Independent variables<br>  1. Susceptibility<br>  2. Severity<br>  3. Cues to action<br>  4. Attitude<br>  5. Subjective norms<br>  6. Intent to have a PPD<br>  7. Intent to have the PPD read | |

PPD, purified protein derivative.

grams by Mexican migrant farm workers. The family survival article, however, is qualitative, and, therefore, its purpose is not prediction. Thus, the variables in the family survival article are not and should not be categorized as independent or dependent. The study has an outcome of interest, what helps Mexican American families survive, but it does not measure specific factors that may predict this survival. Rather, the study explores the meaning of family survival for its participants.

You may also notice in Table 4–1 that the variable "Intention to have a PPD" is identified as both a dependent variable and an independent variable. This is an example of a research term being "gray" rather than clearly "black or white." The TB-screening article attempted to identify predictors of getting screened for TB, which, in this case, was a PPD test that was read 48 to 72 hours after its application. However, experience and theory indicate that an individual's intention to get a PPD is an important step that may predict whether a person gets the PPD. The authors use intent to get a PPD as an important factor that they want to be able to predict, making it a dependent variable in some of the analysis. They then use intent to get a PPD as one factor that predicts getting the PPD. In that part of the analysis, intent to get a PPD becomes an independent variable and getting the PPD is the dependent variable. We discuss types of variables in quantitative research in more detail in Chapter 5.

Creating order or organizing information about only one variable is called univariate analysis. In Chapter 2, we said that multivariate indicates there are more than two variables being discussed, and, in fact, most studies will probably include more than one variable. However, analysis of data at a given point may focus on only one variable, and that is called **univariate** analysis. When you worked with the data from your in-class study, you were doing univariate analysis—that is, you were organizing data about individual variables. Another word that you will often see in results sections is bivariate. **Bivariate** analysis refers to analysis with only two variables. Notice that the words themselves reveal their meanings: "uni" variate or one variable, "bi" variate or two variables, and "multi" variate or more than two variables.

Both qualitative and quantitative studies have variables, but information about the variables for studies using these two approaches differs in how data are collected and how they are organized and reported in the results section of a report. The purpose of qualitative studies is to increase our understanding about some aspects of experiences, so the results of qualitative studies describe what was found, usually by organizing the data into concepts and then providing examples of the specific language used by participants to support and clarify the meaning of those concepts. These results describe findings about single variables, usually without using many numbers. Because quantitative studies use numbers to represent variables of interest and then often apply statistical tests to allow inference, we expect to see mostly numbers in the results sections of a quantitative report.

### Language Describing Results From Quantitative Studies

To discuss the language in results sections of research reports, we must take a closer look at data and data analysis. As mentioned in Chapter 2, data are the information collected in a study. This information may take several forms; it may be numbers, words, or even drawings, and it may be written, spoken, or observed. Once the information is collected, it has to be sorted and organized to be meaningful in answering the questions addressed in the research. In preparation for this chapter, you were asked to try to organize some of the data from your in-class questionnaire to make it easy to understand. What did you do to make the information more understandable?

Probably, your first thought was to create some kind of order in the data. The data you were given consisted of numbers, and a logical way to create order is to list them from the smallest number to the largest (or vice versa). Doing so gives a sense of how alike or different people were in the values of the numbers, such as age or marital status, by showing how many numbers are repeated or close together and what are the largest and smallest numbers. The next thing you may have done is determined what were the most common responses. This could be done by simply counting how many times each response was given, by calculating the percentage for each response out of the total responses, or by calculating an average of all the numbers.

Other approaches to making sense out of a group of numbers include using graphs, bar charts, or pie charts. These approaches provide a visual representation of the data that allows us to see how different the largest and smallest numbers were and what were the most common responses. Figure 4–1 is an example of a histogram (a type of bar chart) that might have been included in the fictional article on students' choices for clinical practice.

Hopefully, you found organizing the data helped you to increase your understanding of what that information meant. No matter which approach you took, the product probably helped you to see two things: (1) how much diversity or difference occurred in the data and (2) what were the most common responses in the data. In

**FIGURE 4-1**    **Histogram for the frequency distribution of students' choices of field of practice based on results in fictional article.**

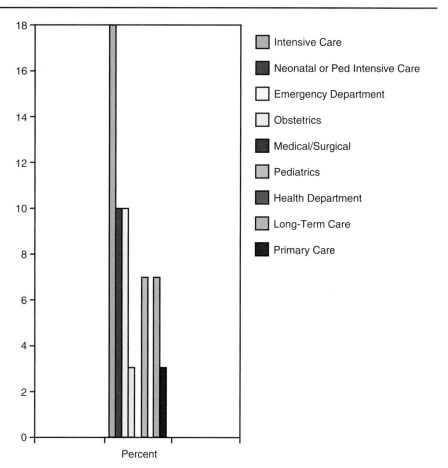

the language of statistics, the diversity in data for a single variable is referred to as the **variance**, which reflects the distribution of values for the variable. The most common or frequent responses in a set of data are statistically described as the **measures of central tendency**. Each is discussed individually.

### *Variance, Standard Deviation, and Distribution*

Variance is a statistic, that is, a number, that can be used to show how much difference or variety exists in a group of numbers. Table 4–2 lists the ages of nursing students from three different classrooms. With short lists like this, you can look at the numbers and determine that there is more variety in the ages of students in classroom 2 than in classroom 1 or 3. But how do you objectively measure the variety or describe that variety in a way that can be consistently understood and interpreted by anyone? Obviously, just saying that classroom 2 has more variety in age than does classroom

| TABLE 4–2 | Ages of Students in Three Different Classrooms With Variation and Central Tendency | |
|---|---|---|
| **Classroom 1\*** | **Classroom 2\*** | **Classroom 3\*** |
| 20 | 20 | 18 |
| 21 | 24 | 20 |
| 20 | 19 | 20 |
| 20 | 21 | 24 |
| 19 | 18 | 20 |
| 21 | 23 | 20 |
| 20 | 18 | 20 |
| 20 | 19 | 18 |
| 19 | 18 | 20 |
| 20 | 20 | 20 |
| $SD = 0.67$<br>$M = 20$<br>Mode = 20<br>Median = 20 | $SD = 2.11$<br>$M = 20$<br>Mode = 18<br>Median = 19.5 | $SD = 1.63$<br>$M = 20$<br>Mode = 20<br>Median = 20 |

\*Age in years.

1 and 3 is nonspecific—how much is "more?" You could also say that the ages range from 19 to 21 in classroom 1, compared with ages ranging from 18 to 24 in classroom 2. This is certainly more specific and gives us a better sense of the differences, but the ages of students in classroom 3 also range from 18 to 24 years, yet there is more variety in ages in classroom 2 than in classroom 3. Therefore, there must be some way to represent the values in between the two numbers that give us the age range.

The variety in a group of numbers is explained statistically by computing a number appropriately, called the variance. The variance is the sum of the squared differences between each value in the set of numbers and the mean (average) of those numbers, divided by how many numbers there were in the set minus one. Using age of students in classroom 1 as an example, the variance is computed by subtracting the average of all 10 students' ages (20) from each student's individual age and squaring the difference, then adding those squared differences and dividing by 9. We square the differences between the mean to avoid negative and positive differences canceling each other. Therefore, the variance statistic is an average of the squared deviations from the mean.

Whether you understand the formula for computing the variance, you can understand that variance tells you how much variety there is within a set of numbers. For example, the variance for the ages in classroom 1 is 0.44 ($s^2 = 0.44$), the variance for the ages in classroom 2 is 4.44 ($s^2 = 4.44$), and the variance in classroom 3 is 2.66 ($s^2 = 2.66$). These statistics reveal that there is more variety in age in classroom 3 than in classroom 1 but less variety in classroom 3 than in classroom 2. Although you can see the variety in the ages by looking at the short list of numbers in Table 4–2, if the list contained 100 numbers or 1000 numbers, it would be much more difficult to get the variety without computing the variance. The variance gives us a specific statistic that represents differences or variety when reporting results for a single variable.

Thus far, we have discussed the variance for a single variable; however, more often the results section of a research report will use a statistic called "standard deviation" instead of the variance. The **standard deviation** is simply the square root of the variance, so it also reflects variety among all the numbers. Remember that to compute the variance we squared differences in values from the mean. This results in the values for the variance being squared units of measurement, such as 6.66 squared years for the variance in classroom 2. The idea of "squared years" however, does not make much sense. If we take the square root of that variance, we get a standard deviation of 2.11 years (not squared years). The standard deviation is, in a sense, the average difference in ages from the overall average age. You can see by looking at the values for the ages in classroom 2 that it makes sense that the variety in ages can be accurately communicated by saying that there is an average of 2 years difference from the overall average. This makes more sense than 4.44 squared years. In contrast, the standard deviation for the ages of students in classroom 1 is 0.67 years (or less than 1 year), and the standard deviation of the ages of the students in classroom 3 is 1.63 years. Standard deviation is usually abbreviated in research reports as *SD,* so a research report giving the standard deviation for classroom 3 would write "$SD = 1.63$". Although classroom 2 and 3 both have a youngest and oldest student of 18 and 24 years, respectively, the average deviation from the overall average age is clearly greater in classroom 2.

Why do we care about variance and standard deviation? To understand the meaning of results for clinical practice, we must understand how much variety there was in the results. For example, if you were reading a research study that examined the effectiveness of an intervention to relieve pain and the report tells you that the average rating of pain on a 10-point scale after the intervention was 2, that sounds good. Suppose that two different interventions each led to an average rating of 2, but the first had a standard deviation of 3.5, whereas the second had a standard deviation of 0.7. Although the first intervention led to the same average as the second intervention, the standard deviation tells us there was a great deal more variety in pain ratings with the first intervention. This means that some of the people who received the first intervention had higher scores or more pain, as well as possibly lower scores or less pain. Although lower scores may be better, our goal in nursing is to consistently improve pain, and higher scores in some of our patients definitely are not desirable. The second intervention led to much less variety in ratings of pain, which means that most of the subjects scored their pain close to a rating of 2 after the intervention. As a clinician who understands standard deviations, you might decide that the second intervention is more consistent in relieving pain because it had a smaller standard deviation, and choose to use that intervention rather than the first one.

A pain intervention study is an example of a study in which we may not want variety, because our clinical goal is to consistently decrease our patients' pain levels. In other cases, however, we may want variety to make the information useful clinically. For example, in the TB-screening article, the authors report that the mean age of the farm workers in their sample was 29, with a standard deviation of 10.7 ($SD$ = 10.7) (Poss, 2000). This means that the average deviation around the age of 29 was only 10.7 years, telling us that the sample consisted of relatively young individuals. The RN in the health department works with Mexican farm workers of all ages, so he must decide whether the more limited variety in ages in this study will affect the clinical usefulness of this study. The range of ages in the TB-screening study was 18 to 67 years, but those numbers alone would not have told us that these results are primarily for younger men. The author of this study has included a sentence specifically stating that 60% of the participants in the study were between 18 and 27 years of age. Now that we understand the meaning of the standard deviation and know that the mean age was 29 years, with a standard deviation of 10.7 years, we understand that many of the subjects were young by just looking at that statistic, even if the author had not told us.

Distribution is another term that is used in results sections to indicate the variety or differences found. In research, **distribution** refers to how the findings are dispersed. The variance and standard deviation for a set of numbers give us a clear sense of the spread of those numbers. However, it is not appropriate to compute the statistics of variance and standard deviation for variables that fit into discrete categories, such as type of job preference, rather than variables that are real numbers, such as age. For simplicity, often a researcher will assign numeric values to categories, such as 1 = professional employment, 2 = blue-collar employment. However, the actual numbers "1" and "2" are not a true measure of type of employment, and adding or subtracting the numbers will not tell us the "average" type of employment.

In cases where the variable is a category, we may find distribution described using a table of percentages, a histogram, or a pie chart. For example, the fictional article shows us the frequency distribution of choices of field of nursing in Table 1. A **frequency distribution** is the spread for how frequently each category occurred or was selected. We see from Table 1 that 60% of the students choose intensive care as their preferred field after graduation, and another 10% choose neonatal intensive care and emergency department fields. Figure 4–1 shows the same frequency distribution in a histogram format. Figure 4–2 shows what the frequency distribution would look like in histogram format if none of the students had selected the neonatal and emergency room fields and instead had selected the health department and long-term care fields. You can see that the distribution of choices would have looked different even with 60% still selecting intensive care. Just as the statistic for standard deviation can tell us about the distribution or variety in a numeric variable, a frequency table or histogram can tell us about distribution and variety in a categoric variable.

**FIGURE 4-2**   **Example of histogram for distribution of field of study choices if health department and long-term care were endorsed more frequently.**

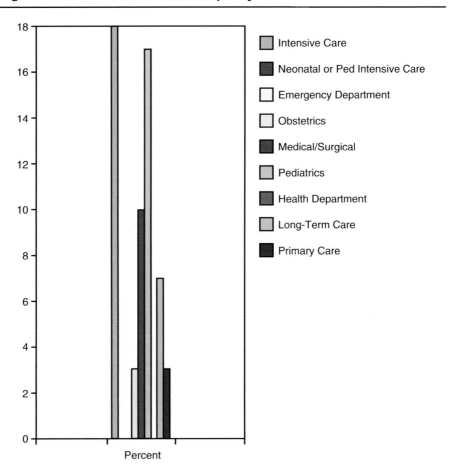

An important statistical concept that you may remember from your statistics courses is the normal curve. A **normal curve** is a type of distribution that is symmetric and bell shaped. Figure 4–3 shows two graphs with distribution curves; the one on the left is the familiar normal curve. Many of the variables in life that we are interested in understanding or using in research are distributed closely to how the normal curve looks. For example, height can range from small, in the case of a neonate, to tall, in the case of a few extraordinary individuals, but most people fall somewhere in the middle, with a relatively even balance on each side of the average height. The normal curve is a theoretical distribution. That means that if we could measure a variable, such as height, for every human on earth and plot all the heights, the result would be this perfectly symmetric bell-shaped curve. One thing that makes the normal curve unique is its symmetry; you can fold the normal curve in half at the center, which is the average, and the two sides will match. On the right side of Figure 4–3, there is an example of a distribution that has a curved shape but is asymmetric. Much

**FIGURE 4-3**    **Examples of a normal curve and a curve that skews to the right.**

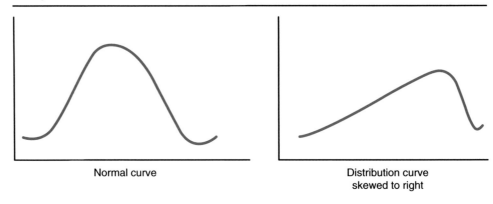

Normal curve

Distribution curve
skewed to right

of inferential statistics is based on the assumption that the distribution of a variable would be normal or bell shaped if all the possible values for the variable were known. This assumption is based on experience with many variables of interest that are normally distributed. Therefore, when reading results, you will find references to a distribution of a variable being "approximately normal."

In summary, one of the important aspects of data that we expect to see described and summarized in the results section of reports is the diversity or variety in the data. We may find this described using a univariate statistic called the standard deviation (or possibly the variance) or a frequency distribution, histogram, or pie chart. In any case, the variety for each study variable is important for us to understand, because it affects the clinical decisions we can make based on the study.

### Central Tendency

In addition to wanting to know about the diversity in a set of numbers for a variable, we almost always want to know what was the most common or average response or value for a variable. In quantitative research, a measure that shows common or typical numbers is called a measure of central tendency. Central tendency measures reflect the center of a distribution, or the center of the spread. The univariate statistics, called the mean, the mode, and the median, are the three most commonly used measures of central tendency. Table 4–2 shows that the mean value for the ages of the students in each classroom is 20 years. The **mean** is simply the average of all the values for a variable—that is, the sum of all the values divided by the number of values summed. The **mode** is the value that occurs most frequently: in classrooms 1 and 3, the mode is 20 years, but in classroom 2, the mode is 18. Although the mean of the ages in the three classrooms is the same, suggesting that the center of the distributions is the same, the center of the distribution of ages in the three classrooms differs when one looks at the mode.

The **median** is the value that falls in the middle of the distribution when the numbers are in numeric order. Although 20 years is the median age in classrooms 1 and 3, the median age for classroom 2 is 19.5 years (the average of $19 + 20$, the two most central values for age in that classroom). Although the mean, mode, and median are all measures of central tendency, comparing the three for a single variable also tells us something about the distribution. Looking at the mean (20 years), mode (18 years), and median (19.5 years) for students' ages in classroom 2, we see that although the average age was 20, more students were younger than 20 years old than were older than 20 years old. The age distribution "leans" toward the younger ages. This "leaning" is described as skew when reporting research results. We have said that the mean, mode, and median are measures of "central" tendency, but if there is a **skew** in the distribution, these three measures will have different value. This tells us that the middle of the distribution is not in the exact center of that distribution, it is off to the left or right of center. The second curve of Figure 4–3 has a skew to the right, which means that the middle of the distribution falls more to the higher range of the possible values. A normal curve does not have a skew. In fact, part of what defines a normal curve is that the mean, median, and mode are all equal.

Now look at Figure 4–4, which shows curves drawn around the distribution of ages for the three classrooms we have been using as an example. Notice that the curve for classroom 1 is perfectly bell shaped and symmetric and that the mean, mode, and median are equal. The curve for classroom 2 is skewed to the left, is not symmetric, and the mean, mode, and median are not equal. The curve for classroom 3 looks similar to that for classroom 1, but it is narrower and not symmetric.

Again, why do we care about measures of central tendency? We care because a long list of numbers for a variable, such as a long list of ages or pain ratings, is difficult to make much sense of without some type of organization. A summary of those numbers that tells us the central tendency and the distribution allows us to quickly understand some important aspects for the individual variable, such as the most common or frequent value and how much variety there was in the values. This, in turn, allows us to better understand how the results may or may not apply to real clinical practice.

The data from the in-class study exercise provides an excellent example of how much more we can learn about a variable when the data are summarized to give us the distribution and the central tendency. A second example is found in the first few sentences of the results section of the TB-screening article. Had the author simply given us a list of the ages of 206 migrant farm workers, it would have been both tedious and frustrating to try to get a sense of their overall ages. However, when the author tells us the range of ages (18 to 67) and the mean and standard deviation for age ($M = 29 \pm SD = 10.7$), we have information that tells us immediately the ages of patients in the study and to whom the results of this study may be applied.

---

# CORE CONCEPT

*Measures of central tendency and distribution are univariate statistics that summarize information about a variable.*

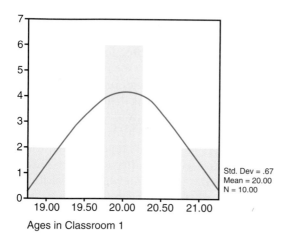

Ages in Classroom 1

Std. Dev = .67
Mean = 20.00
N = 10.00

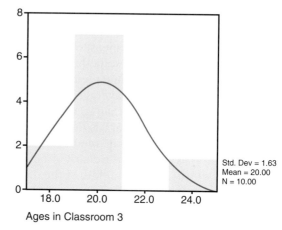

Ages in Classroom 3

Std. Dev = 1.63
Mean = 20.00
N = 10.00

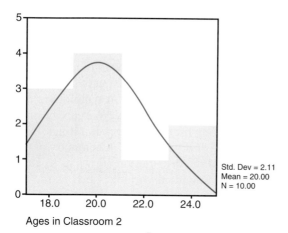

Ages in Classroom 2

Std. Dev = 2.11
Mean = 20.00
N = 10.00

**FIGURE 4-4**  **Frequency distribution histogram and curves for ages of students in three classrooms.**

## Language Describing Results From Qualitative Studies

Thus far, we have discussed language used to describe variables measured in numbers using quantitative methods. If the data you were given in the out-of-class exercise had been words instead of numbers, it would not have been as immediately obvious how to create some kind of order in it. What you might have done is break down the words into units that you could organize, such as individual sentences, paragraphs, or groups of sentences that address the same idea. You could then organize the groups of sentences according to shared ideas and determine how many different ideas occurred and how much agreement there was about the ideas. The goal of data analysis in a qualitative study is the same as that in a quantitative study: to organize the data and create some kind of an order to it so that its meaning can be found.

Box 4–1 lists excerpts of data that might have been collected in response to the question "What experiences in your life have led to your anticipated choice for field of nursing practice?", the question identified in the fictional article as the measure

**Examples of Qualitative Data Collected in Response to the Question "What Experiences in Your Life Have Led to Your Anticipated Choice for Field of Nursing Practice?"**

"I have always loved movies where the nurses save the lives of people during a disaster. I guess, well, it seems like the best place to do that, you know, is, well, the emergency room."

"Nursing is all about caring for people. I mean, I don't know how I would have gotten through my son's illness without the nurses."

"The one thing I remember when I had my tonsils out was the nurse giving me ice cream. It made me feel safe."

"I come from a family of nurses who have all worked in hospitals, mostly the surgical or medical ICU."

"It was the nurse holding my hand when the doctor in the emergency room told me about my brother that made it possible for me to keep going."

"My roommate in college was a nursing student, and she always helped any of us who came to her, whether it was if we were sick or just feeling down."

"Every time I have had to go to the hospital with one of the kids, it was the nurses who really listened to me and made a difference."

"My aunt was a nurse. She always was so strong and sure of herself—I wanted to be just like her."

"The shows I've seen about the flying nurses—that is just such an exciting thing to do, I guess I figured I would never get bored."

"My best friend in high school was in a car accident and I was so scared to go see her. But the nurse, he just really helped me relax and not freak out seeing all the machines and things."

"There was no one like my Grandma Jane—she was the most caring person I ever knew; she nursed about everyone in the family until it was her turn to get sick and die."

used to collect subjective responses to help understand why students chose their fields of practice. Take a moment and read through those responses. Reading data in this form is even less helpful than reading a list of 206 ages. For the qualitative researcher, the organizing, ordering, and synthesizing of the data collected is the heart of the research method. In fact, in most qualitative studies, data are analyzed throughout the process of implementing the study, and the results of this analysis are then used to guide additional data collection. This is in contrast to quantitative studies in which the researcher usually does not analyze the data until it has all been collected, because changing the way or which data are collected undermines the results of the study.

Another difference between data analysis in qualitative studies and quantitative studies is that no absolute formulas, such as that used to compute variance, are consistently applied to the data. Qualitative data analysis requires understanding, digesting, synthesizing, conceptualizing, and reconceptualizing descriptions of feelings, behaviors, experiences, and ideas. Content analysis is often the word used to describe this process of data analysis. **Content analysis** is the process of understanding, interpreting, and conceptualizing the meanings in qualitative data. To do this, the researcher starts by breaking down the data into units that are meaningful and then develops a categorization scheme. A **categorization scheme** is an orderly combination of categories carefully defined so that no overlap occurs. In qualitative analysis, the categorization scheme is developed based on the ideas found in the data, then pieces of data, units that reflect distinct ideas, are put into the categories. This process of breaking down and labeling large amounts of data to identify the category in which it belongs is called **coding** the data or **data reduction**. When this coding or data reduction occurs, the researcher is also refining the categorization scheme and using the categories to guide further data collection.

One might say that there is a spiraling nature to the process of data analysis in qualitative studies, as illustrated in Figure 4–5. The process is not circular, because it does not simply return to where it began but rather evolves to eventually identify key themes or concepts that reflect the meaning of the data. Theme is another word that often is found in the results section of a qualitative report. A **theme** is an idea or a concept that is implicit in and recurrent throughout the data. Themes are not the concrete explicit words contained in the data; rather, they are the underlying ideas behind the words. Qualitative data analysis seeks to categorize and understand the data and the relationships among the categories to eventually conceptualize the data into themes. The spiral occurs, in part, because as categories are developed through analysis, they are used to collect additional data, which is then coded and

**FIGURE 4-5**     **Spiraling process of qualitative data analysis.**

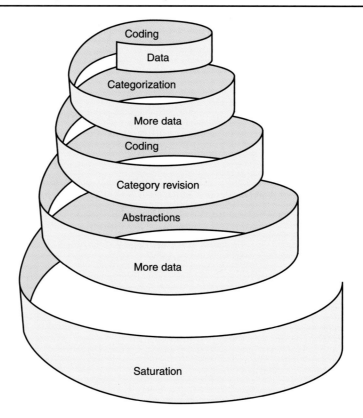

categorized. Eventually data saturation occurs. **Data saturation** in qualitative research is the point at which all new information collected is redundant of information already collected. Data saturation occurs when all new information fits into the now-established coding system, so that the new information is saying the same thing as the data already collected. Therefore, no new information is being generated through continued data collection.

Look again at the data in Box 4–1, which have already been broken down into units, mostly sentences and, in a few cases, more than one sentence that combine to express one idea. Content analysis to develop a categorization scheme might start using a category for "Caring experiences" and another for "Television and movies." As the researcher examines the data and codes them into these two categories, you see that only two of the units fit under the "Television and movies" category, whereas all the rest belong to "Caring experiences." The researcher might then notice that, in some cases, the data under "Caring experiences" suggest a desire to follow in someone's footsteps. This idea can be refined to a category called "Experiences with nursing role models." Once the data that reflects role models are moved into the new category, further analysis of the data that remained suggests that not only caring experiences but also personal caring experiences are being described. Thus, in the end, three themes can be derived from the data. Figure 4–6 shows this process in content analysis in schematic form.

This is a simplified example of how a qualitative researcher might analyze data to identify themes. Notice that the final three themes identified are never explicitly addressed in the actual data. That is, no piece of data says that it was the nurse role model that led to the choice of field of nursing. The themes identified are implicit; that is, the ideas are repeated differently by different people.

The themes or categories derived from qualitative data analysis are usually reported in the results sections of qualitative research reports. The author of a qualitative report cannot provide measures of central tendency or distribution to describe the data. Rather, the themes or categories are described, often using specific examples from the actual data to help make the implicit ideas within the themes clearer. For example, in the family survival article, the author identifies seven aspects of life that were viewed by participants as essential for a family to survive. The first of these is "having secure employment," and the author gives us a direct quote from one of the participants in the study—first in Spanish and then in English. Those words allow us to have a much greater understanding of the meaning of "secure employment" than does the category label alone. Also notice that the participant never directly said the words "secure employment." Secure employment is the conceptual label developed by the researcher to bring meaning to the data.

In summary, the description of the variables in the study is always an important part of the results sections of research reports. Description of data aims to summarize the data in a way that makes it readily understandable and meaningful. Description of only one variable is called univariate analysis, and, in quantitative research, that description almost always includes information to tell us about the distribution and central tendency for the variables. In reports of qualitative research, the entire results section is descriptive, taking units of data (words, pictures, and sentences) and developing categories and themes to describe that data.

FIGURE 4-6 **Schematic.**

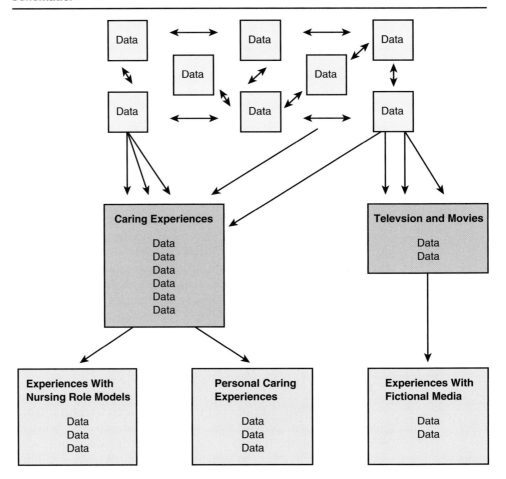

## CONNECTING RESULTS THAT DESCRIBE TO CONCLUSIONS

Because this chapter focuses on understanding descriptive results, and in keeping with qualitative research the results reported in the article about family survival are all descriptive, we focus on that article as we discuss connecting results and conclusions. The RN in our vignette has read the results and conclusions sections of the research report about family survival in Mexican American families. The results started with **demographic** data, descriptive information about the characteristics of the people studied. Both quantitative and qualitative studies almost always include demographic data, although the reports of qualitative studies may not use statistics to describe those characteristics. However, the article found by the RN does include both the mean and the standard deviation for several characteristics of the participants in the study, including age of the mother, father, and children; parents' education level; and family income. From these results we know that the findings from this study reflect the experiences and beliefs of Mexican American families that are relatively young, with both parents having slightly less than a high school education, and with low incomes.

This particular qualitative study used an ethnographic design to examine the research question, and the results include more statistics than may be given in some qualitative studies. Chapter 9 discusses different study designs in more detail. The three broad phenomena that the author explored were family survival, family continuity, and family growth. The results are organized around these three phenomena, and, in each section, the author lists the categories that were derived from the data and the number of participants who gave an answer that fit into each of the categories. For example, in the results for the phenomena of family survival, the category of secure employment was spontaneously identified by most of the families as essential for a family to survive, whereas being healthy was only identified by one family. Yet, when the author put all the categories that were identified on cards and asked families to sort them as to which they saw as essential, being healthy was identified as important by all 23 families, whereas steady employment was not selected by one of the families. An important part of the data analysis in qualitative research is taking the data back to the participants themselves for them to confirm or add to the ideas identified (recall the spiral in Figure 4–5). In this case, an idea that was initially identified by only one family and that might have seemed less important than others was considered essential by all the families when it was brought back to them.

The results reported under the phenomenon of family continuity are detailed, showing specifically which members of the family, in how many families, performed selected tasks, each listed in tables. Unlike for family survival, the author does not describe in the results how she originally identified the specific tasks. In general, the author reports that tasks within the Mexican American families were divided by gender, with women doing inside household tasks and men doing outside household tasks and with a sharing of child-care tasks. Further, there was a fair amount of continuity in both the type of task and the family member who performed the task within the families.

To report results about the third phenomenon studied, the author again reports the number of families who spontaneously identified different categories that they believed affect family growth and then the number of families that endorsed each of these categories when they were all presented to the participants in the form of a card sort. A total of 10 characteristics that participant families identified as important to family growth were affirmed through the card-sorting process, with 7 of the 10 supported by almost all the families. The least affirmed category was "family receiving professional guidance," with only 14 families indicating this was important for family growth.

How do these results connect to the conclusions of this study? As we discussed in Chapter 3, the conclusions of this report start by summarizing the key findings from the study. Now that we have read the actual results, it is clear that what is provided in the conclusion is a summary without the details. The conclusions of this report include a discussion comparing the results from this study to a known theorist's description of family adaptation, such as that by Roy and Andrews (Niska, 2001). Because this is a qualitative study, the author is not testing Roy's theory but wants to build or support existing theory and so explains how the categories of ideas from the study conceptually fit with the modes in Roy's theory. Thus, the results are shown to connect to previous ideas, in this case, ideas from theory rather than from other research.

The author also addresses the clinical implications of her study near the end of the conclusions. She states that because the ideas expressed by the participants in the study conceptually fit with Roy's model of the family, "nurses can be confident in using these characteristics of family survival, continuity, and family growth as a foundation to start their discussion with a family about existing family goals and expected outcomes of nursing interventions that enhance family nurturing, support, or socialization" (Niska, 2001, p. 328). Then the author identifies what future research studies must consider, given the results from the study.

In summary, the specific results described are the basis for the new knowledge identified in the conclusion. Without reading the results, we would not know what the actual characteristics of family survival, continuity and growth, were, making the clinical implications identified in this study difficult to understand. Having read the results section, however, the conclusions generally are clear and make more sense.

## COMMON ERRORS IN THE REPORTS OF DESCRIPTIVE RESULTS

Two kinds of problems may be found when reading the descriptive results in a research report: (1) incomplete information and (2) confusing information. We have emphasized the importance of understanding the distribution and central tendency in variables from quantitative studies to make clinical decisions. One problem that sometimes arises when reading the results is that this descriptive information cannot be found. The authors may fail to provide any univariate statistics about some of the variables in the study, or they may fail to provide all the information needed.

For example, a report may only include a measure of central tendency for an important variable, without giving a range of values or the standard deviation. This absence of information about the variation in the variable makes it difficult to know how to interpret the findings related to that variable and can even lead to incorrect conclusions. The previous example of a study that examined two interventions to help pain whose results are a mean pain score of 2 for both interventions is a good example of this. Given the mean scores alone, one might conclude that the two interventions have exactly the same effect. This conclusion would be incorrect, however, because the standard deviations for the mean pain scores in this example (0.7 and 3.5) were different.

Another example of a report with incomplete descriptive results is the fictional article. One of the variables that the author later indicates was important relative to the students' choices of field of practice was their health rating. Yet, the only univariate information provided about the variable is that 20% of the subjects rated their health as fair or poor. We do not learn how the percentages broke down for ratings of "excellent health" or "good health" nor whether most of the 20% of subjects who rated their health at the lower end chose "fair" or "poor." This lack of information affects our ability to interpret the results that are reported later.

A second problem that may be found in the results section is a confusing presentation of the results. Descriptive results are often reported in tables, and sometimes those tables are not labeled clearly or are organized unclearly. A table may use titles or identify variables inconsistently with the wording used in the text of the report. In fact, sometimes the text of a report fails to refer to the table at all. Another problem is that too much information may be put into the text rather than using a table. For example, the information provided in Table 1 in the fictional article would have been confusing and hard to understand had the author included a paragraph reporting those results as follows:

> Students chose several fields immediately after graduation, with 18 (60%) choosing intensive care, 3 (10%) choosing neonatal or pediatric intensive care, and 3 (10%) choosing emergency departments. One student (3%) chose obstetrics for field of study immediately after graduation, and no students chose either medical/surgical or health department. Two students (7%) chose pediatrics, two students (7%) chose long-term care or nursing home care, and one student (3%) chose primary care.

Although you could probably sort out this information, it is clearer to view it in a table. A similar problem may occur in a qualitative report if the author does not give us clear descriptions of the categories or themes developed from the study. Look at the fictional article again and at the three themes identified that represented the meaning of experiences students identified as affecting their choice of practice. If the author had simply listed the themes as "personal life experience," "experiences with nursing role models," and "experiences with fictional media," it would have been difficult to know how these types of experiences differed. The definitions and examples given in Table 2 in that article make it clear what those themes mean.

## PUBLISHED REPORT—WHAT WOULD YOU CONCLUDE?

Understanding better what to expect in the reports of descriptive results makes it possible for you to know whether the research is something that might apply to your clinical practice. The RN in our vignette began his search with a general interest in gaining a better understanding of how families such as the Hernandez family could be helped to manage the stress of a long-term communicable disease. After reading the results and conclusions sections of the family survival article, the RN has an increased understanding of what young Mexican American families see as essential for survival and growth. In particular, health, being united, being supported from outside family, and steady employment were viewed as essential for family survival, and communication, togetherness, planning, and helping children are viewed as essential for family growth. Given the importance placed on health and employment, the RN now has an increased understanding that the TB diagnosis may be a serious threat to the survival of a family, making it critical to consider the whole family and its functioning when planning care for the individual who has tested TB positive. The RN also knows that task continuity is important to families and that these tasks may be divided along traditional gender lines. He knows that TB may change the tasks performed by family members, but he is not clear about how these tasks were identified in this study, so he cannot readily translate these results and conclusions into actual practice.

Remembering that the aim of a qualitative study is to increase our understanding and not to provide specific detailed plans, the RN is not surprised that he has not found a protocol for developing family strength to support survival. He has gained an increased understanding of potential issues that his clients may face, but several questions remain after reading only the results and conclusions sections. These questions include:

- How were the family tasks identified?
- How well did the study capture the meanings of the participants' answers, given the different language and cultural background?
- Why did the author specifically connect the results to Roy's model of the family rather than some other theory?
- How did these particular families become involved in this study?

To answer these questions, it is necessary to read and understand earlier sections of the research report.

We continue to look at the language of results sections of research reports in the next chapter, trying to add to the knowledge that may help the RN in the health department in planning services for Mexican American clients and their families.

## OUT-OF-CLASS EXERCISE

### Making Inferences About Well-Being and Marriage

Before proceeding to Chapter 5, look at the data collected from your in-class practice study, focusing on two variables: rating of well-being and marital status. Complete univariate analysis of that data to summarize distribution and central tendency. Then determine what the data tells you in terms of answering the question "Do married students have higher levels of well-being than unmarried students?" Answer that question based on the data, and write a statement regarding how you arrived at your answer. If you are not using an in-class study, a practice set of data about well-being and marital status is provided in Appendix E, which you can use for this exercise. Then you will be ready to begin the next chapter.

## References

Bliss, D. Z., Johnson S., Savik, K., Clabots, C. R., & Gerding, D. N. (2000). Fecal incontinence in hospitalized patients who are acutely ill. *Nursing Research, 49*(2), 101–108.

Lipman, T. H., Hayman, L. L., Favian, C. V., DiFazio, D. A., Hale, P. M., Goldsmith, B. M., et al. (2000). Risk factors for cardiovascular disease in children with Type I Diabetes. *Nursing Research, 49*(3), 160–166.

Niska, K. J. (2001). Mexican American family survival, continuity, and growth: The parental perspective. *Nursing Science Quarterly, 14*(4), 322–329.

Poss, J. E. (2000). Factors associated with participation by Mexican migrant farmworkers in a tuberculosis screening program. *Nursing Research, 49*(1), 20–28.

## Resources

Locke, L. F., Silverman, S. J. & Spirduso, W. W. (1998). *Reading and understanding research.* Thousand Oaks, CA: Sage Publications.

Polit, D. F., & Hungler, B. P. (1999). *Nursing research: Principles and methods* (6th ed.). Philadelphia: Lippincott.

Salkind, N. J. (2000). *Statistics for people who (think they) hate statistics.* Thousand Oaks, CA: Sage Publications.

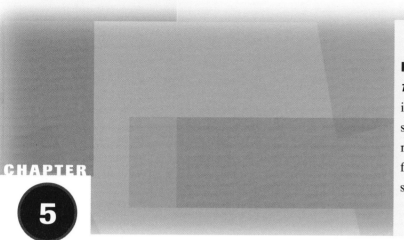

**LEARNING OUTCOME:**

*THE STUDENT WILL* interpret inferential statistical results in relationship to their meaning for the conclusions of the study.

# Inferential Results

## *Why Did the Authors Reach Their Conclusion—What Did They Actually Find?*

**KEY TERMS**

Analysis of variance
Beta (β) value
Confidence intervals
Correlation
Covary
Factor analysis
Nonparametric

Null hypothesis
Parametric
Probability
Regression
Research hypothesis
*t* test

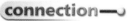

## CLINICAL CASE

The RN works in the tuberculosis (TB) program for the county Health Department. He has recently started working with the Hernandez family because Mr. Hernandez had a positive TB skin test during a routine bimonthly examination at a community-screening clinic and has been confirmed to have active TB. After obtaining a detailed history, it is likely that Mr. Hernandez has had active TB for several months but only participated in the screening program this past month because his mother-in-law wanted to go. The RN is interested in gaining knowledge that will help him work directly with the Hernandez family and also give him ideas about approaches that the Health Department might take to improve overall participation in its TB-screening programs in the Mexican American and migrant worker communities. He found two articles that were relevant to his interests and has read each of them. The first article used a qualitative method to examine factors affecting family survival among Mexican Americans (Niska, 2001). The second article examined factors associated with participation in a TB-screening program for Mexican farm workers (Poss, 2000). This article used a quantitative approach and used several statistical terms in the results section, which the RN must interpret to decide what the results mean for him as he plans future screening programs.

## THE PURPOSE OF INFERENTIAL STATISTICS

Chapter 4 discussed the meaning of the language used in research reports when descriptive results, those that describe or explain a variable or variables, are presented. This chapter continues the discussion of how to understand the results sections of research reports but focuses on inferential results, those intended to explain or predict a variable or variables. Notice that the word "explain" is included in both of these definitions. This is because there is an overlap between simple description, description that explains, and explanation that can be used for prediction. We are looking at a continuum of statistics that build from simple knowing, to understanding, and finally to predicting, as shown in Figure 5–1.

Let's look at a simple example using the results about the ages, gender, and degree status of students in a nursing class shown in Table 5–1. The mean ($M = 27$)

**FIGURE 5-1** **A continuum for the purposes of data analysis.**

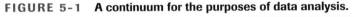

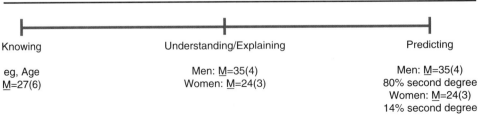

Knowing

eg, Age
$M$=27(6)

Understanding/Explaining

Men: $M$=35(4)
Women: $M$=24(3)

Predicting

Men: $M$=35(4)
80% second degree
Women: $M$=24(3)
14% second degree

| TABLE 5-1 | Fictional Data for Ages, Gender, and Degree Status of a Nursing Student Class | | |
|---|---|---|---|
| **Subject Number** | **Age (y)** | **Gender** | **Degree Status** |
| 1 | 20 | F | 1st |
| 2 | 23 | F | 1st |
| 3 | 33 | M | 1st |
| 4 | 21 | F | 1st |
| 5 | 25 | F | 1st |
| 6 | 40 | M | 2nd |
| 7 | 32 | F | 2nd |
| 8 | 20 | F | 1st |
| 9 | 26 | F | 1st |
| 10 | 25 | F | 1st |
| 11 | 37 | M | 2nd |
| 12 | 26 | F | 1st |
| 13 | 23 | F | 1st |
| 14 | 22 | F | 1st |
| 15 | 24 | F | 2nd |
| 16 | 30 | M | 2nd |
| 17 | 35 | M | 2nd |
| 18 | 21 | F | 1st |
| 19 | 25 | F | 1st |

and standard deviation ($SD = 6$) for the age of the students is an example of simple description. Notice in the figure that these are written with the mean followed by the standard deviation in parentheses. This is often the form used to report a mean and standard deviation in the results of a research report. In this case, these descriptive univariate statistics tell us that the students are relatively old and that there is a fair amount of variation in the ages, but we have no idea why the variation exists. To have some explanation of the variation, descriptive statistics might be used to give us information about the age of the men versus the women in the class. In the example, the mean age for the male students is 35 ($SD = 4$), whereas the mean age of the female students is 24 ($SD = 3$). We now have a partial explanation of the variation in ages: there are both men and women in the class, and the men in the class are older than the women in the class. The variation in age is explained to some extent, but we do not assume we can use students' gender distribution to predict age of students. However, if we find out that 80% of the male students are second-degree students, whereas only 14% of the females are second-degree students, this additional information can potentially be used for prediction. We can speculate that men may be more likely to pursue nursing as a second career and that the more second-degree students there are in a class, the older the students will be. To test whether we can use the number of second-degree students to predict age of students in a classroom, we must use inferential statistics.

Why use inferential statistics instead of just descriptive statistics? Because at this point we do not know if the differences and relationships among variables found in this classroom occurred by chance alone. We know that there are differences in this particular classroom, but we do not know whether, in general, second-degree students are more likely to be men and older. Descriptive statistical results allow us to know and explain variables that we are interested in understanding, but we have to go a step further to use that explanation to predict how those variables may occur in the future. Inferential statistics allow us to build the evidence to support predictions about the future. Inferential statistics are based on the concepts of probability and statistical significance; therefore, to understand results that use inferential statistics, we must understand these terms.

## PROBABILITY AND SIGNIFICANCE

As the RN in our vignette starts to read the section of the report titled "Testing of Hypotheses," he encounters the language of inferential statistics in the statement that there were "significant correlations between intention to have the PPD skin test and all of the TII subscales" (Poss, 2000, p. 23). In Chapter 2, we defined significance as a low likelihood that any relationship or difference found in a statistical test occurred by chance alone. Quantitative research often attempts to take what has been found in a specific situation, that is, one study, and infer that similar results would occur in other similar situations. The RN in the vignette is not only interested in what happened in Poss's study but also wants to predict that the same thing will happen in his screening clinic if he creates the same or a similar situation.

In inferential statistics, we test for relationships, associations, and differences among variables that are statistically significant. We do this by creating distributions of test statistics that reflect variables that have no connection between them, are unrelated, or are not different. In Chapter 4, we said that a distribution refers to how the findings are distributed. A distribution of test statistics shows how the test statistics from hundreds of samples would look if plotted on a graft. Then we compute a test statistic for the results in our particular study and compare what we found in our sample or specific situation to what would be predicted to be found if there was not a relationship or difference in the variables. By convention, researchers say that if the test statistic falls into the range where we would expect 95% of all statistics to fall, given that there is no relationship or connection, then it is a nonsignificant statistic. Stated in the opposite way, if a test statistic falls *out of the range* of values that we would expect to occur 95% of the time if there was no relationship among the variables, then we say it is a statistically significant value.

To illustrate this idea, let's use the statistic reported in the fictional article about the difference in ages of nursing students who choose acute settings versus nonacute settings. The article states that there was a significant difference in age and gives a test statistic of "$t = 2.1$, $P < .05$". The "$t$" value is a test statistic for differences in means between two groups, which we will discuss later in this chapter. In this case, the statistic was computed for the differences in the average ages of students who did and did not select acute care setting for field of practice. Now look at Figure 5–2, which shows a distribution that is a normal curve, in this case a $t$ distribution. Notice that for the $t$ distribution, zero is at the center and the possible values for the $t$ test become larger at either end. A $t$ distribution shows how the $t$ tests for hundreds of different samples of two variables *that did not differ from each other in the real world* would be distributed. Now, returning to age as a variable of interest, if in the real world the ages of two groups are *not* different, then most of the time we would not get a big difference for the ages in any particular sample and the $t$ test statistic would be a small number. However, occasionally, by chance alone, we get a large difference in age between groups in a sample (perhaps because a 12-year-old genius is in a particular sample). Using the example from the fictional article, if in the real world students who did and did not pick acute setting were approximately the same age, then most of the time, if we took a sample of ages of students choosing the two types of setting and computed a $t$ test, the value would be plotted on the distribution some-

**FIGURE 5-2** **t-distribution for differences in two means in a sample when there is really no difference in the "real" world; green zone shows where 95% of values will fall, and two red zones show where 2.5% of the values will fall.**

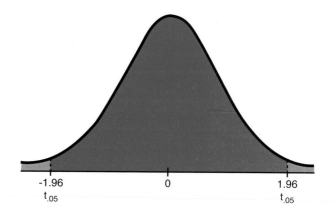

-1.96          0          1.96
$t_{.05}$                  $t_{.05}$

where toward the middle, in the green zone. In fact, the green zone marks where a *t* test value will fall 95% of the time, if, in the real world, the two variables tested are *not* different. The red zones at either end of the normal curve are the areas where the *t* values will fall by chance alone 2.5% of the time if, in the real world, the two variables tested are not different. When we say that a test statistic is significant, we are saying that only a small percentage of the time will we get that test statistic *if,* in the real world, there was no difference or connection between the variables.

Ignoring the meaning of "correlation" for now, when the RN in the vignette reads that intention to have a purified protein derivative (PPD) skin test and all the TII subscales were significantly correlated, he knows that what was found in this study *probably* did not happen by chance. How much "probably" means, or what the probability is that whatever was found happened by chance is reported by a *P* value. The *P* value represents the **probability** and is defined as the percentage of the time the result found would have happened by chance alone. If the RN looks at Table 2 in the report, he will see *P* values reported for each of the statistics given in the table. A *P* value of .05 translates to 5%, which means that the statistic reported would only happen 5 out of 100 times by chance alone. If the *P* value were .01, then the statistic would only occur by chance 1 out of 100 times (1%), and if the *P* value were .001, the statistic would only occur by chance 1 out of 1000 times (1/10 of 1%). Statistical significance, no matter what statistical test has been used, means that the results are unlikely to have happened by chance alone. Therefore, we infer from the finding of statistical significance that the difference, association, or relationship that we tested statistically is one that really exists in the real world because we were unlikely to get our test statistic by chance alone. Remember that inferential statistics are only used in quantitative methods because only in quantitative studies do we assume that the absolute truth or single real answers can be found.

Statistical significance is also sometimes described in the results sections of research reports in the form of confidence intervals. **Confidence intervals** state the range of actual values for the statistic we are computing (such as the difference in the mean ages of nursing students who do and do not choose acute care settings) in which 95 out of 100 of the values would fall. A confidence interval for the differences in ages between nursing students choosing the two types of settings might be 0.8 to 6.2, and a research report might state that the differences in the means of ages for the two groups was 4.2, with a 95% confidence interval (0.8, 6.2). This means that given the difference found in the study, 95 out of 100 times the difference in ages between the two groups of students will fall between 0.8 years and 6.2 years. Notice

---

## CORE CONCEPT

*Inferential statistics are used to report whether the results found in the specific study are likely to have happened by chance alone. Statistical significance is* not *an absolute guarantee that the values are really different or related in the real world. Rather, statistical significance means that there is less than a 5% chance that the amount of relationship or difference found happened by chance.*

| TABLE 5-2 | Comparison of *P* Values and Confidence Intervals | |
|---|---|---|
| | **P Value** | **Confidence Interval** |
| Assumption | The relationship or difference tested is zero | The relationship or difference is that found in the data |
| Meaning | Gives the percentage of the time that we would get the test statistic by chance alone | Gives the range of values (biggest and smallest numbers) that would occur 95% of the time for the relationship or difference found |
| Interpretation | The smaller the value, the less likely that the test result occurred by chance alone | The smaller the range, without zero in it, the more confident we can be that the test statistic reflects the "real" world |

that this range does not include zero, so there is a low likelihood that there is zero or no difference.

Confidence intervals are almost always stated for the 95% range, whereas the probability of getting the result reported if there really was no difference or relationship is usually reported as one of three possible percents, 5% ($P < .05$), 1% ($P < .01$), and 0.1% ($P < .001$). Table 5–2 summarizes the differences between $P$ values and confidence intervals.

Returning to the TB-screening article and the report of significant correlations between intention to have a PPD and all of the TII subscales, we now know that whatever a correlation is, it was unlikely to have happened by chance. We will talk more about what a correlation is shortly.

## PARAMETRIC AND NONPARAMETRIC STATISTICS

Before we begin to discuss some of the specific statistical tests that you are likely to find reported in the results sections, we must understand the difference between parametric and nonparametric statistics. These terms refer to the two broad classes

### C ORE  C ONCEPT

*Whether the report includes* P *values or confidence intervals, the authors are telling you how likely it is that the results from the study happened due to chance and, therefore, how likely it is that these results can be used to infer that there would be similar results in future similar situations.*

of inferential statistical procedures that can be applied to numeric results from studies. **Parametric** statistics can be applied to numbers that meet two key criteria: (1) the numbers must generally be normally distributed—that is, the frequency distribution of the numbers is roughly bell-shaped, and (2) the numbers must be interval or ratio numbers, such as age or intelligence score—that is, the numbers must have an order and there must be an equal distance between each value. **Nonparametric** statistics are used for numbers that do not have a bell-shaped distribution and are categoric or ordinal. Categoric or ordinal numbers represent variables for which there is no established equal distance between each category, such as numbers used to represent gender or rating of preference for car color.

Understanding the difference between parametric and nonparametric statistics is important for two reasons. First, although it is the researcher's responsibility to decide which type of inferential statistics should be used, as an intelligent reader of research you must understand that the decision is not always clear cut. In fact, whole books are written about which types of statistics should or should not be used with selected data. Therefore, the author of a research report may include a sentence or two stating that either parametric or nonparametric statistics were used and the rationale for that decision. Second, types of statistical tests used in research differ depending on the kind of numbers in the results. Therefore, more than one type of statistical procedure is needed to look for the same kind of relationship. For example, often research is looking for differences between two groups. If the variable that we expect to be different in the two groups has interval or ratio numeric values (and is distributed roughly normally or bell shaped) such as age, then the researcher can use a *t* test. But if the variable that we expect to be different for the two groups is a category, such as choice between red or green cars, then the researcher cannot use a *t* test and may use a Kruskal-Wallis one-way analysis of variance (ANOVA) test. The *t* test is a parametric statistical test, and the Kruskal-Wallis is a nonparametric test, but both help us look for differences between groups. As we discuss some of the more common statistical tests that may be described in the results section of a research report, we will identify parametric and nonparametric statistics so that you will recognize and understand some of each class of statistical procedures.

## BIVARIATE AND MULTIVARIATE TESTS

The RN in our vignette is not interested in becoming a statistician, but he does want to know which factors may be important in planning TB-screening programs that target the Mexican American and migrant communities. The statement that there was a significant correlation between intent to get a PPD and scores on the TII subscales indicates that the authors found something that was not likely to be a chance

---

C O R E   C O N C E P T

*Researchers use different types of statistics to test for the same kind of relationship depending on the form of the data collected. The research report may tell you why a particular type of statistical test was applied.*

occurrence and that might be useful in understanding or predicting use of TB-screening programs. To understand what was found, we must understand the meaning of "correlation," as well as several other statistical terms. Table 5–3 summarizes some of the most common statistical tests used in nursing research by three general purposes for tests. In general, we use statistical tests to: (1) look at differences

| TABLE 5–3 Common Statistical Procedures Categorized by Type of Relationship Tested and Number of Variables Included | | |
|---|---|---|
| **Type of Relationship Tested** | **Two Variables—Bivariate** | **Three or More Variables—Multivariate** |
| **1. Differences—are groups unlike one another on a given variable or variables?** | | |
| Independent groups | ■ *t* test (parametric)<br>■ Sign test or median test (nonparametric)<br>■ Mann-Whitney *U* (nonparametric)<br>■ Wilcoxon rank test (nonparametric)<br>■ Fisher Exact test (nonparametric) | ■ ANOVA (parametric)<br>■ ANCOVA, MANOVA, One-way ANOVA (parametric)<br>■ Kruskal-Wallis one-way ANOVA (nonparametric)<br>■ Chi-square for independent samples |
| Related groups usually over time | ■ Paired *t* test (parametric)<br>■ McNemar change test (nonparametric) | ■ Repeated measures ANOVA (parametric)<br>■ Friedman two-way ANOVA (nonparametric) |
| **2. Relationships between variables—is there a natural connection between two or more variables?** | ■ Pearson's *r* (parametric)<br>■ Spearman rho (nonparametric)<br>■ Kenndall tau (nonparametric)<br>■ Contingency coefficient (nonparametric) | ■ Multiple regression (parametric)<br>■ Canonical correlation (parametric)<br>■ Path analysis (parametric)<br>■ Structural equation modeling (parametric)<br>■ Discriminant analysis (parametric)<br>■ Logistic regression (nonparametric) |
| **3. Relationships within a variable—is there a structure within a variable?** | | ■ Factor analysis (parametric)<br>■ Cluster analysis (nonparametric) |

ANOVA, analysis of variance; ANCOVA, analysis of covariance; MANOVA, multiple analysis of variance.

between groups for one or more variables, (2) look at relationships among two or more variables, or (3) look at relationships of factors within a variable itself. Each of these general purposes addresses a different type of question. When we perform statistical tests to look at differences, we are asking some version of the question "Are groups unlike one another on a given variable or variables?" When we perform statistical tests to look at relationships among variables, we are asking some version of the question "Is there some natural connection between two or more variables?" Finally, when we look at relationships within a variable, we are asking some version of the question "What are the natural components that make up a variable?" The statistical tests used when we are only looking at two variables or two groups are different from those we use with three or more variables or groups. We will first look at bivariate statistics, statistical tests that are used with just two variables.

## Tests Looking for Differences Between Two Groups

In our discussion of significance and probability, we used an example from the fictional article in which the author wanted to explain or predict choice of field of practice. To do so, the author divided the students in the study into two groups: those who chose an acute care setting and those who did not. The author then looked for variables that were significantly different between the two groups, hoping that they might help us to understand and predict which students will select nonacute practice settings. A *t* test was used to test for significant differences. A ***t test*** computes a statistic that reflects the differences in the means of a variable for two different groups or at two different times for one group. The two different groups being tested can consist of anything of interest to nursing, such as men and women, single-parent families and two-parent families, those who quit smoking and those who did not, or hospitals with level-one trauma centers and hospitals without them. In all of these examples, one variable differentiates the two groups. Alternately, the two "groups" can be the same unit at different points in time, such as families before and after a divorce, smokers before and after a smoking cessation program, or hospitals before and after they add a level-one trauma center. The variable tested can be anything that can be measured as a continuous number, such as age, family functioning, self-efficacy, or cost per patient visit.

The fictional article reports the results of two *t* tests. The two groups for both of these tests were the same: those who chose an acute setting and those who did not choose an acute setting. However, the tests looked for differences in two different variables. In the first test, the researcher tested to see if age differed between the two groups, and, in the second test, the researcher tested to see if health rating differed between the two groups. In both cases, there was a statistically significant difference between the groups on the variables. The author also tells the reader that "there was no significant . . . differences in number of years of post-secondary education and field of study." Because the test was not statistically significant, no test statistic is reported here, but the author believes it is important to tell you that the possibility of this difference was tested and found not to be present. When using research in clinical practice, it is just as important to understand a result telling you that a difference or relationship was *not* significant as it was significant. Findings that there were no significant relationships or differences help us to rule out factors that will affect our clinical care.

Other statistical tests that examine differences between two groups are mostly nonparametric and include: Fisher exact test, Mann-Whitney test, Wilcoxon signed rank test, McNemar test, and sign or median test (Table 5–3). It is not necessary for you to understand exactly how these tests are chosen and applied. You must understand that whenever one of these tests is reported in the results section of a report, it is being used to examine differences between two groups. If the *P* value that is reported with the test is less than .05, then there was a difference between the groups that probably did not occur by chance alone.

## Tests Looking at Relationships Between Two Variables

Often in nursing research we are looking for relationships or connections between two variables. When two variables are connected in some way, they are said to covary. Two variables **covary** when changes in one are connected to consistent changes in the other. For example, height and weight covary in healthy growing children. As the height of a child increases, the weight usually increases as well. Another example of covariance is found between the amount of practice of a procedure, such as urinary catheterization, and the number of errors. In this case, as the variable "amount of practice" increases, the variable "number of errors" consistently decreases. The statistical test used to examine how much two variables covary is called a **correlation**.

Two things are important to notice about a correlation statistic, also called a correlation coefficient. First, it is important to notice whether the number is negative or positive. In the example of the correlation between height and weight in children, the number for the correlation will be positive because the two variables move in the same direction; that is, they both increase. In the second example, the correlation between practice and errors will be negative, because the two variables move in opposite directions. Figure 5–3 shows two graphs that can represent the two examples. Notice that in the first graph the points all fall along a line that moves diagonally from the bottom to the top of the graph. This shows that there is a positive connection or relationship between these two variables, because as one goes up, the other goes up. In contrast, on the second graph, the points fall along a line that moves diagonally from the top of the graph toward the opposite end. This shows that there is a negative connection or relationship between the two variables, because as one goes up, the other goes down.

Second, it is important to notice the magnitude of the number for a correlation coefficient. Because of the way a correlation coefficient is calculated, it can only have a range of values from −1 to +1. A relationship between two variables that is "perfect," that is, as one goes up the other goes up or down in exactly the same amount, will have a value of either −1 or +1. The lines drawn in the middle of the two graphs in Figure 5–3 show what perfect correlations look like. In real life there is almost never a perfect correlation. Returning to the example of height and weight in children, some children will get taller and not gain very much weight, and some children will get heavier but only a little taller. Therefore, there will not be a consistent increase in weight each time there is an increase in height. That is why we see the scatter plot in Figure 5–3, in which each spot represents one child, and the spots do not all fall along a perfectly straight line. However, the bigger the value of the correlation coefficient, the more consistent and stronger the relationship is between the two variables.

**FIGURE 5-3**  **Scatter plots showing a positive relationship between height and weight in children and a negative relationship between practicing a procedure and number of errors.**

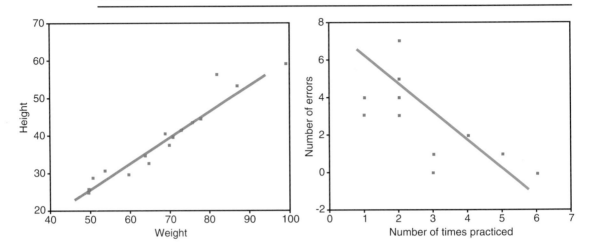

To test whether or not two variables covary, a correlation statistic is computed and tested to see if the computed value is likely to have occurred by chance. In the TB-screening article, the author tested whether the Mexican Americans' report of their intention to get a PPD was related to several beliefs and attitudes. The first sentence in the results section of this article tells us that the descriptive statistics for each of the TII subscales are shown in Table 1. Although we do not yet know much about this TII measure, when we look at Table 1, we see that the names of the subscales are listed and include "behavioral beliefs," "susceptibility," and "general attitude." We now have a greater understanding of the sentence "Pearson correlation coefficients between the model variables revealed significant correlations between intention to have the PPD skin test and all of the TII subscales (Table 2)" (Poss, 2000, p. 23). We know that a "correlation" is a statistic looking at covariance or relationships between two variables and that there was a relationship that probably did not occur by chance alone between reported intention to get a PPD and factors such as behavioral beliefs and susceptibility.

If two variables covary, then they are connected to each other in some way. However, correlation does not tell us how the two variables are connected or whether one of the variables causes the change in the other. For example, if we had no other information besides the correlation statistic for height and weight of children, we would be left wondering whether weight causes growth in height, height causes increased weight, or both tend to increase because of some other factor we have not considered, such as age or nutrition. Therefore, correlations are inferential statistics that explain about relationships but cannot be used to predict because they do not tell us anything about which variable "causes" the other variable to change.

> ## CORE CONCEPT
>
> *A correlation between two variables only tells us that they are connected in some way, not the cause of that connection.*

If we look at Table 2 in the article, we see a matrix of numbers that shows the correlation statistic for each of the possible relationships between different pairs of variables. If we want to know whether there was a relationship between education and intention to get a PPD, we can look at the first column, third row, and find a statistic of 0.53**. The two asterisks next to the statistic are decoded at the bottom of the table and indicate that this statistic had a $P$ value of .01. This means that in only 1 out of 100 chances would we get a statistic of 0.53 for the relationship between education and intention to get a PPD, *if there really was not such a relationship.* Therefore, we decide that there is a relationship between education and intention to get a PPD, and will expect to find such a relationship in other groups of Mexican Migrant farm workers. We also learn from this number that the connection or relationship between education and intention is positive, meaning that as education goes up, an individual's intention to get a PPD goes up as well. Finally, we know the strength of the connection is moderate, because .53 falls approximately halfway between zero, which indicates no connection at all, and one, which indicates a perfect connection.

Numerous types of correlation statistics can be computed between two variables, but the one you will probably find most frequently is the Pearson's product-moment correlation, which uses the symbol "$r$" to represent the value of the bivariate relationship. Besides the Pearson's product-moment correlation, other types of correlation statistics include the Spearman's rho, the Kendall's tau, and the Phi. In all cases, the statistic gives the strength of the covariance between two variables.

The results section of the TB-screening article presents two different tables with correlations. Looking at these tables, we see that all of the correlations that are reported are positive, so we know that in all cases the relationships between the variables were that as one increased the other also increased. Because the size of the correlation coefficient reflects how strong the connection was between the two variables, we see that there was a strong relationship between the variable "intention to have a PPD" and the variable "PPD given" ($r = .84$, $P < .01$). This is in contrast to the correlation between education and behavioral beliefs ($r = .20$, $p < .05$). Although both of these connections are statistically significant, the strength of the relationships is different. What we understand from these statistics is that although education and behavioral beliefs are connected to each other, the connection is not that strong, whereas there is a strong connection between intention and action in terms of getting a PPD.

## Tests Looking for Differences Among Three or More Groups

Frequently, nursing research addresses questions to more than just two groups. For example, we might be interested in comparing patients who smoke, patients who have never smoked, and patients who have quit smoking for their rates of respiratory complications after cardiac surgery. We can perform three different *t* tests to examine differences in complication rates between smokers and those who have never smoked, then between smokers and former smokers, and then between those who have never smoked and former smokers. Keeping up with these comparisons makes one's head whirl, and, obviously, the number of comparisons required would get more complicated with the more groups we have. In addition, each time we get a result that is statistically significant, a small chance remains that we are wrong in our decision that the result did not happen by chance. These chances of being wrong add up when we do multiple statistical tests to answer just one question, making our chance of an error in our decision much larger when we do three or more tests on the same set of variables. The alternative is to use a different type of statistical test called an analysis of variance (ANOVA).

An **analysis of variance** tests for differences in the means for three or more groups. Although it is not necessary that you do the calculations for an ANOVA, it may be helpful to know what the test does, which is reflected in its name. The ANOVA compares how much members of a group differ or vary among one another to how much the members of the group differ or vary from the members of the other groups. In other words, the test analyzes variance, comparing the variance within a group to the variance between groups. For example, an ANOVA test of respiratory complications in three groups of patients who are categorized by smoking status calculates how much variation in respiratory complications there is within the patient group that smokes, the patient group that never smoked, and the patient group that formerly smoked. It then calculates the amount of variation in respiratory rate between the smoking patients, the patients who never smoked, and the former smokers. Finally, the test compares the variation *inside* the groups to the variation *between* the groups to see their differences or similarities. The test statistic in ANOVA is usually an "*F* ratio" value, and, like other statistical tests, the final test statistic is then compared to a set of statistics one would get if there were no differences between the groups. The *F* ratio compares the variation between groups to that within groups, and the larger the *F* ratio the more variation between groups. However, the value of *F* ratios differs depending on the number of groups compared and the number of people studied, so it is not possible to make general statements about the meaning of the *F* ratio, except within the context of significance testing. If the *F* ratio value for a particular study falls into the area of statistics that have less than a 5% chance of occurring by chance, then we decide there is a statistically significant difference between the groups. In the example of respiratory complications, if the *F* ratio was significant, we would be able to decide that smoking and smoking history affect the rate of those complications.

Neither the fictional article nor the TB-screening article used an ANOVA, because neither study needed to compare the means of three or more groups. However, in reading nursing research results, you often find this statistical test, or a variation of it, reported in the results section. Other versions of the ANOVA allow the addition of more variables and various interconnections among variables into the ANOVA. Some of the most common are analysis of covariance (ANCOVA), multiple analysis of variance (MANOVA), and one-way ANOVA. For each of these, the basic purpose of the test is to compare means of an independent variable among three or more groups. Some of the most common nonparametric statistical tests that also test for differences among three or more groups are Kruskal-Wallis, and the Chi square test (*see* Table 5–3).

In addition to comparing three or more groups, we often want to look for differences within groups during three or more time points. Continuing with the example of patients who smoke and their respiratory complication rates, suppose that instead of comparing them to patients who never smoked we compared smoking patients' respiratory complication rates before and after pulmonary toilet care over a 3-day period. In this case, we are not comparing different groups, but the same group over time. The statistical test used in this type of situation is a repeated measures ANOVA. Like the other ANOVA tests, it calculates differences in variance within the group at each time point, but compares those variances to the variances between the time points. Commonly used nonparametric tests for differences within groups at three or more points in time include Friedman tests and the Cochran's *Q*.

### Tests Looking at Relationships Among Three or More Variables

Just as we are often interested in differences among three or more groups, we also are interested in how a group of more than two variables covaries. For example, in the TB-screening article, the authors are interested in how a whole set of variables, such as education, behavioral beliefs, subjective norms, and susceptibility, all covary in relation to an individual's intention to get a PPD. If each of these variables is connected to intention to get a PPD but is also connected to each other somewhat, how much does each variable independently contribute to the variation that happens in intention to get a PPD? Our goal is to understand what factors or variables connect to the different intention scores and in what direction and to what extent, so that we can use our knowledge of those connections to increase the potential that Mexican farm workers will intend to get a PPD in the future. If Mexican farm workers' scores reflecting their intention to get a PPD were a big pie, each of the factors studied might be a piece of that pie, although those pieces of pie will overlap somewhat, as shown in Figure 5–4. We are interested in seeing not just how much each factor by itself connects, but how the factors overlap, so that we know which of the many factors might be the most useful to focus on when planning future programs. The statistical procedure that we use to look at connections among three or more variables is called regression. **Regression** measures how much two or more independent variables explain the variation in a dependent variable. The regression procedure allows us to predict future values for the dependent variable based on values of the independent variables.

Let's apply this to the specific case that the RN in our vignette is reading. The researchers in the TB-screening study know that individuals' intentions to get a PPD is strongly related to whether they get one. Therefore, one goal in nursing is to increase an individual's intention to get a PPD. The researchers have chosen to measure several factors that they believe may affect intention. The bivariate statistics reported in Table 2 (Poss, 2000, p. 24) indicate that statistically significant relationships exist between intention and seven factors (behavioral beliefs, education, susceptibility, severity, normative beliefs, general attitude, and subjective norm). The table also shows a relationship between intention and the act of getting a PPD, but that is not a variable that would predict intention because getting the PPD occurs

**FIGURE 5-4** **Illustration of overlapping factors that are part of why an individual intends to get a purified protein derivative (PPD). Purple shows overlap between susceptibility and education, blue shows overlap between education and subjective norm, and dark violet shows overlap between subjective norm and general attitude.**

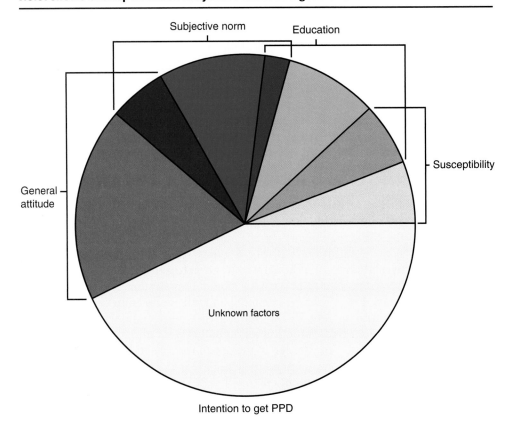

after one intends to get it. Remember that bivariate correlations do not indicate causation, only covariation. However, if we know that one variable by definition occurred before another, we can rule out that the later variable caused the earlier one. By definition, intention to get a PPD was not caused by getting the PPD.

Knowing that seven variables are connected to intention to get a PPD is helpful, but it will be more useful for the RN to know which factor makes the biggest difference so that he knows where to focus his efforts. A regression analysis gives the information needed to know how much different factors independently contribute or connect to a dependent variable. In the TB-screening article, the researchers used a type of regression called logistic regression. When regression is used, one of the first things tested is which variables independently significantly contribute to explaining the variance (differences) in the dependent variable. A significant contribution means that the amount of variance in the dependent variable that is explained by the independent variable in the study is great enough that we would not have gotten the result we did by chance alone in 95% of samples. In the results section of the article, the authors describe which tests they used to determine which of the seven variables worked best to predict intention. You do not need to understand all of those tests to understand that their overall purpose was to determine which of the seven independent variables made a difference in individuals' intentions to get a PPD by eliminating the overlap that existed among the variables. Once this was done, only four independent variables remained: education, subjective norm, susceptibility, and general attitude. These are the factors included in Table 4 of the article (Poss, 2000, p. 25) where the regression results are reported.

Table 4 in the article has several columns, but we are only going to focus on two of them: the columns labeled "Sig" and "Exp(B)." The *P* value is reported under the heading "Sig," which, in this table, stands for significance. Even if we do not understand logistic regression, we can see that the *P* values for education, subjective norm, susceptibility, and general attitude are all less than .05, which means that the findings did not likely occur by chance. "Exp(B)," which heads the last column, is the symbol for how much the particular variable is connected to the dependent variable. In logistic regression, the "B" value reflects the odds that if the independent factor is present, the dependent variable will occur. In other types of regression a **beta (β) value** is given, which tells us the relative contribution or connection of each factor to the dependent variable. In either case, what you should understand is that each variable in a regression analysis is tested to see whether it is independently connected with the dependent variable. If it is connected, a test of how much or to what extent it is connected is provided. Knowing this, the RN in the vignette can see that education had the strongest connection to intention to get a PPD (Exp(B) = 9.927) and that subjective norm had the second strongest, but definitely smaller, connection (Exp(B) = 1.702). The authors also point out that they cannot say that education *causes* an increase in intention, because this test only identifies covariance, not causation. A study's design is what allows us to infer causation and is discussed in Chapter 9. We do know from these results, however, that a TB education program was the most important factor in understanding whether an individual intended to get a PPD.

In addition to regression analysis, numerous statistical procedures examine relationships among three or more variables. The names of some of the most common types of procedures that you may see used in nursing research are listed in Table 5–3 and include canonical correlation, path analysis, structural equation modeling, and discriminant analysis.

### Tests Looking at the Structure or Components of a Variable

We have now discussed bivariate statistical tests that look for differences between two variables and tests that look at relationships between two variables. We also have discussed multivariate tests that look at differences or relationships among three or more variables, and we have identified several parametric and nonparametric statistical tests for each purpose. The last general purpose for statistical procedures is to look at the structure or components within a variable of interest. These types of statistical tests are used when the variable of interest is complex and not easily measured using a single measure or question. The researcher may collect information about the complex variable using several different questions or measures and then want to find out what are the connections among the questions or measures. For example, a nurse researcher might be interested in studying patient satisfaction with care. Several aspects of care may influence satisfaction, such as availability of care, communication with providers, cost of care, and whether expectations for care are met. The researcher might develop 60 statements that each speak to some aspect that may affect satisfaction to be used in a survey. Responses to the survey may be scores on a scale to indicate the respondents' level of agreement with each of the statements. Scores to all 60 statements can be added together to produce a single score for satisfaction, but this does not help us understand what were the important components of satisfaction that make up that score. Statistical procedures, called **factor analysis**, can be used to look for discrete groups of statements that are more closely connected to each other than to the other statements. Factors are the components or discrete groups of measures or statements that covary closely. In our example, the researcher might find that statements about paying bills, insurance, and difficulty getting referrals all covary more closely then statements about communication. These statements might be said to reflect a factor that could be called "barriers to satisfaction." Factor analysis will identify groups of measures of a single variable that are connected closely enough that the connections are not likely to happen by chance. In clinical practice, a study that uses a factor analysis procedure has the potential to provide knowledge about what are some of the components or parts that comprise a health-related concept, such as fear, pain, or denial. The nonparametric statistical test that may be used to look at structure within a variable is called cluster analysis.

To summarize, several specific statistical procedures are used to test for differences and relationships. The types of tests differ depending on the type of data and whether two or more than two variables are to be tested. When any of these tests are applied to specific data, they produce a test statistic that will be symbolized in a unique manner, such as a "$t$" statistic, "$F$" statistic, or "$r$" statistic. The specific statistic from the study is compared to a distribution of statistics that would occur in similar data by chance alone if there were really no relationship or difference. If the statistic from the data falls into the range of values that would only occur less than 5% of the time, if there was really no relationship or difference, the result is statistically significant. Often, the level of statistical significance is specifically stated in the form of a $P$ value or a confidence interval.

## HYPOTHESIS TESTING

The results section of the TB-screening article uses the heading "Hypothesis testing" before it gives results of inferential statistical tests. In Chapter 2, we defined hypotheses as predictions regarding the relationships or effects of selected factors on other factors. Inferential statistics are used to test whether the predictions in hypotheses are "accurate," so hypotheses direct which statistical procedures are used with the data. The results for two types of hypotheses may be described in a research report. The first type, a **research hypothesis**, is a prediction of the relationships or differences that will be found for selected variables in the study. The TB-screening article, for example, used seven different research hypotheses, predicting that each of seven variables would be positively and significantly related to intention to get a

PPD. This is a clear prediction that not only will there be a relationship but also that it will be positive. The author indicates in the conclusions that all of these hypotheses were supported.

The second type of hypothesis is a statistical hypothesis, often called the null hypothesis. A **null hypothesis** predicts that there will be no relationship or difference in selected variables. Remember that, in general, researchers want to be cautious about jumping to conclusions based on the results of their particular study. This is why researchers agree that statistical test results are acceptable only when they would occur by chance less than 5% of the time. Otherwise, even if we find a difference or relationship in the data, we decide that it was just a chance happening and does not prove there is a "real" relationship. The null hypothesis reflects this same thinking by stating our prediction about relationships or differences in the negative, predicting no relationship or difference. The researcher then must find enough evidence to reject that prediction, a statistically significant test result being the evidence that is required.

In summary, a research hypothesis is stated in the positive and predicts the nature and strength of a relationship or difference among variables. The researcher hopes that the results of the study support the prediction. A statistical hypothesis is stated in the negative, and the researcher hopes that the statistical tests are significant so that the null hypothesis can be rejected. Not all quantitative research studies use hypotheses, but if there are one or more hypotheses, they are usually identified in the section of the report that describes the research problem. Chapter 10 discusses hypotheses in more detail.

## IN-CLASS STUDY DATA

To illustrate the use of inferential statistics, let's look at the data that were collected in your in-class study. If you are not using an in-class study, you can refer to a sample set of data that could have been collected in a nursing class included in Appendix E for this section of the chapter. Suppose that before this data were collected, you had observed that your fellow students who were married were generally healthier than those who were not married. You wonder whether this is true and realize that the data from your in-class study could be used to test this idea, because a question about marital status and a question about overall health were included. This means there are two variables of interest: (1) marital status and (2) rating of health. The question of interest concerns differences between two groups and might be stated as "Is there a difference in health rating between married and unmarried nursing students?"

To use the in-class data to answer this question, you must first divide the health ratings into two groups: the health ratings of students who indicated that they were married and the health ratings of students who indicated that they were single, divorced, or widowed. Once you do this, you can easily get an average health rating for the two groups and see if they are different. If they are exactly the same, or close, you probably do not have to look any further for a tentative answer to your question based on this data. If there is a difference, the next question is whether the difference is in the direction you predicted and whether it is big enough that you can believe that it did not happen by chance alone. Looking at the average health ratings will tell you whether single students seemed to have higher or lower health ratings. However, you cannot judge whether the findings prove or disprove your hypothesis, because the ratings may have been simply chance findings. This is where inferential statistics come in, because if this information is entered into a statistical computer program, you can run a *t* test to calculate differences in the means for rating of health of married and unmarried students.

If you are using an in-class study, predict whether some difference found in your class data will be significant before your professor runs an independent *t* test to determine the *t* value for your in-class data. For the fictional data in Appendix E, the computer computes that the mean health rating for single students is 3.1 and the mean rating of health for married students is 2.3. These ratings look different, and are opposite from what was predicted before data were collected. When we do a *t* test, we get a *t* value of 2.7 ($P = .011$), so there is a significant difference in health ratings between single and married students. However, from this data, we can conclude that the evidence does not support the hypothesis that married students are healthier; instead, it supports the opposite idea. In this fictional study, single nursing students had significantly higher ratings of their health than did married nursing students. That it was a statistically significant difference tells us that we can be sure that the difference did not happen by chance alone.

## CONNECTING INFERENTIAL STATISTICAL RESULTS TO CONCLUSIONS

There are several important connections between results and conclusions of reports that have used inferential statistics. When inferential statistics have been used, we know that the goal of the researcher is to generalize the findings of the study to similar situations or groups in the future. Therefore, we expect to find in the discussion/conclusions statement both how the results can be applied to similar situations or groups in the future and what aspects of the study may limit our ability to draw conclusions about future situations or groups. In the fictional article, for example, the author summarizes the findings and then concludes that "Nursing programs that are particularly concerned about shortages in non-acute settings may be able to expand this work force by focusing their recruitment efforts on older students and by further developing or expanding RN to BSN and LPN to BSN programs." The author is saying that in the future, age and type of program of study are likely to be connected with choice of field of study, just as they were in the study. Although the author fails to give any statement of the limitations of the conclusion, the size of the sample—one class of 30 nursing students—might be a reason to consider limiting it.

If the results of a report included hypothesis testing, we also should expect a statement in the conclusions of the report about whether the hypotheses were rejected or accepted. Most important, the meaningfulness of statistically significant results should be discussed in the discussion and conclusion section. Throughout this chapter, we talked about statistical significance; however, the presence of statistical significance does not necessarily indicate that the results are meaningful for clinical practice. Conversely, lack of statistical significance does not necessarily mean that there is no clinical significance in the results. The presence of statistical significance depends on several factors, one of which is the number of cases in the study. This is logical, given that we are trying to use probability to help us to infer connections or differences in the real world. If the study only includes a few cases or subjects, then the chances of a "weird" or unusual case affecting the average result is pretty high. The test distribution for a study with only a few cases results in a large "green" zone and a small "red" zone because there is a good chance that a single odd case will change the actual test statistic (*see* Figure 5–2).

A study that has a large number of cases has a high likelihood of finding statistically significant findings, simply because whatever is found is not going to easily be affected by the chance that an odd case fell into the sample. However, the difference or connection that is found may not be large enough to have meaning for clinical practice. The author of the fictional article, for example, does not give the average ages of students who selected acute and nonacute settings. It is possible that the difference in age was only 1 or 2 years. A difference of this size may be statistically significant but may be too small to have any meaning when one is trying to recruit individuals to nursing.

A clinical example of the difference between statistically significant and clinically meaningful findings might be a study of ratings of pain, such as the one discussed in Chapter 4. Suppose that this study had 500 subjects and that after one group receives an intervention, the mean ratings of pain are 2.5 (1.3) for patients getting the intervention and 2 (1.5) for patients not getting the intervention. In Chapter 4, we used an example where the standard deviations were different although the means were the same. In this example, the means are different, whereas the standard deviations are similar. The researcher might report that there was a statistically significant difference in pain ratings between the group that did and did not get the intervention. This means that the difference in ratings was not likely to happen by chance. However, if you look at the difference, it is not large and may not, in fact, be clinically meaningful. You must decide whether a difference of only one half of a point is large enough to warrant your implementing the intervention, even though you may believe that this difference is unlikely to have occurred by chance. Thus, statistical significance does not necessarily imply clinical significance.

We would expect, therefore, that the conclusions of a research study that used inferential statistics would address whether the statistically significant findings were also meaningful findings. We also would expect that the conclusions would address whether findings that were *not* statistically significant might still warrant further consideration because they appear to be clinically meaningful.

## COMMON ERRORS IN RESULTS SECTIONS

As with the reports of descriptive results, two kinds of problems may be found when reading inferential statistic results in a research report: (1) incomplete information and (2) confusing information. Incomplete information occurs when the results section of reports gives us the statistical test results, including the $P$ value or confidence interval, but does not give us the descriptive results needed to interpret the statistically significant result. For example, suppose that the author of the fictional article had told us that there was a significant difference in health rating ($t = 2.1$, $P < .05$) among students who chose acute versus nonacute fields of practice. The test statistic alone does not tell us which group had the higher health rating, so it is impossible to interpret the meaning of this statistically significant difference.

Another example of incomplete information might be a research report that includes a statement that there was a statistically significant finding but does not provide the test statistic. Because some of the statistics tell us a great deal, the lack of the statistic can limit our understanding of the results. If the author of the TB-screening article, for example, had only told us that there was a significant relationship between intention to get a PPD and getting a PPD, we would have no idea about either the direction of that relationship or the strength of that relationship. It would be conceivable that those who intended to get a PPD actually got a PPD less often then those who did not intend to get one. That would be a negative relationship, and the value for "$r$" would be negative. Of course, the author does give us all of the correlation coefficients, so we know that the $r$ value was .84, which tells us that there was a positive relationship and that it was strong.

A third type of incomplete information is a failure to test for relationships or differences that might be meaningful for understanding the results of the study. The fictional article reports in the results section that age and health rating were both different in students who chose acute versus nonacute fields of practice. One might wonder whether age and rating of health are related. This is a logical question, given what we know about aging and health, and the answer would help us better understand the meaning of the results of this study. However, the author does not test for a relationship between these two variables, so we are left wondering about the possibility of this relationship.

In addition to incomplete information, research reports may present results in a manner that is unclear or unnecessarily confusing. The titles of tables should clearly identify the content of the table and should be referenced within the text of the results section. Labels for columns in a table should be consistent with the use of language in the text and with accepted language for reporting statistical results. The author of the TB-screening article does a good job of ensuring that her tables are understood by stating in the text that the "statistic labeled Exp(B) in Table 4 is the odds ratio" (Poss, 2000, p. 25). The concept of an odds ratio, that is, the probability that a dependent variable will change when an independent variable changes, is commonly understood, but the label Exp(B) is not always used to identify this ratio. However, due perhaps to an editing error, the labels for the columns in Table 4 of this report are not lined up with the columns in the table, and this makes reading the table confusing. Although editing errors will inevitably occur, anything that makes a research report confusing contributes to difficulty in using that research in practice.

## PUBLISHED REPORT—WHAT WOULD YOU CONCLUDE?

The RN in our vignette now has an increased understanding of the results and conclusions of the study examining factors associated with Mexican American farm workers' use of TB-screening programs. He knows that there were several statistically significant relationships among different factors in the study. He also knows that when relationships among groups of those factors were examined, an education program, subjective norm, susceptibility, and general attitude all had significant independent connections to intention to get a PPD, whereas intention and susceptibility were the significant factors connected to getting a PPD and having that PPD read. The author has stated that all her hypotheses were supported and that the results are limited to settings where migrant farm workers do not have to travel to get their health care.

The RN might decide that he could plan programs that take PPD screening to the Latino population in his area and can probably use the results of this study. However, he does not know much about the particular farm workers who were included in this study. In particular, the RN does not know whether those who were in the study were typical farm workers or a subgroup of farm workers who were willing to be in a study. To find out how closely the farm workers in the study represent Mexican farm workers in general, the RN will have to read the "Sample" subsection of the methods section in the research report. Chapters 6 and 7 address samples and how they affect the conclusions we can draw from research.

Looking at the size of the odds ratio for the connection between intention and getting a PPD (Exp(B) = 4.468) and having it read (Exp(B) = 3.806), the RN can interpret that this is a meaningful connection. The odds of getting a PPD applied are four and a half times higher if the farm worker intends to get it, and the odds of having the PPD read are almost four times higher if the farm worker intends to have it read. Therefore, the clinical question now might be: How does one influence farm workers' intentions? This question requires the RN to understand better what is meant by factors such as "educational program," "subjective norm," and "susceptibility." In addition to reading the part of the methods section that describes how the sample was acquired, the RN must read the part of the methods section that describes the measures used in the study to understand better what the factors in the study actually mean.

## OUT-OF-CLASS EXERCISE

### What Do You Want to Know About Samples?

The next two chapters focus on the process of sampling and the meanings of different types of samples. In preparation for reading the next chapter, think about your in-class study sample. Write a list of the information you would like to have about the characteristics of the sample for this study, including a rationale for why you would like that information next to each item. Then think about what you know about the composition of your class and assume that an interesting result that has implications for nursing education was found in the in-class data. If you were writing the conclusions of a report about this finding, how would you describe the group of individuals to whom the results might be applied in the future? Write a short paragraph describing this group, including to whom the results probably apply and to whom they probably do not apply. After you complete this preparation, you are ready to begin Chapter 6.

If your class did not use an in-class study, you can do this exercise by simply pretending that a study was conducted using your class group. List what you would want to know about the people in the study and why. Then, given what you do know about those in your course group, write a short paragraph describing to whom the results of a study with this course group probably would apply and to whom they probably would not apply.

## References

Niska, K. J. (2001). Mexican American family survival, continuity, and growth: The parental perspective. *Nursing Science Quarterly, 14*(4), 322–329.

Poss, J. E. (2000). Factors associated with participation by Mexican migrant farmworkers in a tuberculosis screening program. *Nursing Research, 49*(1), 20–28.

## Resources

Field, A. (2000). Discovering statistics using SPSS for Windows. London: Sage Publications.

Locke, L. F., Silverman, S. J., & Spirduso, W. W. (1998). *Reading and understanding research.* Thousand Oaks, CA: Sage Publications.

Pedhazur, E. J., & Schmelkin, L. P. (1991). *Measurement, design, and analysis: An integrated approach.* Hillsdale, NJ: Lawrence Erlbaum Associates.

Polit, D. F., & Hungler, B. P. (1999). *Nursing research: Principles and methods* (6th ed.). Philadelphia: Lippincott Williams & Wilkins.

Salkind, N. J. (2000). *Statistics for people who (think they) hate statistics.* Thousand Oaks, CA: Sage Publications.

Talbot, L. A. (1995). *Principles and practice of nursing research.* St. Louis: Mosby.

**CHAPTER**

**6**

# Samples

## *To What Types of Patients Do These Research Conclusions Apply—Who Was in the Study?*

**KEY TERMS**

Bias
Cluster sampling
Cohort
Convenience sample
Criteria for participation
Generalizability
Matched sample
Nonprobability sampling
Population
Power analysis
Probability sampling
Purposive sample

Quota sample
Random assignment
Random sample
Randomly selected
Sample
Sampling frame
Sampling unit
Saturation
Snowball sample
Stratified random sample
Systematic sample

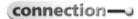

## CLINICAL CASE

The four different RNs in the four vignettes that we discussed in previous chapters each had a clinical question and sought an answer through published research. As we reviewed what they could conclude about their questions, in each case we had to wonder whether the results and conclusions of the study could be applied to the patient or patients of concern to the RN. Specifically, we were left wondering:

1. Could the conclusions from the study of cardiovascular risk factors for children with insulin-dependent diabetes mellitus (IDDM) be used to guide discharge planning for M.K., the 16-year-old patient who had been admitted to the intensive care unit (ICU) in insulin shock?
2. Could the conclusion from the study of fecal incontinence in acutely ill patients be applied to planning care for J.K., the 68-year-old man with Parkinson's disease and a history of fecal incontinence on previous admissions?
3. Were the conclusions of two studies of homeless patients relevant, and could they be used to plan a program about HIV and unwanted pregnancy

prevention that would be meaningful to patients such as C.R., the 32-year-old homeless woman seen in the emergency room (ER)?
4. Were the conclusions and results of two studies of Mexican Americans relevant to the Latino population seen at the health department where the Hernandez family was being treated?

Rather than introducing a new clinical case, we will revisit these four clinical cases (and the six research articles found by the RNs) as we look at samples and determine how understanding them helps us to know how to use research in clinical practice. Whether we are concerned with using research to guide discharge planning or to direct care planning, education planning, or program planning, it is important to answer the question, *To what types of patients do these research conclusions apply?* We must consider this question, because a study may address a clinical problem of interest to you, but it may not have used a sample that reflects your patients. You must understand the implications of different sample types to use study results effectively in clinical practice.

## SAMPLES VERSUS POPULATIONS

As discussed, research is rarely able to include in one study all the cases that might be affected by the research question. The study of cardiovascular risk factors in children with IDDM, for example, could not study every child with diabetes, and the study of homeless patients' perceptions of satisfaction with care could not study every homeless person. All of the studies discussed so far were interested in understanding something about a larger group of patients than those included in their actual studies. The larger group about whom these researchers were interested in gaining knowledge is called the study **population**. The population for any particular study is defined by specific common characteristics. For example, the population of interest in the fecal incontinence study had three common characteristics; they: (1) were adults, (2) were acutely ill, and (3) were not cognitively impaired. The population of interest in the tuberculosis (TB)-screening study was adults who were in the community, were Mexican, and were farm workers. The population for the homeless-patient-satisfaction study was adults who were homeless and had used primary health care. Notice that it is possible to clearly identify the common characteristics that comprise each population.

Of course, none of these studies included every member of the population of interest. The subset of the overall population that is included in a study is called a **sample**. To understand whether a study applies to your clinical situation, you will have to consider three questions about the study sample and the related population:

1. Does the population for this study reflect the types of patients or situations that I am interested in understanding?
2. Does the sample in the study reflect or fit with the population of interest?
3. Does the approach taken to choosing the sample limit how much I can use the results of the study?

Most of this chapter addresses the third question, but the first and second questions are also essential to answer to understand and use research in clinical practice.

### Does the Population for This Study Reflect the Types of Patients or Situations of Interest?

To decide whether a study addresses a population that is relevant or clinically similar to the patient group you are interested in understanding, you must identify the common characteristics of your patient population. Nurses occasionally have a problem using research because they look for studies that exactly fit the specific patients with whom they are working. In the case of M.K., the 16-year-old with diabetes, for example, had the RN searched CINAHL for a study that specifically addressed discharge care for female adolescents with IDDM that also addressed health behaviors, she would have likely found little or nothing. The combination of gender, age, diagnosis, health behavior, and discharge care patient characteristics is so specific that no one may have implemented a study focusing on that population. By broadening the characteristics that define the population to only adolescents with IDDM and risk factors, however, the RN found a study that could potentially apply to her specific patient care situation. Yet, too broad a definition of the population might have found studies with populations that were different from M.K., making them useless in planning her care. For example, a literature search that only used the words *diabetes* and *risk factors* would yield a large number of studies of cardiovascular risk factors in adults with non-IDDM. Although there may be some overlap between the concerns of the population of adults with non-IDDM and the population of adolescents with IDDM, clearly there are some important differences that affect how useful studies with adults will be to understanding M.K.'s case.

How do you find out what the population of a study may be? Several places in a research report should identify the population for the study, but, in this chapter, we focus on the section of most reports that is labeled *Sample, Sampling Methods,* or something similar. It is in this section of the report that the author identifies how individuals were selected for the study and lists the criteria for participation in the study. The **criteria for participation** describe the common characteristics that define the target population for the study. In the fecal incontinence study, for example, the authors state that their study included "184 adult patients in acute and critical care units . . . 92 tube-fed who began nutritional support solely by tube feeding and a **cohort** of 92 non–tube-fed patients" (Bliss, Johnson, Savik, Clabots, & Gerding, 2000, p. 102). This tells us that the target population was acutely ill adults who, in at least half the cases, required nutritional support. The RN caring for J.K. might have preferred to find a study with a population that consisted of patients with Parkinson's disease, but a study about adults who are acutely ill does match J.K.'s characteristics. Although it might have been applicable to J.K., a study that was limited to patients with Parkinson's disease would have significantly narrowed the potential usefulness of the study for general clinical practice. In summary, it is important to identify the criteria for study participation to understand the target research study population and to decide on its applicability to your clinical practice.

### Does the Sample in the Study Fit With the Population of Interest?

At first glance, this question may appear to be the same as the first question, but it is not. Once a study defines the population of interest—that is, the larger group we are interested in gaining knowledge about—the researcher must find a way to recruit or get a sample of individuals who are members of that population. This is sometimes more difficult than it might seem. Occasionally, it is not ethical to ask members of the population to submit to the study, occasionally it is difficult to get members of the population to agree to be in a study, and, occasionally, there are limits inherent to a setting that make it difficult to get members from the population of interest. We discuss each of these potential problems in getting study samples later in this chapter and in Chapter 7. For now, it is important to realize that a researcher may define the population of interest for a study one way and end up with a sample that does not fit that planned population.

We discovered an example of a sample that does not completely fit the population of interest when we discussed the limitations of the fecal incontinence study. The population of interest for that study was adults who are acutely ill, but the sample ended up comprising only adult *men* who were acutely ill. This probably occurred because the setting for the study was a Veterans Affairs Medical Center and the veterans in the United States are primarily men. Fortunately for the RN, J.K is a man, so although the actual sample for the study did not entirely fit with the population of interest, the population that was studied still fits with the one about which the RN wanted to learn.

If the RN had been caring for a female patient with Parkinson's and found this article, it would initially have appeared that the study was likely to be highly applicable. Yet, once the RN answered the question, *Does the sample for the study fit the population of interest?,* she might have hesitated to apply the results to her female patient. The RN might also decide that gender does not make a great deal of difference when considering the problem of fecal incontinence and that the study results still could be applied to a female patient. In either case, to intelligently read and use research, it is important to identify your population of interest, the population of in-

---

C ORE  C ONCEPT

*A researcher may define the population of interest for a study in one way but end up with a sample that differs from that defined population.*

terest for a particular research study, and whether the sample reflects that population of interest.

QUALITATIVE

When reading qualitative research, understanding whether the sample fits the population of interest is essential, because the subjective experiences of the sample are at the heart of the study. Suppose, for example, that the researchers in the study of homeless patients' satisfaction with care had interviewed individuals in a transition housing program, where formerly homeless individuals were staying temporarily while they developed resources for permanent housing. The population of interest in that study was homeless individuals to understand better their experiences with health care. The meaning of those experiences for formerly homeless individuals is likely to be different from the meanings for those who are currently homeless. Because the goal of the satisfaction research was to inform our practice by increasing our knowledge about the overall experience of receiving primary health care as a homeless person, a sample of formerly homeless individuals would not have been appropriate and, in fact, would have entirely changed the population for the study.

QUANTITATIVE

In a qualitative study such as the satisfaction study, the goal is to broadly increase our understanding of the population of interest, recognizing that each piece of the picture that we collect gives us a better sense of the whole phenomenon. In a quantitative study such as the fecal incontinence study, however, the goal is to generalize the findings from the sample to the population of interest, expecting that what works or happens with the smaller sample will also work or happen with the larger population. Remember that **generalizability** is the ability to say that the findings from a particular study can be interpreted to apply to a more general population. Although both qualitative and quantitative research have populations and samples, only quantitative research has the goal of generalizability.

### Does the Approach Taken to Choosing the Sample Limit the Usefulness of the Study Results?

The third question to consider when determining to what types of patients a research study applies concerns how the researcher obtained his or her sample and whether that approach limits how you can use the study conclusions in clinical practice. To address that question, we first must discuss some of the unique language that is used in research to describe samples.

The language describing the process of obtaining a study sample, or sampling, differs between qualitative and quantitative studies, because the general purposes of the two types of research differ. Sampling in qualitative and quantitative studies differs in two broad areas: (1) constraining versus enriching the complexity of samples and (2) rigidity or flexibility in sampling. We start by discussing the sampling in qualitative studies.

#### *Sampling in Qualitative Research*

One of the first things that differentiates a qualitative sample from a quantitative sample is the language used to describe the people in the study. In qualitative research, the individuals that comprise a sample are often called *participants, volunteers, members,* or *informants.* These terms reflect the perspective that the individuals are an active part of the research process and are sharing their knowledge and experiences with the researcher.

The qualitative researcher is looking for the most content and the most contextually rich sources of data available to understand the meaning of the experiences of interest. Immersion in the experience with as much of the real complexity as possible is critical in understanding these realities and experiences. Therefore, the qualitative researcher wants each participant or case to be different and unique to lend additional insight into the richness of a particular phenomenon. The researcher seeks ways to find individuals who are deeply involved and a part of the phenomenon being studied. In the study of Mexican American family survival, for example, the researcher lived in an area with Mexican American families so that she could experience life in the community. The families in the study were diverse, with no constraints placed on them other than being Mexican American. Under the "Findings" heading, the author reports that there were a range of parents' ages, a range of number and ages of children, variation in whether mothers worked outside the home, and variation in the father's employment status. There was no attempt to limit the sample to one type of family; rather, acquiring a sample that reflected diversity was the goal. The type of sample used in this study is called a **convenience sample** because it includes members of the population who can be readily found and recruited.

Qualitative research may also use an approach called snowball sampling. A **snowball sample** starts with one participant or member of the population and uses that member's contacts to identify other potential participants for the study. The next few participants then share other contacts who may have useful experiences to share, thus ever increasing the sample. Snowball sampling helps the researcher to find participants who might otherwise not be identified easily and often allows the inclusion of several views or experiences.

A snowball approach to sampling might be useful, for example, in a study of the experience of smoking cessation among Appalachians. The researcher would initially find an individual from Appalachia who is trying to quit smoking. During the interview, that participant might mention that she knows some people who found it easy to quit smoking and some who really struggled. The researcher would be interested in understanding the experiences of both groups and might ask the participant to contact those individuals to see if they would talk with the researcher. Then, perhaps, an individual who describes quitting as easy might mention his use of family support and prayer, leading the researcher to want to explore further these two sources of assistance with quitting. Perhaps this participant knows several other people from his church who have quit smoking and agrees to ask them to speak with the researcher. At the same time, the individual who had difficulty quitting might identify several other people who have been unable to quit and agree to ask them to talk with the researcher.

Two things are happening in this case. First, the sample is gaining momentum and growing (like a rolling snowball) as each participant identifies others who might have experiences that will help the researcher to understand smoking cessation. Second, the researcher begins to have an understanding of the quitting experience that leads to searching for participants who can fill in or add to particular aspects of that understanding, such as the use of prayer to quit.

Another type of sampling used in qualitative research is purposive sampling. A **purposive sample** consists of participants who are intentionally selected, because they have certain characteristics that are related to the purpose of the research. The characteristics sought in the sample will vary, depending on the approach taken by the researcher. Occasionally, a researcher's goal is to obtain as much diversity as possible in the sample, but sometimes the goal is to focus intently on a particular aspect of the phenomenon under study. Although the research report of the homeless patients' satisfaction with care does not specifically use the term *purposive*, the researchers probably used that type of sampling strategy to acquire participants who reflected numerous experiences with homelessness and health care.

### Sampling in Quantitative Research

The sampling approaches in quantitative research focus on acquiring subjects who match as closely as possible the population of interest. To accomplish this goal, sampling strategies in quantitative research either attempt to remove as much extraneous variation as possible from the study subjects or use strategies that prevent the sample from being limited to any particular group or characteristic. In general, quantitative studies that seek to describe and understand some aspect related to health and health care use sampling strategies that lead to a sample that represents as closely as possible the target population. Studies that seek to predict or to test predictions use sampling strategies focused on eliminating factors that might confuse the results of the study. For example, a quantitative descriptive study of the process of smoking cessation should include subjects who have the different economic, educational, racial, and gender backgrounds that are found in the general community of interest. In contrast, a study of the effectiveness of a smoking-cessation program that compares a group using the intervention to a group not using it should ensure that the groups did not differ in factors such as race or education. If these factors differed, they might affect quitting success and make it difficult to determine whether the intervention itself made a difference.

In either case, one of the goals in sampling is to avoid bias. **Bias** occurs when some unintended factor confuses or changes the results of the study in a way that can lead to incorrect conclusions. We say that a bias distorts or confounds the findings in a study, making it difficult or impossible to interpret the results.

The goal of limiting or avoiding the introduction of bias into the study sample is reflected in the use of the term *subjects* to describe the members of the sample. *Subjects* is intended to convey that the researcher is separate and as removed as possible from those in the sample. The distance and impersonal tone implied in *subject* is intended to help the researcher to avoid introducing any of the researcher's own expectations or interests into the study findings.

### Nonprobability Sampling

Quantitative studies with the purpose of describing or increasing our understanding usually use nonprobability samples. **Nonprobability sampling** uses approaches that do not necessarily assure that everyone in the population of interest has an equal chance of being included in the study. These types of sampling strategies usually are used because they are easier or less costly or because it is not possible to identify everyone in the population. Some of the types of nonprobability samples may sound familiar, because they include convenience samples, purposive sampling, quota sampling, and matched samples.

The same processes are used to obtain a convenience sample in quantitative research as in qualitative research. A convenience sample consists of subjects who meet the participation criteria and who can be readily identified and recruited into the study. For example, the TB-screening study used a convenience sample of 206 Mexican migrant farm workers. The criteria for participation in the study were being a Mexican migrant farm worker without a history of a positive purified protein derivative (PPD) skin test or active TB. Any farm worker in the 20 different camps that the researcher could access could be included in the study. The pool of all potential subjects for a study is also called a **sampling frame**—that is, the pool of all individuals who meet the criteria for the study and, therefore, can be included in the sample. When the study tells us that the sample was one of convenience, we know that subjects from the sampling frame were included because they could be conveniently accessed, often on a first-come first-serve basis. This means that those who heard about the study first, were most open to being in a study, or happened to be nearby when the researcher came to do the study were the subjects recruited. Because there was not an equal chance for every Mexican farm worker in the 20 camps to participate in the study, the sample was a nonprobability sample. Similarly, the study of risk factors for persons with IDDM used a convenience sample of the 149 patients in the endocrinology section of one hospital.

Purposive sampling also is used in quantitative research, particularly when the population of interest is unusual or difficult to access. Remember that purposive sampling is the careful and intentional selection of subjects for a study based on specified characteristics. Although purposive sampling is used relatively frequently in qualitative research, it is used less often in quantitative research, because the potential for introducing unintended bias into the sample can be high. None of the quantitative studies discussed so far used a purposive sample. A purposive sample might be used in quantitative research if the researcher were interested in describing family adaptation when a member survives a highly lethal health problem. The researcher might intentionally seek out the families of individuals who have survived ovarian and pancreatic cancers, because they are two of the most lethal types of cancer. Clearly, other highly lethal conditions occur in health care, but the categories of ovarian and pancreatic cancer are readily identifiable and consistently have low survival odds. Therefore, the researcher might purposely select for the sample families with survivors of these two conditions.

Quota sampling is another type of nonprobability sampling in which every member of the population does not have an equal chance of being included in the study. In a **quota sample**, one or more characteristics are identified that are important to the purpose of the study and used to establish limits on or quotas for the number of subjects who will be included in the study. The goal is to make the sample more representative of the population in a situation in which all of the members of the population cannot be identified. For example, the researcher studying nursing students' choices of field of practice might have decided that gender would be an important factor to consider. After discerning that the known percentage of male nursing students in her state was 16%, she might have used quota sampling to ensure that her sample would have a similar gender composition. She might have done that by setting a goal of recruiting 21 female nursing students and 4 male nursing students, so that 16% of the sample would be male.

The last type of nonprobability sample that often is used in nursing research is a matched sample. In a **matched sample**, the researcher plans to compare two groups to explain or understand something that differentiates them but knows that some other important characteristics could confuse or bias understanding what is under study. To prevent the other important characteristic(s) from making comparison difficult, the researcher intentionally selects subjects whose important characteristics are the same, or matched. The report of the study of fecal incontinence indicates that the original sample for the study comprised 92 tube-fed and 92 non–tube-fed patients who were matched on risk factors for *Clostridium difficile.* The researcher wanted to compare tube-fed and non–tube-fed patients in terms of how often they developed diarrhea and did not want the groups to differ on their risk for *C. difficile,* which can also cause diarrhea. Therefore, the specific factors that put a patient at risk for *C. difficile* infection, such as exposure to antibiotics, illness severity, nutritional status, or duration of hospitalization, were identified before the study and subjects were recruited into the study who were similar on those characteristics but differed on whether they were tube-fed. This matched the subjects—that is, they had the same risk factors for *C. difficile* within each group. Again, all acutely ill patients did not have an equal chance of being in the study, because they only were included if they had risk factors for *C. difficile* that were similar to those of another subject who differed from them in terms of being tube-fed. Thus, at the beginning of the study, for each subject in the tube-fed group, there was a subject who matched him or her in risks for *C. difficile* in the non–tube-fed group. The author of the fecal incontinence study also states that because of loss of subjects from the study, this matching was no longer in effect for the study that she is now reporting. This becomes important because the author must include tests to see whether risks for *C. difficile* caused diarrhea in the study subjects.

### Probability Sampling

Quantitative studies whose purpose it is to predict are more likely to use **probability-sampling** strategies than nonprobability strategies. Probability-sampling strategies ensure that every member of a population has an equal opportunity to be in the study. The most common types of probability-sampling strategies are simple random sampling and several variations on simple random sampling: stratified random sampling, cluster sampling, and systematic sampling.

Although simple random sampling is familiar to most people, the principles involved in this type of sampling are important to understand. In a simple **random sample**, all the members of a population of interest must be identified and listed and each member of the population is assigned a number. Therefore, to select a random sample, all members of the population must be part of the sampling frame. After deciding how many members of the population will be in the study, the researcher uses some device, such as a random number table (see Figure 6–1) or a computer

**FIGURE 6-1**    **Random number table of 200 numbers between 0 and 99.**

| | | | | | | | | | | | | | | | | | | | |
|---|---|---|---|---|---|---|---|---|---|---|---|---|---|---|---|---|---|---|---|
| 79 | 75 | 64 | 48 | 5 | 70 | 28 | 68 | 79 | 66 | 64 | 40 | 6 | 59 | 30 | 11 | 42 | 29 | 97 | 9 |
| 65 | 25 | 22 | 58 | 19 | 27 | 80 | 36 | 63 | 16 | 25 | 20 | 12 | 93 | 47 | 1 | 38 | 42 | 19 | 79 |
| 58 | 13 | 92 | 29 | 56 | 10 | 51 | 38 | 16 | 0 | 97 | 76 | 65 | 40 | 67 | 34 | 20 | 39 | 86 | 79 |
| 18 | 97 | 73 | 96 | 28 | 54 | 85 | 80 | 9 | 77 | 43 | 47 | 89 | 13 | 24 | 61 | 6 | 63 | 86 | 99 |
| 91 | 70 | 17 | 84 | 26 | 21 | 82 | 24 | 42 | 32 | 51 | 94 | 89 | 35 | 93 | 10 | 15 | 28 | 71 | 98 |
| 81 | 78 | 61 | 93 | 75 | 27 | 17 | 39 | 20 | 18 | 66 | 98 | 12 | 73 | 96 | 88 | 31 | 3 | 57 | 72 |
| 9 | 7 | 49 | 77 | 38 | 53 | 87 | 86 | 52 | 42 | 12 | 14 | 37 | 5 | 50 | 68 | 80 | 4 | 90 | 15 |
| 50 | 28 | 27 | 49 | 31 | 67 | 53 | 91 | 15 | 48 | 23 | 83 | 90 | 65 | 25 | 69 | 31 | 14 | 79 | 82 |
| 72 | 66 | 0 | 83 | 52 | 25 | 93 | 26 | 39 | 23 | 10 | 73 | 44 | 58 | 13 | 85 | 21 | 24 | 22 | 79 |
| 59 | 27 | 90 | 21 | 52 | 41 | 73 | 40 | 83 | 49 | 93 | 97 | 81 | 40 | 49 | 51 | 7 | 44 | 56 | 39 |

program, to select who will be in the study. The researchers arbitrarily pick a number from a random number table, which consists of rows and columns of numbers, and then continues in any direction in the table to select numbers. Because all possible numbers are represented in the table, it is by chance alone that the number of any particular member of the population is chosen. Therefore, to obtain a random sample of nursing students in Tennessee, a researcher must identify and list every individual who is a nursing student in the state. If the researcher wanted a sample size of 200 nursing students, the researcher would assign numbers to every student in the state, pick a number in the random number table, and continue to read off numbers going down, up, or diagonally through the table, until the numbers of 200 students have been picked. Because the goal of quantitative research is to generalize and to avoid bias, a simple random sample is considered the best type of sample, because the only factors that should bias the sample would be present by chance alone, making it highly likely that the sample will be similar to the population of interest.

In **stratified random sampling**, the population of interest is first divided into two or more groups based on characteristics that are considered important to the purpose of the study and then members within each group are **randomly selected**. If a researcher were interested in studying some aspect of nursing students in Tennessee that may be significantly different for undergraduates and graduate students, the population of all nursing students could be stratified—that is, divided according to level of study. Then the students in each stratum would be listed and assigned a number, and the selection of a random sample would be carried out twice, first with the undergraduate students and then with the graduate students. This strategy is similar to the nonprobability sampling strategy of quota sampling, except that in stratified sampling, members in each stratum have an equal opportunity to be in the sample.

Cluster sampling is a third type of probability sampling that can make it easier to acquire a random sample. **Cluster sampling** occurs in stages, starting with selecting groups of subjects who are part of a larger element that relates to the population and then sampling smaller groups until eventually individual subjects are selected. A cluster sample of nursing students in Tennessee might start by listing every National League for Nursing (NLN)-accredited undergraduate and graduate program in Tennessee. A random sample of 10 of these programs might be selected, and then a random sample of 200 students could be selected from a list of every nursing student in those 10 programs. Every student in Tennessee still had an equal opportunity to be selected for the sample, but the researcher did not have to identify and list every student to select that sample. Instead, the larger element of universities with accredited programs was sampled, followed by sampling from those universities.

The last type of probability sample that may be used in nursing research is a **systematic sample**. This strategy is similar to the random sample because the members of the population are identified and listed. However, rather than using a random digit table to select members of the population for the sample, members are selected at a fixed interval from the list. The selected interval may be every tenth member, every fifth member, or any other interval that will lead to a sample of the size desired. When using a systematic sample, it is important to ensure that the members of the population are not listed in some order that creates a bias in the sample. For example, the students from every NLN program of nursing in Tennessee might always be listed starting with undergraduate students followed by graduate students. If the researcher were using systematic sampling, taking every fifth student for a total of five subjects from each program, the students selected might all be undergraduates because only the top part of each list would be included in the sample. If, on the other hand, the students in each program were listed alphabetically, selecting the fifth student for up to five subjects would lead to a sample that was likely to consist of undergraduate and graduate students in the proportion that exists in the population as a whole. Table 6–1 summarizes the types of samples used in qualitative and quantitative research. The same strategy is described using slightly different language depending on whether it is used in a qualitative or quantitative study.

## DIFFERENCES IN QUALITATIVE AND QUANTITATIVE SAMPLING

We said at the beginning of this section that qualitative and quantitative sampling differ in their overall goal and approach. This is important to understand, because it allows you to understand better how a sample and the approach taken to obtain that sample affect the usefulness of the research for your practice.

**TABLE 6–1    Sampling Strategies for Qualitative and Quantitative Research**

| Qualitative Research | Quantitative Research |
|---|---|
| **Convenience sample:** Participants who are readily available and represent the phenomenon of interest are included in the sample. | **Convenience sample:** Members of the population who are easily identified and readily available are included in the sample; a nonprobability sample. |
| **Snowball sample:** Participants who are known to and recommended by current participants are identified and included, building the sample from a few participants to as many as are needed. | **Quota sample:** One or more criteria are used to ensure that a previously established number of subjects who fit those criteria are included in the sample; a nonprobability sample. |
| **Purposive sample:** Participants who are intentionally selected because they have certain characteristics that are related to the purpose of the research are included in the sample. | **Purposive sample:** Subjects in the sample are limited to those who have certain characteristics that are related to the purpose of the research; a nonprobability sample. |
| | **Simple random sample:** Subjects are selected by enumerating all members of the population, and a completely random process is used to identify who will be included; a probability sample. |
| | **Stratified random sample:** Members of the population are grouped by one or more characteristics, and subjects are selected from each group using a completely random process; a probability sample. |
| | **Cluster sample:** Groups of the population are enumerated and selected by a completely random process, then individual subjects from within these groups are randomly selected; a probability sample. |
| | **Systematic sample:** The members of a population are enumerated and every $k^{th}$ member at a fixed interval is selected as a subject; a probability sample. |

## CORE CONCEPT

*Sampling strategies in qualitative and quantitative research differ in their goals and approaches even when they are using a similar strategy.*

QUALITATIVE

In general, sampling strategies in qualitative research seek to identify participants who will bring to the study detail and complexity. Even when a researcher uses a purposive sample to focus on a particular type of experience, the goal remains to have as much depth and detail as possible. As a result, sampling in qualitative research is usually driven by the data collection itself and changes as the study progresses. The researcher collects data and analyzes them concurrently, using insights from the data to guide further participant recruitment and the information that is sought from those participants. Qualitative sampling strategies are fluid and flexible and are intentionally and thoughtfully revised as the data analysis suggests new avenues to explore or aspects that need additional focus. These strategies are used to seek a detailed and rich understanding of the aspect under study. This process continues until the information shared by participants has become redundant and no new information is being added; at this point, the researcher identifies that saturation has occurred. **Saturation** of data is the point in qualitative research data collection at which the data become repetitive and no new information is being added.

QUANTITATIVE

In contrast, the goal of quantitative sampling strategies is to acquire a sample that is as representative as possible of the population of interest so that the findings from the study can be generalized. To accomplish this goal, quantitative studies control and limit differences in the sample that may bias or distort the study results. Quantitative research does not necessarily want everyone in the study to be exactly alike: the goal is that the sample be similar to the population of interest. Nonprobability approaches, such as quota sampling and matched sampling, limit variations that may bias a study. For example, it is generally recognized that the people who are most likely to agree to participate in research studies are white and educated. There are several social and historical reasons for this, but, as a result, researchers may implement sampling strategies that specifically target underrepresented groups using a quota or matched sample approach. Probability sampling's goal is to ensure that every member of a population can be in the study, so that no systematic factor defines the sample and makes it different from the population. Quantitative sampling often limits or controls the variety that qualitative sampling seeks.

The other important difference between quantitative and qualitative sampling strategies is the flexibility of the process. Researchers in quantitative studies remove themselves from the selection of subjects to eliminate personal bias. Therefore, in quantitative research, a sampling plan is identified and strictly followed and analysis of data usually is not started until the entire sample is identified and recruited. If the sampling plan includes stratifying or matching, then selected characteristics of the sample are identified and analyzed throughout the selection process, but the findings regarding the variables of interest are not examined until the entire sample is in place. Although a qualitative study will thoughtfully change sampling strategies in response to data analysis, a quantitative study will usually follow a clearly identified plan that is determined before sampling has started and that is not modified during the sampling process. A summary of the differences in sampling approaches between qualitative and quantitative research is provided in Table 6–2.

| TABLE 6–2 | Differences in Sampling Approaches Between Quantitative and Qualitative Research | |
|---|---|---|
| **Sampling Approach** | **Qualitative Research** | **Quantitative Research** |
| *General goal of sampling* | To include as many sources as possible that add to the richness, depth, and variety of the data | To ensure that only the variables of interest influence the results of the study by limiting extraneous variations in the sample |
| *Approach to sampling* | Usually driven by the data as it is collected; therefore, flexible and evolving as the study develops | Established before beginning the process of sampling and followed strictly to avoid introducing bias into the sample |
| *Language for those in the sample* | Participants, volunteers, and informants | Subjects |

## STRENGTHS AND WEAKNESSES OF DIFFERENT SAMPLING APPROACHES

QUALITATIVE

Because the goals of sampling in qualitative and quantitative research are different, the strengths and weaknesses of the different strategies for each approach differ as well. A convenience sample for a qualitative study has the advantages of being relatively easy and inexpensive to acquire but may have the disadvantage of yielding a group of participants that is not as diverse and cannot provide as rich a detail about the phenomenon of interest as desired. For example, a convenience sample of homeless people from just one shelter may yield individuals who have been homeless for only a short time because of the location of the shelter.

QUANTITATIVE

A convenience sample for a quantitative study also has the advantages of being easy and inexpensive, but has the disadvantage of lack of control over factors that may bias the study. A convenience sample will consist of those subjects who happen to be at the right place at the right time to be included in the sample. What brings those people to the "right" place and time may have to do with their age, economic status, education, illness, or history—factors that may then bias the results of the study.

QUALITATIVE

Similarly, purposive sampling has different advantages and disadvantages depending on whether the study is qualitative or quantitative. A purposive sample in a qualitative study actively seeks to enrich the data by including participants who have a particular type of experience or understanding to share. The potential disadvantage to purposive sampling in qualitative research is the possibility of prematurely focusing the data collection on some particular experience or understanding and missing the broader range of data that may come from a convenience sample.

QUANTITATIVE

In quantitative research, purposive sampling is used to identify a sample that has certain characteristics that are relevant to the population of interest in the study. The advantage is that selected factors are clearly defined and identified in the sample, but the disadvantage is that the greater a sample is limited and defined by selected characteristics, the less likely it is to reflect the population at large. In the example of a purposive sampling of families with a member who has survived ovarian or pancreatic cancer, for example, both of these cancers occur in relatively young individuals, leading to their families being relatively young, making the results less applicable to older families. A second bias that may be introduced in this sample is that cancer may make unique demands on families that other highly lethal conditions, such as a severe closed head injury or acute pancreatitis, do not.

In quantitative research, nonprobability sampling strategies are usually more likely to allow bias to enter a sample and make it less likely to be representative of the population of interest. This is because all nonprobability samples have the potential for some outside unidentified factor directing who is and is not included in the study. By definition, probability samples eliminate the potential of some outside factor systematically entering into the sample because all of the members of the population have an equal chance of being included. However, probability-sampling strategies have the disadvantage of being complex, costly, or not feasible, given the population of interest. For example, it would not be possible to enumerate all of the homeless individuals in any particular state as one might enumerate all of the nursing students, making a probability sample more difficult. However, it might be possible to enumerate all homeless shelters in a state and use cluster sampling to randomly select shelters and then randomly select residents of these shelters. This would yield a probability sample of homeless people who are housed in shelters within the state—but not of all homeless people, because many homeless individuals do not use traditional shelters.

QUANTITATIVE

One approach that is taken to decrease the potential for a bias in a sample using quantitative methods is to assign subjects randomly to different groups that are going to be in a study. This is not truly a sampling strategy, but more of a research method that is used to offset a potential problem that can occur from nonprobability sampling. **Random assignment** ensures that all subjects in a study have an equal chance of being in any particular group within the study. The sample may be one of convenience or purposive, so there may be some bias influencing the results. However, because that bias is evenly distributed among the different groups to be studied, the bias will not unduly affect the outcomes of the study.

Obviously, random assignment is only an option when a study is going to include more than one group of subjects, because the process requires giving each subject in the sample an equal chance to be in any particular group. The HIV-prevention study, for example, used random assignment of different shelters to try to decrease any bias that might have been present in the convenience sample of homeless women's shelters that comprised the sample. Randomly assigning women to the three possible HIV-intervention groups would have been desirable but was not feasible, because the interventions needed to be easily available. Randomly assigning the whole shelter to an intervention group allowed the interventions to be given to all the women in a shelter at one time in a convenient manner. Table 6–3 summarizes the advantages and disadvantages of different sampling strategies.

The HIV-prevention study brings up an important point about samples: not all samples consist of individuals. A **sampling unit** is the element of the population that will be selected and analyzed in the study. The sampling unit depends on the population of interest and can comprise individuals and can also be hospitals, families, communities, or outpatient prenatal care programs. Occasionally, samples consist of more than one sampling unit, as in the HIV study. The first sampling unit in the HIV study was emergency and sober-living shelters, and the sample was a convenience sample of those whose directors agreed to be in the study. These shelters were randomly assigned to the three HIV program options, and the women in the shelters and their intimate partners were followed over time. The women and partners were the second sampling unit for this study, as well as the unit used for the analysis. Another example of a sampling unit other than individuals is the sample of Mexican American families in the family survival study. This study asked mothers and fathers to each provide information as individuals, but it used both parents' data to reflect the family as a sampling unit and the unit of analysis.

## SAMPLE SIZE

QUALITATIVE

In addition to understanding how the approach taken to sampling will affect which patients the results of the study will apply to, it is important to understand how the sample size affects the ability to draw conclusions from a study. Similar to sampling strategies, sample size is usually dictated by the process of data analysis in qualitative research; data saturation is an example. The size of the sample in a qualitative study is dictated by the method of study and the complexity of the phenomenon of interest. The researcher continues to collect data until all new information is redundant of previously collected information. Because the data collection methods in qualitative research yield much data from each participant, the sample sizes in qualitative research are usually smaller than in quantitative research. The composition and richness of the setting and participants, rather than the sample size, tell us how useful the results of a qualitative study may be with our own patients.

QUANTITATIVE

The sampling strategy and the complexity of the phenomenon of interest also dictate sample size in quantitative research. In quantitative research, however, the goal of generalizability drives the sample size. Probability samples often can be smaller than nonprobability samples, because probability samples control for bias through the random selection process. Nonprobability samples must be larger in general, so that any unusual or systematic factors that could bias the

| TABLE 6–3 Advantages and Disadvantages of Sampling Strategies in Qualitative and Quantitative Research | | | | |
|---|---|---|---|---|
| | Qualitative Research | | Quantitative Research | |
| **Sampling Strategy** | *Advantages* | *Disadvantages* | *Advantages* | *Disadvantages* |
| Convenience sample | Easier to identify participants; often provides a breadth of information | May "miss" a source of information that is not readily available | Inexpensive; easier to recruit subjects | Most likely to include biases that make it difficult to generalize |
| Purposive sample | Focuses research on the potentially richest sources of information | Only likely to become a disadvantage if the sampling becomes too narrowed | Locates a sample that is hard to recruit or identify | Likely to include many unique characteristics that limit the ability to generalize |
| Snowball sample | Allows the researcher to locate sources of information that might otherwise not be identified or available | Could lead to focusing the research and understanding prematurely | | |
| Quota sample | | | Allows the researcher to control the sample on selected characteristics, so that it more closely resembles the population of interest | Open to systematic variations that can bias the sample |
| Simple random sample and stratified random sample | | | Eliminates likelihood of a systematic bias in the sample, so that results are more readily generalized | Time-consuming; costly; may not be feasible to enumerate the population |

| TABLE 6-3 | Advantages and Disadvantages of Sampling Strategies in Qualitative and Quantitative Research (Continued) | | | |
|---|---|---|---|---|
| | **Qualitative Research** | | **Quantitative Research** | |
| **Sampling Strategy** | *Advantages* | *Disadvantages* | *Advantages* | *Disadvantages* |
| Cluster sample | | | Same advantages as a simple random sample, but more efficient | Population of interest may not be readily grouped or the groups identified may narrow the population |
| Systematic sample | | | Can be easy to implement | May introduce a bias if there is some systematic factor imbedded into the list that occurs at regular intervals |

study will be canceled out by the number of subjects in the study. For example, if the study of the risk factors in children with IDDM had only included 20 children, there would be a good chance that some of those children would have unusual circumstances that might bias the results, such as having parents who are marathon runners or who have a physical disability that limits their children's options for activities. Even 1 or 2 of the 20 children having unusual circumstances or characteristics would have had a significant effect on the study's results. With 140 children in the study, however, the effects of only 1 or 2 children with unusual circumstances will not be as great. Therefore, in general, the larger the sample size in a quantitative study, the more likely that the sample will be representative of the population of interest and the more likely that the study will apply to our clinical situations.

In addition to the logic inherent in obtaining larger samples to eliminate the effects of odd or unique cases, sample sizes in quantitative research are determined by the goal of applying inferential statistics to the data. Remember that inferential statistics are used to calculate a test statistic that is then compared to a distribution for test statistics that would occur by chance alone for that particular sample size. The larger the sample size, the more likely we are to get results that are statistically significant—that is, that did not happen by chance alone. However, it is always costly to recruit and implement a study with many subjects, so it is useful for the researcher to know how large a sample is likely to be needed to be able to apply inferential statistics accurately to the data. Quantitative researchers often use a process called power analysis to determine how large a sample they will need. **Power analysis** allows the researcher to compute the sample size needed to detect a real relationship or difference in the phenomenon under study, if it exists. You may see a written statement that power analysis indicates that a specified sample size was adequate. In this way the authors tell you why they used the size sample that they did.

## COMMON ERRORS IN REPORTS OF SAMPLES

QUALITATIVE

The most common error that occurs in study reports of sampling is a lack of adequate detail to allow us to decide intelligently whether the types of subjects or participants allow us to apply the results of the study to our clinical situation. In qualitative research, this error will most likely take the form of an inadequate description of the study setting and participants. For example, to understand the meaning of the homeless satisfaction with care study, we must have information about the settings from which the participants came. Had the study only used participants who were housed in substance-free shelters, the understanding gained from the study would be less complete than the understanding we gain from a study of participants from several settings, including a clinic, a soup kitchen, and different shelters. The authors have adequately described the setting and sample for their study, allowing the reader to intelligently relate the findings from the study to clinical practice. The qualitative study of family survival also provides some useful information about the setting for the study, such as the population count for the rural area where families in the study lived. However, more information about the composition of the community, its economic status, and the length of time that the different families lived in the United States would have further increased our understanding about to whom the results of this study may relate.

QUANTITATIVE

In quantitative studies, the information that may be missing or inadequate in a research report usually involves the process of acquiring the sample. To judge the representativeness of a sample or whether the sample reflects the clinical population you are interested in learning about requires knowing the sampling strategy, the sampling criteria, and how the sampling strategy was implemented. For example, a convenience sample of nursing students exiting a college of nursing building at lunchtime is more likely to be representative of the nursing students in that college than a convenience sample of students from any one particular classroom, because students exiting the building are more likely to reflect a range of levels of study, whereas a single class will mostly consist of students all at the same level.

Similarly, a random sample of homeless shelters that then takes a convenience sample of homeless individuals is less likely to yield a representative sample of homeless than a random sample of all homeless staying at all shelters on a particular night. To use information about sampling intelligently, we must know the setting where the study occurred and the process of implementing the sampling plan. We also must be given the descriptive statistics that relate the characteristics of the final sample acquired. For example, consider the sample for the fecal incontinence study. Nothing in the sampling plan for that study indicates an intention to limit the study to males. Even though we know that veterans' hospitals are likely to serve men predominantly, not until the authors report that only two subjects in the study were women do we learn that the results of the study only reflect men.

In summary, information about the sampling strategy and the actual sample are important in understanding to whom results of a study may apply. Unique language is associated with the sampling process for both qualitative and quantitative research. Sampling in qualitative research gathers as rich and complete a set of data as possible, and sampling strategies are guided by and may change based on the concurrent data analysis. Sampling in quantitative research eliminates potential bias and gathers information from a subset of the population that resembles the actual population as closely as possible. Sampling strategies in quantitative research are carefully planned, with important characteristics defined and used to limit or control the subjects in the study. Probability samples are considered better than nonprobability samples in quantitative research because they eliminate systematic bias, but they are also more difficult and costly than nonprobability sampling. Sample size depends on the strategy and methods of the study, with qualitative samples generally being smaller than samples for quantitative studies.

## CONNECTING SAMPLING TO THE STUDY RESULTS AND CONCLUSIONS

We started this chapter by asking whether the results and conclusions from the six different studies used so far could be used to guide practice in the different clinical situations described in previous vignettes. Sampling strategies connect to the results of a study in several ways. In both qualitative and quantitative studies, the characteristics of the sample affect the meaning of the results. The appropriateness and focus of sampling in a qualitative study both are driven by and drive data collection, and the detail and complexity of the resulting themes or theory will reflect that sampling. In quantitative studies, the sampling strategy dictates how certain we can be that the results found represent what exists in the real population. Along with sample strategy, sample size also affects the believability of the study results. In the clearest connection between sampling and the potential results of a study, a certain sample size is required even to use some inferential statistical procedures.

Sampling should also be connected to the conclusions of a study. The nature of the study sample and the sampling strategies used may be either a limitation of the study or an aspect that needs further study. For example, the TB-screening program identified the setting for their study as one in which all the components of a screening program were made available on site. To determine whether the theory that was tested in this study applies to TB screening in general, another study is needed. That study must have a sample of subjects who were potentially using a program that required them to visit an outside location at a designated time. Similarly, the conclusions from the family survival article reflect factors of importance to young families and cannot be used to guide practice with families with older children or children who have left home.

In addition to sampling strategies being directly connected to results and conclusions, understanding the language and meaning of sampling in research adds one more piece to the puzzle of reading and understanding research for use in practice. Once you have decided whether the population for the study reflects the type of patients or situations that are of interest to you, whether the sample reflects that population, and whether the approach taken to choosing the sample limits the meaning of the study, you are well on your way to knowing whether the results of the study can be applied to your clinical question.

## PUBLISHED REPORTS—HAVE YOU CHANGED YOUR MIND?

Let's go back and review the four clinical vignettes discussed in this book so far. Start with the case of M.K., who has IDDM, is 16 years old, smokes, does not wear her seatbelt, and does not have good glycemic control. The RN wanted to identify what would be the most effective focus for discharge teaching with M.K. and found a study of cardiovascular risk factors in children with IDDM. This study of risk factors was not limited to adolescents, but predictors of cardiovascular disease (CVD) are relevant for patients of all ages. The criteria for exclusion from this study included presence of ketosis, diabetes as a secondary disease, or a known lipid abnormality. After reading these criteria, the RN decides that the target population is relevant to M.K. and that the sample reflects the target population. The RN also recognizes that there may be limits to how representative the sample is, because it is a convenience sample from just one institution. She knows that health care facilities often serve a particular segment of the population that is economically or geographically able to access the facility. Not being told about the socioeconomic status of these children may be a limitation. Finally, the sample size of 140 children is likely adequate to decrease the chance of one or two unusual cases creating a bias in the study (Lipman et al., 2000). Overall, the RN working with M.K. decides that nothing in the sample precludes her from using the results of this study in her practice.

The RN working with J.K., the 68-year-old man with Parkinson's disease who has been admitted with pneumonia, is interested in learning what she might do to prevent J.K. from developing fecal incontinence and associated skin breakdown. The discussion on sample in the article on fecal incontinence does not directly identify the sampling strategy, except to say that the study was a "secondary data analysis" and that the original sample was a matched sample of tube-fed and non–tube-fed acutely ill patients. Secondary data analysis is a research method that uses already existing data that were not collected for the specific purpose for which they are now being used. We discuss secondary data analysis, as well as other research methods, in Chapter 9. The RN understands the idea of a matched sample and that the author of this article tells us that the matching effect was lost due to subjects being excluded from the study. We have to assume, then, that we now have a purposive sample of 152 acutely ill adults. We have already discussed that this sample comprises 150 men and only 2 women, but this does not concern the RN because her patient is a man. Review of the diagnoses of the subjects in the sample indicates that several acute illnesses, including neurologic and pulmonary disorders, were represented, suggesting that these patients were similar to J.K. The author of the study states that the final sample had average ages of 70 and 65, depending on whether they had fecal incontinence, so the RN knows that the sample for this study fits with J.K. However, one piece of information about the sample may be of some concern: none of the sample had a history of fecal incontinence (Bliss et al., 2000). Although this might have been a criterion to be in the study, the authors do not directly tell us that. In any case, J.K. does have a history of fecal incontinence, and the RN will have to decide if that makes J.K. different enough from the study sample to make its results inapplicable to J.K.'s care.

The third clinical vignette concerns an RN who works in the ER and has taken care of C.R., a homeless woman who has used the ER for care of several episodes of sexually transmitted disease and is now concerned that she may be pregnant. The RN is interested in developing and teaching an HIV-prevention and pregnancy-prevention program to homeless women such as C.R. who use the local women's shelter. She has found two articles that she hopes will help her to plan this program. The qualitative article about homeless patients' satisfaction with care tells the RN that 17 homeless individuals were interviewed for the study, of whom only 3 were women. The homeless individuals came from several settings, but none of them is identified as a shelter housing exclusively for women, such as the one to which the RN wants to apply the results of the study. The RN must decide if homeless women and men are likely to have different experiences and, therefore, if the ideas about satisfaction and the meaning of homelessness that are presented in this article are likely to reflect the experiences of women who are homeless. The RN does note that the authors work in a clinic for the homeless, which supports their ability to implement this type of research, because they are familiar with the contextual factors relevant to homelessness. The authors also indicate that data collection continued until data saturation was achieved (McCabe, Macnee, & Anderson, 2001). This tells the RN that the data from the three women who were included in the study did not differ a great deal from that of the men or else more interviews with women would have been required to achieve data saturation. Overall, the RN decides that she can use the findings of this study to increase her understanding of the experience of being homeless and receiving health care, but she will continue to look for studies about experiences that may be unique to homeless women.

The second study found by this RN was quantitative and used a convenience sample of homeless women and their intimate partners. The large sample size of this study gives the RN some confidence that systematic bias will be decreased. However, only 35 shelters are represented and used in the random assignment to the different types of programs tested. Knowing that different shelters house different types of women and seeing that the women ended up differing in age and education level does raise some concern about bias. The criteria for eligibility are clearly spelled out in this report, and although the age and homeless status are obvious matches with C.R., the requirement of having an intimate partner willing to participate in a study may not fit C.R. or other women in the local shelter (Nyamathi, Faskerud, Leake, Dixon, & Lu, 2001). Again, the question becomes how much the RN believes that this requirement changes or colors the results of the study, potentially making it less useful for the RN's purposes. The RN in this vignette suspends judgment about the usefulness of this study in helping her to develop a program for the homeless women until she has a better understanding of what information was collected and what was actually included in each of the programs tested.

The last clinical vignette involved an RN in a health department who was trying to find research to help him work with the Hernandez family and to plan future TB-screening programs for the Latino population in his community. The qualitative article he found about family survival used a sample of 23 Mexican American families. The ages of the parents in these families and the composition of the families are reported and fit well with the Hernandez family. However, as indicated, the author does not tell us how recently these families came to the United States, and that may make an important difference regarding to whom the results of this study can be applied. Because data in this study were collected for 3 years, the RN knows that the families have been in the United States for that long by the end of the study (Niska, 2001). The RN decides that he must consider the methods used in this study more closely before deciding about its usefulness for him.

The second article found by this RN also uses a convenience sample, this time of 206 Mexican migrant farm workers from 20 different migrant camps. The number of subjects and that they came from several migrant camps increase the RN's confidence that the sample is relatively representative of Mexican migrant farm workers. That the farm workers are predominantly young and men does not surprise the RN, because this is what he has found to be the case in his area (Poss, 2000). The biggest concern that the RN has about the sample is that it can mainly be applied to migrant workers and not as much to the Latino population that has settled in his area. Again, the RN decides that he must understand better the variables in this study before he can decide how much he might use the results of the study.

Overall, then, the RNs in our vignettes have not so much changed their minds as acquired a better sense of how useful these research studies will be for their practice. Understanding the language of sampling and the meaning of the sampling strategies helped make it clearer what the relationship was between the sample and the results and conclusions of the study. This chapter focused entirely on the language and process of sampling in quantitative and qualitative research. What we have not discussed is what can go wrong in this process that can make a sample not fit with the target population. Nor have we discussed the important subject of the rights of individuals who participate in research. These two topics interrelate and are discussed in the next chapter.

## OUT-OF-CLASS EXERCISE:

### Free Write

Before you move on to the next chapter, take a moment to think about the in-class questionnaire that you may have completed or about some past occasion when you were asked to participate in some type of research. Write a paragraph describing how the study or questionnaire was explained to you and what you were told about having or not having to fill it out. Then write your thoughts about whether your rights, safety, and privacy were protected. Finally, think about and write down any types of individuals on whom research should not be done or situations in which research should not be done. What makes you believe that these individuals or situations should or should not be included in research? Keep these paragraphs to refer to as you read Chapter 7.

## References

Bliss, D. Z., Johnson S., Savik, K., Clabots, C. R. & Gerding, D. N. (2000). Fecal incontinence in hospitalized patients who are acutely ill. *Nursing Research, 49*(2), 101–108.

Lipman, T. H., Hayman, L. L., Favian, C. V., DiFazio, D. A., Hale, P. M., Goldsmith, B.M., et al. (2000). Risk factors for cardiovascular disease in children with Type I Diabetes. *Nursing Research, 49*(3), 160–166.

McCabe, S., Macnee, C. L., & Anderson, M. K. (2001). Homeless patients' experience of satisfaction with care. *Archives of Psychiatric Nursing, 15*(2), 78–85.

Niska, K. J. (2001). Mexican American family survival, continuity, and growth: The parental perspective. *Nursing Science Quarterly, 14*(4), 322–329.

Nyamathi, A., Faskerud, J. H., Leake, B., Dixon, E. L., & Lu, A. (2001). Evaluating the impact of peer, nurse case-managed, and standard HIV risk-reduction programs on psychosocial and health-promoting behavioral outcomes among homeless women. *Research in Nursing & Health, 24*, 410–422.

Poss, J. E. (2000). Factors associated with participation by Mexican migrant farmworkers in a tuberculosis screening program. *Nursing Research, 49*(1), 20–28.

## Resources

LoBiondo-Wood, G., & Haber, J. (1998). *Nursing research: Methods, critical appraisal, and utilization* (4th ed.). St. Louis: Mosby.

Locke, L. F., Silverman, S. J., & Spirduso, W. W. (1998). *Reading and understanding research.* Thousand Oaks, CA: Sage Publications.

Pedhazur, E. J., & Schmelkin, L. P. (1991). *Measurement, design, and analysis: An integrated approach.* Hillsdale, NJ: Lawrence Erlbaum & Associates.

Polit, D. F., & Hungler, B. P. (1999). *Nursing research: Principles and methods* (6th ed.). Philadelphia: Lippincott.

**LEARNING OUTCOME:**

*THE STUDENT WILL* evaluate the sampling process considering legal and ethical principles and potential problems inherent in that process.

# Sampling Errors and Ethics—What Can Go Wrong?

INFORMED CONSENT
PROBLEMS WITH THE SAMPLING PROCESS
PROBLEMS WITH SAMPLING OUTCOMES
COMMON ERRORS IN THE REPORTS OF
   SAMPLING

PUBLISHED REPORTS—WHAT DO THEY SAY
   ABOUT CONSENT AND THE SAMPLING
   PROCESS?

**KEY TERMS**

Anonymous
Assent
Bias
Coercion
Confidentiality
Five human rights in research

Informed consent
Institutional review board (IRB)
Response rate
Risk:benefit ratio
Selectivity
Withdrawal

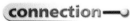

For additional activities go to
http://connection.lww.com/go/macnee.

## CLINICAL CASE

As the RNs in the four vignettes that we have discussed in earlier chapters consider what they can conclude about their clinical questions based on research studies, they have considered the sampling approaches used in those studies. In addition to knowing about the sampling approach taken, they also must understand the factors that affect who can and cannot be included in a sample and what types of problems can occur in even the best planned sampling approaches. As professional nurses, they also must be aware of the legal and ethical principles that guide the implementation of research studies in today's world, because they may be asked to participate directly in implementing research. To help us see the connections between legal and ethical principles and sampling, let's consider a modified version of the clinical vignette from Chapter 2.

Suppose that after the RN in Chapter 2 admits J.K. (the 68-year-old man with Parkinson's who is being admitted for pneumonia), she realizes that J.K. fits the criteria for a research study that is being implemented on her unit. The study describes fecal incontinence in acutely ill adults, replicating an earlier study but using a sample of patients who have a history of fecal incontinence. The researcher for the study has met with all the staff on the unit and oriented them to the study protocol, including the informed consent process that must be completed before any patient is enrolled in the study. The RN certainly wants to help with any research that will eventually serve patients, but she also wants to be sure that she does not cause J.K. any harm or introduce additional stress by asking him to decide whether to participate in a study if the study is not worthwhile. This chapter first discusses how the RN can determine that more good than harm should come from the study of fecal incontinence and that the study has a likelihood of contributing to our knowledge. The chapter then describes some of the problems that can arise when recruiting a sample for a study and how that can affect the usefulness of the study for clinical practice.

## INFORMED CONSENT

The RN in our vignette has been oriented to the study that is being carried out on her unit and realizes that a patient's consent to participate in a study is important. She decides to review the consent form so that she can plan how she will explain it to J.K. and his wife, if they have questions. As she reads through the consent form in preparation for discussing it with J.K., she realizes there are three distinct components to the consent form: (1) a description of the study, including what will be asked of the subject; (2) a description of any risks and/or benefits to participating in the study; and (3) a description of the patient's rights if he or she chooses to be in the study. Each of these sections of an informed consent relates to at least one of the **five human rights in research** that have been identified by the American Nurses Association (ANA) guidelines for nurses working with patient information that may require interpretation:

1. Right to self-determination
2. Right to privacy and dignity
3. Right to anonymity and confidentiality
4. Right to fair treatment
5. Right to protection from discomfort and harm (ANA, 1985)

Table 7–1 defines each of these rights, and we discuss each of them as they relate to the process of research.

**Informed consent** is the legal principle that an individual or his or her authorized representative only makes a decision about participation in a research study after being given all the relevant information needed to make that decision and being given a reasonable amount of time to consider that decision. The written consent form is a legal document indicating that the principle of informed consent has been adhered to. The informed consent document, along with a relatively detailed description of the study, is generated by a researcher before beginning a study and is reviewed and approved by an **institutional review board (IRB)**. An IRB is a board

| TABLE 7-1 | Definitions of the Five Rights of Human Subjects in Research (ANA, 1985) |
|---|---|
| **Right** | **Definition/Description** |
| Right to self-determination | Individuals are autonomous and have the right to make a knowledgeable, voluntary decision that is free from coercion as to whether or not to participate in research or to withdraw from a study. |
| Right to privacy and dignity | Individuals have the right to the respect of choosing what they do and what is done to them and to control when and how information about them is shared with others. |
| Right to anonymity and confidentiality | Individuals should be afforded the respect of having information they share or that is gathered about them kept in a manner that does not connect them to the individual information and the respect of choosing for themselves who knows that they are participating in a research study. |
| Right to fair treatment | Individuals have the right to nondiscriminatory selection of participants in a study, to nonjudgmental treatment that honors all agreements established in the consent, and to resources to address any concerns or problems that should arise during participation in the research. |
| Right to protection from discomfort or harm | Individuals have the right to be protected from exploitation and to be assured that every effort is made to minimize any potential harm from a study, while maximizing the potential benefits of the study. |

created for the explicit purpose of reviewing any proposed research study to be implemented within an institution or by employees of an institution. The individuals on an IRB always represent several backgrounds and interests, usually including members who are researchers, lay members from the community, and individuals, such as ministers, who have a special knowledge and interest in ethics. The variety of the member's backgrounds helps to ensure that a proposed research study is evaluated from numerous different perspectives.

The establishment of IRBs occurred in response to incidences of unethical and dishonest research practices in the past. Best known examples include the Nazi medical experiments during World War II and the Tuskegee "Study" that withheld treatment for syphilis from men from a poor black community in the South without their knowledge to study the progression of the disease. In addition, although the majority of researchers are honest and ethical, there have been occasions when researchers have falsified data or failed to report adverse events that have occurred during their research. IRBs have been instituted to guard against these types of unethical and dishonest practices.

The purpose of an IRB is to ensure that the research project includes procedures to protect the rights of its subjects. The IRB is also charged with deciding whether the research is basically sound to ensure potential participants' rights to protection from discomfort or harm. Any research study that asks anything of individuals is, at a minimum, using their time. A study that is not well planned or has a major flaw that will make the results meaningless wastes its participants' time and effort, so it is the IRB's responsibility to ensure that this is unlikely to happen.

Beyond assuring the basic soundness of a research study, the IRB must ensure that potential participants will be protected from harm or discomfort during their participation in the research project. They do this by reviewing the proposed research to identify any risks or potential risks that would occur if someone participated in the study. The IRB also reviews the potential benefits of the study and then looks at the relative balance between the actual and potential risks and the potential benefits. This evaluation of the risk:benefit ratio is integral to ensuring the right to protection from discomfort and harm. A **risk:benefit ratio** is a comparison of how much risk is present for subjects compared to how much benefit there is to the study.

Researchers are obligated to identify any potential risks to participation in their study and describe how they will try to prevent these risks, how they will monitor for their occurrence, and what they will do if they occur. If the researcher's plan is considered inadequate, the proposed research will not be approved. Some studies entail risks to life or health that simply are too great, no matter what the potential benefit is and despite efforts made to minimize them. In such a case, the risks are said to outweigh the benefits and the research is not approved for implementation.

## CORE CONCEPT

*It is unethical and illegal to implement a research study using animal or human subjects without institutional review board approval.*

> ## CORE CONCEPT
>
> *The goal of research with human subjects is always to minimize the risks and maximize the benefits.*

One of the risks to potential research participants that is considered so important that it is viewed as a separate right is the risk of a breach in anonymity, confidentiality, or both. A participant in research is **anonymous** when no one, including the researcher, can link the study data from a particular individual to that individual. **Confidentiality** is related to anonymity because, although the researcher knows the identity of the participant, it ensures that the identities of participants in the research will not be revealed to anyone else nor will the information that participants provide individually be publicly divulged. Because many nursing studies examine sensitive areas, such as abusive relationships or sexual function, merely being identified as a participant in a study can reveal personal and private information about an individual. A study that follows individuals over time cannot ensure anonymity until the study is complete, because the researcher must know who the participants are to stay in touch with them throughout the study. However, researchers can ensure that participation in the study and the responses of individuals in the study are kept confidential. Once a study is completed, all links between individuals and specific data can be destroyed; this ensures that future work with the research data will be anonymous. As with any of the potential risks in a study, a researcher must tell the IRB, in writing, how the confidentiality and anonymity of subjects in the study will be ensured.

The IRB members address the subject's right to fair treatment by reviewing the researcher's plan for recruiting subjects. A subject recruitment plan must give all the members of the population of interest an opportunity to participate in the study and may not target vulnerable groups simply because it is "easier" to get their participation. Vulnerable populations include such groups as prisoners, because they are available and may feel compelled to participate as a show of good behavior, or the homeless, who may be unduly influenced to participate because of such incentives as payment rather than from a true willingness to participate. Therefore, a study must include women and children, as well as men, if appropriate to the research question, and must include individuals with several economic and racial characteristics. A researcher must justify to the IRB the location for the study, the strategies used to recruit subjects into the study, and any criteria for participation in the study.

In Chapter 6 we discussed that the criteria for participation in a study define the population and are used to either purposely seek diversity or to limit and control for factors that may confound the study findings. In the fecal incontinence study, only adults were recruited. It is likely that the researcher presented an argument that the gastrointestinal (GI) systems and toileting habits of children and adults are different, so that including both children and adults in one study would provide confusing data. Similarly, the article about that study indicated that individuals with a diagnosis of dementia were excluded from the study. The researchers did not do this because of a lack of concern for those with dementia, rather because the presence of dementia could lead to incontinence, making it difficult to separate that factor from the variables under study. Whatever the criteria for inclusion in a study, they will be reviewed carefully by the IRB to ensure that they are fair.

Ensuring the right to self-determination and the right to privacy and dignity are also the IRB's responsibility. The rights to self-determination and to privacy and dignity are reflected in the informed consent document by providing a clear explanation of the study, what will be required of the individuals who participate, and the actual or potential risks and benefits of participation. The intent is that a potential research subject can make a knowledgeable decision based on the information provided in the consent form. In addition, respect for the potential subject is indicated through ensuring them the freedom to decide what they will or will not do or share. Self-determination is also included as a direct right within any study consent form in a statement that says that the subject has the right of **withdrawal** from the study at any time, without penalty, until the study is completed. Once a study is complete, all data become anonymous and it is no longer possible to withdraw information received from any specific individual. All research consent forms are expected to inform subjects that if they start a study and change their minds, that they retain the right to determine what will happen to them by withdrawing from the study.

Another aspect of self-determination is the right to decline participation in a study without consequences. A researcher must assure the IRB that individuals who decline to participate in research will not be punished. This is particularly relevant if the study is being conducted in a health care setting where it is possible that a patient might feel direct or indirect coercion to participate in a study. **Coercion** involves some element of controlling or forcing someone to do something. In the case of research, coercion would occur if a patient were forced to participate in a study to receive a particular test or service or to receive the best quality of care. Even if a patient is not forced to agree to participate in a study, if he or she believes that he or she will not get the best care possible unless agreeing to participate in a study, the participant is experiencing coercion. Therefore, any consent form for a study in which withholding or modifying treatment would be possible will include a clear statement that treatment and care will not be influenced by whether the individual participates in the study.

The right to privacy and dignity also is related to the right to anonymity and confidentiality. A researcher must inform a potential subject if participation in a study will involve invasive questions or procedures, again ensuring the potential subject the respect of being in charge of deciding what they will or will not share or be exposed to. However, in addition, the potential participant is assured that whatever he or she does share in the research will not be disclosed to others without his or her approval. This reflects the participant's right to privacy. Clearly, once data become anonymous, there is no longer a risk of breaching someone's privacy, but until that point, it is the responsibility of the researcher to ensure that right to privacy.

The last aspect of informed consent that reflects the right of the subject to self-determination is a statement about the rights of the participant to care if some *untoward* effect should occur from participating in the research and the provision of the specific names and telephone numbers of the researcher(s) and an IRB representative. These sections of an informed consent form give the potential participant access to both the researcher and an independent resource (the IRB representative) if he or she has questions or problems. Individuals who agree to participate in a study should be given a copy of the consent form so that they can contact the researcher or IRB representative as needed throughout the research and after it is completed.

Throughout this section, we have discussed the responsibilities of IRBs. IRBs are in place to guarantee an organization that any research carried out within that organization or by employees of that organization ensures and respects the rights of their subjects. Although IRBs have the responsibility for review, it is always the primary responsibility of the researcher both to plan for the protection of subjects and to ensure that this protection occurs. If a nurse researcher were to plan a research study in which no IRB review was provided, it would still be the ethical and legal responsibility of that researcher to ensure the protection of subjects.

Let's return to the RN in our vignette. Box 7–1 shows an informed consent form that might have been developed had a researcher chosen to perform a replication of the fecal incontinence study. As discussed in Chapter 2, a replication study essentially repeats an earlier study with a different sample to see if the same results are found. Having reviewed the informed consent form that she will be presenting to J.K., the RN recalls that for this study to have been approved by her institution's IRB, the board must have reviewed the basic soundness of the study in addition to its risk:benefit ratio. This provides her with some assurance that J.K.'s participation in the study would not be a waste of his time or effort. It also provides some assurance that the risks to J.K. of being in this study are probably reasonable, given the potential benefits from the study.

When reviewing the first section of the informed consent, the RN sees a description of the purpose of the study, duration of the study, and procedures that will affect J.K. The first thing the RN notes is that the consent clearly states under the purpose that participation in the study is voluntary and will not be connected to J.K.'s care in any way. She knows that this is an important point to convey to J.K. and his wife, so that J.K. does not feel coerced to participate in the study. She also notices that *fecal incontinence* has been defined as loss of bowel control and that the language of the consent form is generally not technical. Despite this, the RN realizes that she may need to explain to both J.K. and his wife what is meant by *examine your stools each time you have a bowel movement* and that some patients might not understand what is meant by *bowel movement*, so she will need to be prepared to use more common language if necessary. The RN also knows that the idea of rectal swabs will be unpleasant to most patients. She must find an approach to explaining the use of this procedure in the study that gives a fair and impartial explanation but also allays any unreasonable fears that J.K. or his wife may have.

---

# C ORE  C ONCEPT

*The five human rights in research are first and foremost the responsibility of the researcher(s).*

**Box 7-1   Fictional Informed Consent Form for Participation in a Study of Fecal Incontinence**

**Hospital XYZ**
**INFORMED CONSENT**

PRINCIPAL INVESTIGATOR: Jane J. Doe, RN, PhD

TITLE OF PROJECT: Replication study of factors predictive of fecal incontinence in acutely ill adults.

PURPOSE: The purpose of this study is to understand how often patients develop the inability to control their bowels, which we call fecal incontinence, and to examine the relationships among fecal incontinence and several factors that may lead to the development of loss of bowel control, including a history of fecal incontinence.

DURATION: Volunteering for this study will involve being monitored throughout your hospitalization, however long that may be. Participation in this study is entirely voluntary, and deciding not to participate will not affect your care now or in the future in any way.

PROCEDURES: Participation in the study means allowing the nursing staff to examine your stools each time you have a bowel movement and telling the staff if you have a bowel accident. If you are in this study, samples of your stools will be routinely tested for bacteria that can cause diarrhea and, possibly, loss of bowel control. These tests will be free to you. The tests will be done on your stools if possible, but there may be a need to do a rectal swab. A rectal swab involves the insertion of a cotton tipped applicator into your rectum for 2 to 3 seconds to get a sample of stool. In addition, participation in this study means that the researcher will collect some information from your chart about your diagnoses, medications, and test results.

POSSIBLE RISKS/DISCOMFORTS: Bowel function is a private aspect of each person's life, and, therefore, discussion of your bowel control and examination of your stools may be embarrassing to you. If it is necessary to take a rectal swab to get a stool specimen to check for bacteria that can cause diarrhea, there may be some slight discomfort during this procedure. There are no other known risks to participation in this study.

POSSIBLE BENEFITS: The possible benefit to participation in this study is free routine screening for a bacterial infection that may cause diarrhea and, possibly, loss of bowel control. The other possible benefit is the knowledge that you are contributing to a study that may help ill people like yourself in the future.

CONTACT FOR QUESTIONS: If you have any questions or problems, you may call Jane J. Doe at 423-965–0811 or Bob L. Smith at 423-965-0912. You may call the Chairman of the Institutional Review Board at 423-965–7777 for any questions you may have about your rights as a research subject.

CONFIDENTIALITY: Every attempt will be made to see that your study results are kept confidential. A copy of the records from this study will be stored in the Department of Acute Nursing, Room 100, at XYZ University for at least 10 years after the end of this reseat. The results of this study may be published and/or presented at meetings without naming you as a subject. Although your rights and privacy will be maintained, the Secretary of the Department of Health and Human Subjects, the XYZ University Institutional Review Board, the Food and Drug Administration, and the Department of Acute Nursing have access to the study records. Your records will be kept completely confidential according to current legal requirements.

COMPENSATION FOR MEDICAL TREATMENT: XYZ University will pay the cost of emergency first aid for any injury that may happen as a result of your being in this study. It will not pay for other medical treatment.

| **Box** **7-1** | **Fictional Informed Consent Form for Participation in a Study of Fecal Incontinence (Continued)** |

VOLUNTARY PARTICIPATION: The nature, risks, and benefits of the project have been explained to me as are known and available. I understand what my participation involves. Furthermore, I understand that I am free to ask questions and withdraw from the project at any time, without penalty. I have read and fully understand the consent form. I sign it freely and voluntarily. A signed copy has been given to me.

Your study record will be maintained in strictest confidence according to current legal requirements and will not be revealed unless required by law or as noted.

_____

SIGNATURE OF VOLUNTEER OR LEGAL REPRESENTATIVE & DATE

_____

SIGNATURE OF INVESTIGATOR & DATE

By considering these aspects of explaining the consent form, the RN is honoring the rights to self-determination, dignity, and protection from discomfort. Only by fully and correctly understanding the purpose and procedures of the study can J.K. make a knowledgeable decision, ensuring his self-determination. Ensuring that he fully understands the nature of the procedure that may be performed and the reasons for that procedure protects his rights to dignity and protection from discomfort.

When the RN reviews the sections describing the possible risks/discomforts and benefits, she finds that these are clearly stated and include an explicit acknowledgment that bowel function is a private aspect of an individual's life and body. The consent form neither exaggerates nor minimizes the risks and benefits of this study for J.K. The next two sections of the consent form directly address J.K.'s rights by providing him with the names and telephone numbers of the researchers and of an independent source of information, the chairman of the IRB. The consent form also tells J.K. that his records will be kept confidential and exactly where and for how long they will be kept.

Finally, the consent form tells J.K. that he has a right to compensation for any emergency care that he might need due to participating in the study. This statement may cause alarm in either J.K. or his wife, because nothing in the form has suggested that there could be a need for emergency care. The RN knows that she must explain that this is a legally required statement that probably has limited applicability for this particular study. However, the RN also should acknowledge that there is an unlikely chance that a rectal swab could injure an individual's rectum, perhaps causing the need for some type of emergency care.

The last paragraph of the consent form confirms that J.K. has read and understands the study and that he will always have the right to withdraw from the study, if he chooses to do so. The right to withdrawal without any consequences is as important as the right to decline to participate, and assures the patient the right to self-determination and fair treatment throughout participation in a study. Table 7–2 summarizes the links between the five human rights in research and the specific sections of the consent form that we have discussed. After a careful and thoughtful review of the consent form, the RN is prepared to approach J.K. and his wife professionally for their consent to participate in the study.

One last point must be understood about informed consent. So far, we have been discussing informed consent to participate in a study, meaning agreement based on a full understanding that assumes the ability to understand and make rational decisions. Occasionally, in research, the potential subject is not able to understand fully and make rational decisions regarding participation, as is often the case for children and persons with cognitive disorders or severe mental or physical illness. Under those circumstances, a researcher is obligated to seek consent from a designated legal representative of the potential subject, such as a parent, guardian, or other relative.

**TABLE 7-2**    **The Five Basic Rights and Relevant Components of the Informed Consent Form**

| Basic Right | Components of Informed Consent |
|---|---|
| Right to self-determination | Description of purpose of study<br>Description of procedures in study<br>Description of possible risks/discomforts<br>Description of possible benefits<br>Statement of right to withdraw from study<br>Statement of voluntary nature of participation without consequences if person chooses to not participate<br>Information about contacts for questions |
| Right to privacy and dignity | Description of possible risk/discomfort<br>Description of confidentiality |
| Right to anonymity and confidentiality | Description of confidentiality |
| Right to fair treatment | Description of purpose of study<br>Description of procedures in study<br>Description of any compensation for medical treatment |
| Right to protection from discomfort and harm | Description of procedures<br>Description of potential risks/discomforts<br>Description of potential benefits |

However, the subject may have a level of function that allows the researcher to seek his or her assent. To **assent** means to agree or concur and, in the case of research, reflects a lower level of understanding about the meaning of participation in a study than consent. Assent is often sought in studies that involve older children or individuals who have a level of impairment that limits their ability but does not preclude their understanding some aspects of the study. Suppose that J.K. were so ill that he could neither read the consent form nor discuss it in any detail with the RN. Because J.K.'s wife is legally designated as his representative if he becomes unable to participate in decisions about his own care, the RN would explain the study and review the consent form with J.K.'s wife. Her signature would be needed to include J.K. in the study. However, both the RN and J.K.'s wife could seek J.K.'s assent to be in the study by asking him briefly if he would mind helping in a study that looks at bowel control and involves the nurses closely monitoring his bowel movements. If J.K. agrees, we would consider that J.K. has assented to participate in the study: he has agreed without completely understanding all the aspects of the study, and it will be his wife who will make the knowledgeable decision, assuring J.K.'s full rights.

## PROBLEMS WITH THE SAMPLING PROCESS

As we discussed the consent form that might have been used in a replication of the fecal incontinence study, it may have crossed your mind that many patients could be put off or intimidated by the details in the consent form and simply decide that the easiest decision is to decline to participate in the study. This reluctance is a reality of research with human subjects and reflects a tension between the goal of ensuring the rights of individuals who participate in research and the goal of implementing research that uses a sample that is representative of the population at large. Researchers know that the process of seeking informed consent can **bias** a sample because of some systematic characteristic that causes certain individuals to decline to be in a study. Studies of who generally agrees to participate in research studies show that those who are more educated are more likely to participate than those who are less educated. Thus, in research, such as the fecal incontinence study, the sample may have more highly educated patients than those with less education, simply because the consent process is intimidating or because research is not viewed as valuable by those with less education. Clearly, the obligation to ensure that the basic human rights of potential subjects are protected supersedes the concern that consent processes may limit study enrollment, but researchers must consider this factor as they examine the results of their studies.

An associated problem that can occur in sampling is the withdrawal of subjects part way through a study. Individuals who agree to be in a study may withdraw from it for any number of reasons, such as personal problems or a lack of time or even physically moving out of an area. A researcher will usually plan for subject withdrawal by attempting to include more subjects in a research study than are actually needed. However, if there is some consistent reason why subjects withdraw, then the ability to generalize results of the study is limited. For example, if subjects in the fecal incontinence study who developed nausea and vomiting decided consistently that they no longer wanted to be in the study (perhaps because the rectal swabs and stool counts became more bothersome, given the additional symptoms of nausea and vomiting), then the final sample in the study would not reflect the general population of acutely ill patients. It would have failed to represent adequately patients who have problems associated with nausea and vomiting.

Withdrawal from a study is an active statement of a decision to no longer participate in that study. In some studies, however, subjects do not formally withdraw but simply drop out without notification or are lost to follow-up. In this case, the subject simply cannot be found to complete a study or does not return study materials. For example, in studies of smoking cessation, there is always a concern that the subjects who do not succeed in quitting may drop out of the study due to discouragement. This can lead to the final sample for the study including a higher proportion of successful quitters than is really the case, biasing the results by yielding an artificially inflated success rate.

Whether a potential subject declined to be in a study or a subject withdrew or was lost to follow-up in a study, it is important to know as much as possible about what happened during the sampling process to make intelligent decisions about the use of the results in clinical practice. Therefore, as an intelligent user of research, you should expect that the sampling section of a research report will tell you enough about the process of acquiring the sample that you could judge how that process affected the results. Often, that information includes a statement about the number of potential subjects who declined to be in a study, withdrew, or dropped out. When subjects withdraw or drop out of a study, usually some information is given about them. Therefore, researchers can use this information to compare the subjects who stayed in the study to those who did not and may be able to tell us whether there is some important difference between those who did and did not stay in a study. Usually, this is not possible to do with potential subjects who decline to be in a study, because there will be almost no information available about them.

In addition to concern about who agrees to be in a study and stays in a study, another problem that can affect the sampling process is the exclusion and inclusion criteria. As discussed in Chapter 6, sample criteria define the population for the study. Criteria for exclusion or inclusion are opposite sides of the same thing: a criterion for exclusion is a characteristic that makes the potential subject ineligible for the study, and a criterion for inclusion is a characteristic that makes the subject eligible for the study. Researchers choose to focus on inclusion or exclusion depending on the nature of the sample being sought. In a convenience sample in which numerous subjects are being sought, a researcher will generally discuss exclusion, because most individuals will be eligible to be in the study and only a few will be excluded. A study that aims for a tightly controlled sample will more likely describe criteria for inclusion, because the focus is on who can get into the study.

In either case, these criteria define the population for the study and may limit how you can use the results of a study in practice. For example, for an RN working in a long-term care facility on an Alzheimer's unit, the problem of fecal incontinence would certainly be relevant to practice. However, the study on fecal incontinence excluded subjects who were diagnosed with dementia, thus excluding the population of interest in this RN's situation. To use the results of the fecal incontinence article in practice, an RN on an Alzheimer's unit would need to decide if results with subjects who do not have dementia are meaningful for those with dementia. Because the incontinence article focused on variables that reflect physical factors that may affect incontinence, it is possible that this study will still be useful to someone working with patients who have dementia. Dementia would clearly add a complicating factor to problems with fecal incontinence, but the physiologic variables that affect occurrence of fecal incontinence would be the same for those with and without dementia. However, in some cases in which there is in an attempt to control for external factors that could bias a study, the sample excludes so many types of patients that the results may not be useful to many nurses' practices.

The last problem with the sampling process that we discuss in this chapter is incomplete data. This problem is a problem of data collection, but it is closely linked to how a sample may be changed or limited, affecting how useful it is for clinical practice. Incomplete data refer to partial information about the variables in a study. Although the specific problems that can lead to incomplete data are addressed in Chapter 8, the effect of incomplete data often is that the researcher drops data about selected subjects from the analysis of the results. This raises the question of whether those subjects with incomplete data had some characteristic or characteristics that led to their incomplete data. If so, then a systematic bias will be introduced into the final sample.

Suppose, for example, that some subjects in a smoking cessation study only completed part of a questionnaire used by the researcher and did not answer questions about how much they were smoking after they completed a smoking-cessation program. If the researcher drops these subjects from the analysis (because amount of smoking after the program is a major variable in the study and there are no data available for these subjects), then it is likely that the sample is biased in the direction of subjects who were successful and, therefore, willing to report their smoking status. We do not know why the data were incomplete, but we must be concerned that the reason is connected to the variables under study.

In summary, several aspects of the sampling process can lead to problems with the final study sample. The criteria used to identify who will be included or excluded from a study may narrow the sample to the point that the population represented no longer reflects the characteristics of real patient populations. Subjects in a study may withdraw or fail to follow up for some consistent reason that is related to the purposes of the study itself, limiting what we can learn from the study. Incomplete information may be collected because of some factor that relates to the study, causing some data about subjects to be dropped from the data analysis and changing the actual sample for the study. As intelligent readers and users of research, nurses must understand not only the strengths and weaknesses of different sampling strategies discussed in Chapter 6, but also what can go wrong with the sampling process and how that affects the meaning of the study. Table 7–3 summarizes the problems discussed. Other factors that can lead to problems with samples are discussed in the next section.

| TABLE 7-3 | Potential Problems With the Process of Sampling |

| Problem | Example |
| --- | --- |
| Subject withdrawal from study | After starting in a study, subjects decide they do not want to continue to participate. If some aspect *related to the study* leads to withdrawal, it can bias the sample. |
| Lost to follow-up | After agreeing to be in a study, subjects become unavailable to be in it. This may include not returning questionnaires, missing appointments, moving, or having a change in telephone number. If the subjects lost to follow-up represent a particular characteristic related to the study (perhaps high-income), then the final sample may have a bias. |
| Exclusion/inclusion criteria limit applicability of the sample | If a sample is tightly controlled or restricted to make the research successful, it may lead to the population being so specific that clinical meaningfulness is limited. |
| Incomplete data | Data are not provided, are skipped, or are missed, causing the researcher to drop the subject from the analysis of the results. If there is some systematic reason for the data being incomplete, dropping the subjects can bias the results. |

## PROBLEMS WITH SAMPLING OUTCOMES

In addition to problems with the sampling process, some problems can occur with the sampling outcomes—that is, the final sample itself—that are only indirectly related to the sampling strategy and to the problems that can occur in the sampling process. Previously, we discussed the importance of avoiding bias, an unintended factor that confounds the findings of a study, in a sample. As discussed in Chapter 6, some sampling strategies, such as nonprobability sampling, are more open to a bias, whereas others, such as probability sampling, are less open to it. When a researcher uses a nonprobability sampling strategy, the process may be implemented correctly, but the resulting sample may still be biased.

One type of bias that can be introduced in a nonprobability sample occurs when a researcher fails to recognize or consider some factor about himself of herself or his or her approach that could influence participation in the study. For example, a researcher may be more comfortable approaching either men or women when trying to recruit subjects, thus unconsciously biasing a study in the direction of one gender. Or, a researcher may collect data only at a certain time of the day, such as Monday through Friday between 8 am and 5 pm, preventing anyone who works 12-hour shifts or night shifts from being in the study. If type of work and hours worked is related in some way to what is under study, then a bias has been introduced.

Another kind of bias in the sample may occur as a result of the unique characteristics or perspectives of the person who is actually recruiting subjects. We alluded to this at the start of this chapter when we acknowledged that the RN in our vignette wanted to be sure that she was not causing J.K. any unneeded discomfort. Because the RN's main role is to provide care for J.K., she may not be particularly motivated to provide him with information about the potential to participate in a study, or she may conclude on her own that he does not need to be bothered with a study. An example of a recruiter inadvertently introducing bias into a sample might be a study that is conducted in a clinic that cares for both physical and mental health problems. If the person recruiting subjects primarily works with the mental health patients and recruits familiar patients, then the subjects in the study are more likely to have mental illness than the overall population of the clinic.

A second problem that can occur with samples is selectivity. **Selectivity** is the tendency of certain population segments to agree to participate in studies. In this case, the bias is not introduced by the researcher but by those people who are willing and interested in being in a study. We have already discussed one kind of general selectivity that occurs in all research: the tendency of more educated individuals to agree to participate compared with less educated individuals. However, selectivity can occur that is more specific to the purposes of a particular study. A particular study may attract people who are worried about the problem under study or people who are lonely and want someone with whom they can talk. It may be that mostly women are willing to participate in a particular study or, perhaps, only people with family members who have experienced a particular problem will return a mailed questionnaire. The difficulty for the researcher and for the user of research is to determine whether some aspect of the study may have led to selectivity in the sample and how this, in turn, affects the knowledge gained from the study.

Limited response rates can be another problem with samples. **Response rate** is the proportion of individuals who participate in a study divided by the number who agreed to be in a study but did not participate in it. Response rate is not a significant problem when the study occurs in a controlled setting, such as a hospital, because those who agree to be in a study are essentially a captive group. However, in almost any research survey in which subjects are recruited and asked to return a questionnaire or provide data by appointment, some individuals do not return the questionnaire or keep the appointment. As with the other problems that affect samples, the question regarding response rate is who are the people who did not respond and why did they not respond. If they did not respond due to a factor that is related in some way to the study, this could bias the sample. In the types of research in which subjects may fail to respond, the research report should tell you the response rate so that you have an idea of whether a large or small number of possible subjects did not participate in the study. Withdrawal and dropping out of a study are two reasons why response rates can be low.

All of the problems in samples we have discussed occur in recruiting subjects for any type of study, but they will cause more problems in nonprobability samples than in probability samples. Although the potential bias of a low response rate can affect a random sample, the effects of selectivity and researcher bias are mostly offset in a random sample, because the entire population is enumerated and all members of the population have a chance of being included in the study. Therefore, it is common to find more detail describing the sampling process and the final sample when nonprobability sampling was used, because the researcher wants to ensure the reader that steps were taken to prevent the potential biases that may be present in the final sample.

In summary, three factors are related to both sampling strategy and the sampling process that can lead to problems in samples. The first is bias introduced by the researcher or the individual recruiting the sample that reflects the beliefs or characteristics of that researcher or recruiter. The second is self-selection by individuals within the population that can lead to a bias. The third is a limited response rate that makes us wonder what were the characteristics of those who did not respond and how they differ from those who did. Table 7–4 summarizes these three types of problems with samples.

**TABLE 7-4**    **General Potential Problems With Samples**

| Problem | Example |
| --- | --- |
| Bias in subject recruitment | Some aspect of the recruitment process allows an unidentified factor to enter into the identification of subjects requested to participate in the study. Examples include time of day of sampling or recruiter comfort level with selected subjects. |
| Selectivity | Certain subjects volunteer to be in the study due to some characteristic that could relate to the problem being studied. Examples include subjects who are older and lonely being more available or subjects who care about a particular problem volunteering. This can lead to over-representation of one segment of the population in the sample. |
| Response rate | Many potential subjects or actual subjects do not participate in the study. If a study has a low response rate, then the ability to generalize the results of the study to the entire population of interest is limited. |

## COMMON ERRORS IN THE REPORTS OF SAMPLING

Both informed consent and the problems that can arise in samples can affect the answer the question "To what types of patients do these research conclusions apply—who was in the study?" The most common error found in a sampling report is the failure to tell us enough to let us judge the occurrence of potential problems. Almost every study report will include some descriptive information about the sample, and most will indicate the source of the subjects or the location of the study subjects. However, this information may not be adequate for evaluating the sampling process. The research report for the study of fecal incontinence, for example, does not mention whether some patients declined to participate in the study. Because the original study used matching of subjects and was making conclusions based on comparing those two groups, the effect of refusing to participate was not likely to be too great. Yet, once the two matched groups were combined into one sample, that some individuals potentially refused to participate may create a bias in the sample, because we do not know if those individuals had unique characteristics that could have affected the study results. The authors of the study do, however, provide a clear explanation for why 32 subjects were excluded from the study analysis that is helpful to us in evaluating the sample.

Another example of a study in which additional information about the process of sampling would have been useful is the TB-screening study (Poss, 2000). The author tells us that the 206 participants were "chosen" from 20 migrant camps and lists an important criterion for exclusion: a history of a positive PPD skin test or active TB. The author also includes some important information that assures us that the rights of these research subjects were ensured by using a verbal consent in Spanish that was approved by the researcher's university IRB. However, we do not know what "chosen" meant and must be concerned that the researcher may have introduced some type of a bias, because she was the only one selecting whom to approach about participating in the study. We also are not told how many, if any, potential subjects refused to be in the study.

The information that is missing from this report that is probably most important is whether the subjects who did get a PPD skin test differed from those who did not in their demographic characteristics. This is not a question of who is in the sample but rather of how those in the sample differed in characteristics that may have influenced the results of the study. Approximately one fourth of the subjects did not get a PPD, and, although factors that were included in the study, such as attitudes, certainly explain some of that difference, the author never tells us whether she considered age, marital status, gender, or education level as factors affecting whether the subject had a PPD skin test (Poss, 2000). In this case, thinking about the sample has led us back to the results sections and identified an issue that has not been addressed in the research report.

QUALITATIVE

In this chapter, we have focused primarily on the problems with sampling that occur in quantitative research, because many of the problems that can occur relate to bias and the ability to generalize to a population, which is not a goal in qualitative research. However, withdrawal from a study, subjects declining to participate in a study, or subjects being lost to follow-up can all affect the meaning of results of a qualitative study as well.

For example, the authors of the article on homeless patients' satisfaction with health care do not state whether they experienced any difficulty in convincing homeless individuals to agree to be interviewed. If many of the homeless in the different locations that were used to get a sample were unwilling to have a tape-recorded interview about their experiences, it might suggest that an underlying concern about privacy or safety was part of the context for this study. Because knowledge from a qualitative study comes from a full exploration of the experience or perspective of the participant, hesitancy or many refusals to participate would be meaningful information and, therefore, data for the study. The absence of any information about refusal suggests that it was not an issue and did not comprise a part of the data collected.

Similarly, refusal or drop-out rates in an ethnographic study are important to consider. The author of the ethnographic study of Mexican American family survival depended on being able to meet with the same families over time for her data collection. She states that one of the families was lost to follow-up and that two were excluded from the analysis she is reporting because they were working outside the region when data were collected. This information allows us to understand that the results of the study reflect data from the majority of the families who started in the study, which, in turn, suggests that the researcher had a good connection with these families that facilitated an ongoing relationship. Because qualitative research depends on the openness and trust of those providing the data, the evidence for an ongoing relationship helps assure us of the quality of the data collected.

## PUBLISHED REPORTS—WHAT DO THEY SAY ABOUT CONSENT AND THE SAMPLING PROCESS?

As we look at the research studies that the RNs in our four vignettes found, it is important to realize that in sampling, the clinical nurse often is the expert. We have discussed the meaning of several different terms used in research to describe sampling strategies and actual samples, and these are important for understanding the conclusions of a research study. What we have not discussed is that often it is the practicing nurse who most readily recognizes the limits to a sampling process, because those in practice understand their patients' needs and characteristics. If the nurse researcher is not directly involved in patient care with the population of interest, he or she may not realize that a certain segment of the population is not represented in the sample. Therefore, once the RNs in our vignettes understand the sampling language and process, they are likely to be the best judges of whether a study sample reflects real patient populations.

Looking at the research reports used by the nurses in the four vignettes, we can now fully evaluate the sampling process used in these studies. In the sample of the study of risk factors for cardiovascular disease in children with IDDM, the authors specifically state that 149 patients were asked to participate in the study and that 140 consented. Both criteria for inclusion (age) and exclusion (ketosis, renal disease, etc.) also are specified. We have already mentioned that this sample is limited by being a convenience sample that was recruited exclusively from one tertiary center. Looking at the response rate of 140 out of 149, we can believe that even if there was a systematic reason for declining to be in the study, at least only a few members of the population were not represented for that reason. What we do not learn is how many potential patients would have qualified for this study. If the endocrinology section cares for only approximately 150 to 160 children, then almost every potential subject was approached to be in the study, but, if it cares for 2000 children, then it would help us to know how the 149 who were approached were chosen. This information would help us to evaluate whether some type of researcher bias might have occurred in the sample. The research report clearly assures us that the study had IRB approval and that, although parents provided consent for all children, older children provided assent. Overall, the sampling strategy and process for this article is described clearly, but it does leave the RN with a question or two (Lipman et al., 2000).

The report of the study of fecal incontinence found by the RN in our vignette does not directly mention informed consent, probably because there was nothing exceptional about this sample. It is expected and assumed that any research study will have been reviewed and approved by an IRB and that informed consent will have been acquired before enrolling subjects in a study. If the subjects do not represent a particularly vulnerable group, such as children or prisoners, then a report may not specify review by an IRB. In general, we have decided that this study's sample is reasonably representative of the population of men who would be acutely ill and at risk for fecal incontinence (Bliss, Johnson, Savik, Clabots, & Gerding, 2000).

Two articles about homelessness were found by the RN working in the emergency room. The quantitative study that compared HIV programs had a large sample and describes the sampling process in detail. Because this study tested the usefulness of different interventions and has the goal of generalizing the results, it is important that the authors give us adequate information to evaluate how the sample relates to the results and conclusions. As mentioned in Chapter 6, the study used random assignment of shelters to the intervention programs, a strategy that helped to decrease the risk of bias in the study. We also identified that the inclusion criterion of having an intimate partner somewhat limits the population to which this study applies. The report tells us that informed consent was sought for this vulnerable population and that subjects were offered an incentive to participate in the research. Although it is not stated explicitly, we can conclude that the small payment to subjects may have helped the researchers acquire a more diverse sample (Nyamathi, Flaskerud, Leake, Dixon, & Lu, 2001).

The satisfaction with care study does not provide as much detail about the sampling process, but it does provide more detail about the settings from which the sample was recruited. This is in keeping with an emphasis on a naturalistic process of data collection within qualitative research, where the context or environment is much a part of the overall data for the study. Although this report does not mention informed consent, it is assumed that is was obtained. We have already discussed that comprehensiveness rather than generalizability is the goal of this study, and the description of the sample suggests that diverse and, therefore, rich sources of data were used. We might have liked to have known, however, whether the researchers had difficulty recruiting any particular group of subjects, because that information would add to our understanding of the homeless individuals' experiences (McCabe, Macnee, & Anderson, 2001). For example, if women were more hesitant about being interviewed than men, it would suggest that there is something different about the experience of homelessness and seeking health care for women compared to men.

In this chapter, we already have discussed the two research reports that the RN from the health department found. The qualitative study of Mexican American family survival does not make any statements about informed consent. As with the homeless patient satisfaction study, the goal here was not so much to generalize as it was to generate theory. The author does provide some information about the context in which the data were collected and about the three families that were dropped from the data analysis for this report. We do not know if a particular type of family might have declined to participate in the study, and this slightly limits our understanding of the meaning of the results (Niska, 2001).

We have identified that the TB-screening article does include a statement about IRB approval to use a verbal consent approach. Because studies usually use a written consent form, the use of a verbal consent is noteworthy. This information also helps us know that subjects were not excluded from the study either because they could not read or by self-selection because they were intimidated by the consent form. The lack of information about the process of selecting subjects is something we have already mentioned as a limit to our ability to judge whether a bias may have occurred in the sampling process (Poss, 2000). Overall, however, the description of the sample fits the types of patients with whom the RN has worked, giving him some assurance that the sampling process yielded an appropriate sample.

The RNs in all four vignettes now have a much greater understanding about to which types of patients these studies can be applied. Legal and ethical principles have been considered and applied appropriately in all of the studies, and all of the samples have strengths, as well as some limitations. The next challenge for the RNs in these vignettes is to reach a better understanding of why and how data were collected from the individuals in these samples. Just as the sample affects the meaningfulness of a study for practice, the measures used and approach taken to getting data for the study can affect the knowledge gained from the study. For example, the RN in the health department is still unsure about the meaning of variables such as *susceptibility* or *normative beliefs* and wonders how information about such subjective beliefs was collected. The RN who works in the emergency department wonders about the specific components of the different programs tested in the HIV program evaluation study and how the researchers collected information about personal factors, such as sexual behaviors, in a way that produced honest answers. To answer questions such as these, the RNs must read the section of the report that describes the data collection procedures, which is discussed in the next chapter.

## OUT-OF-CLASS EXERCISE:

### What Goes Into a Questionnaire?

Before proceeding to Chapter 8, look at the in-class questionnaire that you completed at the beginning of your course. If you did not have an in-class study, look at the questionnaire included in Appendix D. As you read the questionnaire, write down your impressions regarding the following questions.

1.  As you look at each question, what do you think was the variable on interest?
2.  Do some of the questions fit together to measure just one variable? What variable? Do you think the questions are all logically connected?

3. What about the questionnaire makes it easy to read and answer?
4. What about the questionnaire makes it confusing? Are any particular questions more confusing than others? Why?
5. Do any aspects of the organization of the questionnaire or the wording of questions make it difficult for some people to answer the questionnaire?

After you have written your answers to these questions, to which there are no correct or wrong answers, then you are ready to read Chapter 8.

## References

American Nurses Association (ANA). (1985). *Code for nurses with interpretive statement.* Kansas City, MO: ANA.

Bliss, D. Z., Johnson S., Savik, K., Clabots, C. R., & Gerding, D. N. (2000). Fecal incontinence in hospitalized patients who are acutely ill. *Nursing Research, 49*(2), 101–108.

Lipman, T. H., Hayman, L. L., Favian, C. V., DiFazio, D. A., Hale, P. M., & Goldsmith, B. M., et al. (2000). Risk factors for cardiovascular disease in children with Type I Diabetes. *Nursing Research, 49*(3), 160–166.

McCabe, S., Macnee, C. L., & Anderson, M. K. (2001). Homeless patients' experience of satisfaction with care. *Archives of Psychiatric Nursing, 15*(2), 78–85.

Niska, K. J. (2001). Mexican American family survival, continuity, and growth: The parental perspective. *Nursing Science Quarterly, 14*(4), 322–329.

Nyamathi, A., Flaskerud, J. H., Leake, B., Dixon, E. L., & Lu, A. (2001). Evaluating the impact of peer, nurse case-managed, and standard HIV risk-reduction programs on psychosocial and health-promoting behavioral outcomes among homeless women. *Research in Nursing & Health, 24,* 410–422.

Poss, J. E. (2000). Factors associated with participation by Mexican migrant farmworkers in a tuberculosis screening program. *Nursing Research, 49*(1), 20–28.

## Resources

LoBiondo-Wood, G., & Haber, J. (1998). In *Nursing research: Methods, critical appraisal, and utilization* (4th ed.). St. Louis: Mosby.

Locke, L. F., Silverman, S. J., & Spirduso, W. W. (1998). *Reading and understanding research.* Thousand Oaks, CA: Sage Publications.

Polit, D. F., & Hungler, B. P. (1999). *Nursing research: Principles and methods* (6th ed.). Philadelphia: Lippincott.

**LEARNING OUTCOME:**

*THE STUDENT WILL* relate the data collection methods of a study to the meaning of the results and conclusions of a study.

CHAPTER

**8**

# Data Collection Methods

*How Were Those People Studied—*
*Why Was the Study Done That Way?*

**KEY TERMS**

Audit trail
Confirmability
Construct validity
Content validity
Credibility
Criterion-related validity
Error
Field notes
Group interviews

Instrument
Internal consistency reliability
Interrater reliability
Items
Likert-type response scale
Member checks
Operational definition
Participant observation
Questionnaire

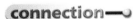

For additional activities go to
http://connection.lww.com/go/macnee.

Reliability
Rigor
Scale
Test-retest reliability
Theoretical definition
Transferability

Triangulation
Trustworthiness
Unstructured interviews
Validity
Visual analog

## CLINICAL CASE

S.G. is an 18-month-old boy who was born at 32 weeks of gestation with a severe spinal bifida that has led to irreversible deficits in both his neuromotor and sensory function. He was admitted yesterday to the pediatric intensive care unit (ICU) in acute respiratory failure secondary to aspiration pneumonia. S.G. has been intubated and is on a respirator, is receiving antibiotics intravenously, and is scheduled to have a percutaneous endoscopic gastrotomy (PEG) tube reinserted tomorrow. This is his twelfth admission since birth, and he and his parents have become well known to the staff on the unit. The admitting RN noted that S.G.'s parents were anxious and had difficulty allowing the nursing staff to provide care to S.G., asking many questions and attempting to "help" with all procedures. This surprised the RN, because the parents have experience with all the equipment and procedures that are currently being used with S.G. The RN knows that S.G.'s prognosis is uncertain

and wonders what she can do to assist his parents during this difficult time. She also wonders if there is anything she can do to make life easier for these parents who face a strenuous uphill battle taking care of S.G. at home. When she gets home from work, the RN links to the university's medical library to search for research studies that might give her some insight and ideas for working with this fragile family. She finds two articles that she is able to download: "Trajectory of certain death at an unknown time: Children with neurodegenerative life-threatening illnesses" (Steele, 2000) and "Distress and growth outcomes in mothers of medically fragile infants" (Miles, Holditch-Davis, Burchinal, & Nelson, 1999). Both of these articles are available on the Connection Web site and in Appendix A. Before beginning this chapter, read the two articles so that the examples used throughout this chapter will be helpful to you.

## REVISITING STUDY VARIABLES

The unique language of research associated with data collection is extensive, as a quick glance at the Key Terms listed at the beginning of this chapter shows. The abstracts of the two articles the RN downloaded address questions about family adjustment and coping that may relate to S.G.'s parents. After reading the two articles, however, the RN finds that understanding how such complex aspects of family adjustment as "parental presence" were measured is essential to understand the results and conclusions of these two studies. The RN in our vignette is interested in the health and coping of S.G.'s parents, both for their sake and for the sake of S.G., because they are his primary caregivers. The RN also wants to prevent a problem between S.G.'s parents and the nursing staff that could occur if the parents continue to be perceived as interfering with S.G.'s nursing care. She knows that these parents have dealt with S.G.'s being so ill in the past, so she believes that the current problem is not a lack of understanding or unfamiliarity with the ICU, but rather what this most recent health crisis means to these parents. With a desire to work with S.G. and his parents in mind, the RN begins to read about the data collection in the two studies she has found.

To examine the measurement approaches taken, the RN first has to identify the variables in each study. We discussed variables in Chapters 4 and 5, defining them as some aspect of interest that differs in different groups or situations. Both qualitative and quantitative studies have variables, but only quantitative studies use the categories of independent and dependent variables. Independent variables are those factors in the study that are used to explain or predict the outcome of interest and also are sometimes called predictor variables, because they are used to predict the dependent variable. In the article the RN found about maternal distress, the authors write of predictor variables rather than independent variables. Dependent variables are the variables that depend on other variables in a study or are the outcome variables of interest. The maternal distress article refers to the dependent variables as outcome variables.

The variables studied in both articles on family adjustment to severely ill children are listed in Table 8–1. The article about trajectory of certain death describes a qualitative study that has three variables: (1) families' perceptions and experiences living with a child who has a neurodegenerative life-threatening illness (NLTI), (2) impact on family of living with a child with an NLTI, and (3) factors that influence family care of a child with an NLTI. The study reported in the maternal distress article addressed distress and growth as the two outcomes of interest and examined maternal attitudes, maternal role attainment, child-illness characteristics, and maternal illness-related distress as predictor variables.

**QUALITATIVE**

Before we continue, let's look at how we determine the variables in a study. Although it is logical that variables differ across groups or situations, many research reports will not explicitly identify the study variables. For example, the trajectory of certain death article never specifically lists the variables studied, as is done in Table 8–1. The variables for a study obviously should reflect the topic of interest, which, in turn, should be described in the purpose, background, and research questions for a study, sections of a research report discussed in depth in Chapter 10. Because a qualitative study usually begins with one or more broad questions and uses open-ended approaches to collecting data, the variables of interest often are identified within the research questions. The study variables are not mentioned in the data collection and analysis section of the trajectory of certain death article, only the methods used for that study. The RN in our vignette, therefore, had to read the previous section of the report that described the specific aims of the study to identify clearly the variables under study.

**QUANTITATIVE**

In contrast, reports of quantitative studies should clearly describe the variables included in the study, even if they are not explicitly labeled as such, because the data collection methods in quantitative research are specifically aimed at measuring the variables in the study as objectively as possible.

| TABLE 8-1 | Types and Definitions of Variables From Two Studies of Family Adjustment to a Critically Ill Child | | | |
|---|---|---|---|---|
| **Variable** | **Type** | **Theoretical Definition** | **Operational Definition** |

*Trajectory of certain death at an unknown time: Children with neurodegenerative life-threatening illnesses (NLTIs) (Steele, 2000)*

| Variable | Type | Theoretical Definition | Operational Definition |
|---|---|---|---|
| Experiences living with a child with an NLTI | Conceptual—neither independent nor dependent because approach is qualitative | Sought through the study | Not applicable |
| Impact on family of living with a child with an NLTI | Conceptual—neither independent nor dependent because approach is qualitative | Sought through the study | Not applicable |
| Factors that affect family ability to care for a child with an NLTI | Conceptual—neither independent nor dependent because approach is qualitative | Sought through the study | Not applicable |

*Distress and growth outcomes in mothers of medically fragile infants (Miles, Holditch-Davis, Burchinal & Nelson, 1999)*

| Variable | Type | Theoretical Definition | Operational Definition |
|---|---|---|---|
| Maternal distress | Outcome or dependent | Depressive symptoms | Center for Epidemiologic Studies Depression Scale (CES-D) |
| Maternal growth | Outcome or dependent | Positive or negative developmental impact | Single rating by researchers of developmental impact on a seven-point scale |
| Personal characteristics—three components | Predictor or independent | | |
| 1. Demographics | | 1. Educational level and marital status | 1. Self-report on demographic data sheet |
| 2. Personal control | | 2. Sense of control over problems, life, the future, and change | 2. Sense of Mastery Scale; seven items |
| 3. Satisfaction with family | | 3. Level of satisfaction with aspects of family life | 3. Family Apgar; five items |

**TABLE 8-1**  Types and Definitions of Variables From Two Studies of Family Adjustment to a Critically Ill Child (Continued)

| Variable | Type | Theoretical Definition | Operational Definition |
|---|---|---|---|
| Maternal role attainment—three components | Predictor or independent | Process by which a mother achieves an identity as a parent, establishes her presence with the child, and becomes competent in parental caregiving. | |
| 1. Maternal identity | | 1. The degree to which a mother reports feeling like she is a mother to her infant | 1. Maternal identify scale: critically ill infant |
| 2. Maternal presence | | 2. The amount of physical closeness with the infant | 2. Composite score including: (1) mothers' report of engaging in three types of activities and (2) amount of 4 mother–child inter-active behaviors |
| 3. Maternal competence | | 3. The quality and effectiveness of parenting | 3. Composite score including: (1) 4 interview rating items, (2) the amount of four mother–child interaction items, (3) six subscale scores from the Home Observation for Measurement of the Environment (HOME) |
| Infant illness characteristics—three components 1. Child's health | Predictor or independent | 1. Whether the child had a multisystem diagnosis | 1. Data from medical records collected and confirmed by up to four masters-prepared pediatric nurses |

| TABLE 8-1 | Types and Definitions of Variables From Two Studies of Family Adjustment to a Critically Ill Child (Continued) | | |
|---|---|---|---|
| **Variable** | **Type** | **Theoretical Definition** | **Operational Definition** |
| 2. Level of technology dependence | | 2. Number of technologies used by a child | 2. Number of up to 27 technology procedures being used |
| 3. Level of mental development | | 3. Aspects of infant cognitive abilities and visual/fine motor coordination | 3. Mental Development Index–Bayley II Scale |
| Maternal illness-related distress–two components | Predictor or independent | | |
| 1. Parental stress | | 1. Perceived hospital environmental stress | 1. Parental Stressor Scale: Infant Hospitalization (PSS); 22 items |
| 2. Child health worry | | 2. Distress related to worry about the child's health | 2. Child Health Worry Scale; five items |

The data collection section of a report of a quantitative study should describe how each variable was measured and, in so doing, identify each study variable. The RN in our vignette found both the outcome and the predictor variables specifically identified in the data collection methods section of the report of the study of maternal distress. Had they not been listed under specific subheadings within the article, however, she should still have been able to read the description of the measures used in the study and, thus, identify the study's variables.

Variables also can be identified and discussed in terms of their definitions rather than whether they are independent or dependent. Variables can be defined at two levels: the theoretical level and the operational level. A **theoretical definition** of a variable is one that is described and understood conceptually, not concretely. An **operational definition** of a variable is one that is defined in specific concrete terms of measurement. For example, the variable *stress* can be operationally defined as an individual's perceptions that an event is threatening and that he or she has no way

## CORE CONCEPT

*The measures in a quantitative study should reflect the specific variables under study.*

to manage the threat. This definition is conceptual, giving the reader a clearer idea of what is meant by the word *stress*, but it does not tell us how that variable might actually be measured. An operational definition of stress might be an individual's summed score regarding his or her ratings on a four-point scale of the perceived level of threat from 40 life events. This second definition is concrete and tells the reader exactly how the variable stress is measured.

Although some variables are concrete and may only be defined operationally, many variables of interest to nursing are relatively abstract and may need both a theoretical and an operational definition if they are going to be used in a quantitative study. The primary purpose of some qualitative studies is to develop a clear theoretical definition of a variable, so that it might eventually be operationally defined and concretely measured. For example, a theoretical variable in the trajectory of certain death study was family impact of living with a child who has an NLTI. However, because the purpose of that study was to increase our understanding of family impact, neither a theoretical nor an operational definition was offered. A concrete definition would presume that we already had a relatively clear understanding of family impact and could concretely measure it. Whereas, in fact, the researchers were trying to construct a theoretical definition of family impact that then could be translated into an operational definition.

If a researcher believed that we had a theoretical understanding of the variable of family impact, he or she might break down that variable into one or more concrete components that would then comprise an operational definition. For example, he or she might operationally define, or operationalize, family impact as the family's scores on a stress scale, a relationship satisfaction scale, and a measure of well-being. Alternately, a researcher might operationalize family impact as parental depression scores, economic status, and use of outside resources. Almost any variable can be operationalized, but the correctness and accuracy of that operationalization must be evaluated. If researchers do not have a clear understanding of the theoretical meaning of a concept, then they may be inconsistent in their measurement of that concept, leading to disagreement about what was actually measured and questions about the overall meaning of the study.

You can think of an operational definition, or the operationalization, of a variable as a form of translation: the researcher is translating an abstract theoretical idea into a concrete set of measures.

QUALITATIVE

The trajectory to certain death study report contains three variables: family experiences, impact on family, and factors that influence ability to care. All three variables need theoretical definitions. A study that is using a qualitative approach should examine variables and increase understanding of something that

## CORE CONCEPT

*Operationalizing variables is like translating a phrase from one language to another. The researcher is translating an abstract, theoretical variable into a concrete measure or set of measures.*

is abstract and unknown by asking for, or looking for, specific examples, experiences, or perceptions. However, because a qualitative study does not attempt to measure variables concretely, we do not expect to find operational definitions included in a report of the study methods.

**QUANTITATIVE**

In quantitative studies, variables often are discussed and defined at both the theoretical level and the operational level, because the goal in a quantitative study is to examine discrete factors as concretely as possible. The maternal distress study includes a variable called "maternal role attainment." Because this variable can have many conceptual meanings, the authors provide a theoretical definition: "process by which a mother or father achieves an identity as a parent, establishes their presence with the child, and becomes competent in parental care-giving" (Miles et al., 1999, p. 132). The authors then provide concrete operational definitions that describe how maternal role attainment was measured in their study.

Although all variables in a quantitative study should have an operational definition, not all variables in quantitative research will have a theoretical definition. Concrete variables, such as gender, weight, platelet count, or oxygen saturation, do not have or need a theoretical definition. There is a common understanding of the conceptual meaning of "gender," so it does not need a theoretical definition. But even concrete variables need an operational definition when they are being examined in research, because several approaches can be taken to measure them. For example, we can operationally define gender in at least three different ways: (1) the presence or absence of a Y chromosome, (2) a self-reported characteristic, or (3) an observed characteristic. In most cases, we will get the same result no matter which way we define and measure gender. However, some people perceive themselves to be the opposite gender from that indicated in their chromosomal composition, and some people are androgynous enough that a superficial observation might lead to incorrect categorization. Therefore, even a variable as concrete as gender must be operationally defined, so that we can understand exactly what was measured.

When a variable is not measured with 100% accuracy, we say there is error in the measurement. In research, **error** refers to the difference between what is true and the answer we obtained from our data collection. If we operationalized gender as the data collectors' assessment of gender, that observation might be wrong probably only 1 in 1000 times. However, there would still be some error, because an observational assessment would be wrong occasionally. The difference between the gender of 1000 people and the measurement of gender through observation would be the error in the measurement of that variable. In Chapter 2, we compared qualitative research to creating an artist's rendition of a new home and compared quantitative research to developing the blueprints for that home. An artist can misunderstand the specifications for a new home and create distortions or illusions in a painting, just as an architect can make errors in measurement that can lead to plans that are inaccurate, incomplete, or wrong. In both cases, error in measurement will occur.

If you have experienced having someone translate your words into another language, you know that translation is open to interpretation and even error. Qualitative research does not operationalize variables, because it does not presume to know enough about the variables of interest to be able to select appropriate and accurate concrete measures. Yet, qualitative research does translate specific experiences or observations into theoretical concepts or descriptions of variables during the process of data collection and analysis. Therefore, qualitative research is open to errors in interpretation during the data collection process. Because quantitative research often examines abstract variables that require both a theoretical and an operational definition, the opportunities for error in measurement can be even greater. Error can occur in the translation from theoretical to operational, and it can occur in the operationalized measurement process. Therefore, both qualitative research and quantitative research are open to problems in the translation of variables; we will discuss how those potential problems with translation can affect the meaning of the results of a study for practice later in this chapter.

Before looking at specific approaches used to collect data for studies, let's apply the ideas of theoretical variables and operational definitions to the fictional article about nursing students' choices of field of practice. The author of the fictional article tells us in the first paragraph, under the heading of "Measures," that the questionnaire used in this study had three sections: one that asked about demographic characteristics; one that asked about education, well-being, and career choice; and one that asked about automobile preferences. Demographic variables are usually fairly concrete and commonly understood, so the author does not offer theoretical definitions of them. However, the author does tell us indirectly that these variables were measured by self-report, because they were measured through a questionnaire that was completed by the students. Therefore, the operational definition of age in this study is reported age. The variable *age* then may be translated to be "the subject's report of his or her age in years." Age also could have been operationally defined by asking for the subject's birth date, which the researcher could then have used to compute age to the day using a computer calculation that subtracts date of birth from the current date. The fictional article does not tell us whether the questionnaire asked for age in years or for birth date, so we do not know exactly how the age variable was operationalized.

The second section of the questionnaire was used to operationalize several variables in the study, including educational background, well-being, and student preference for clinical practice after graduation. Educational background was operationalized by two questions: (1) currently licensed to practice as an RN or a licensed practical nurse (LPN) and (2) total number of years of postsecondary education. Well-being was operationally defined as the student's rating of his or her health on a four-point scale. Anticipated field of choice was operationally defined as choice from a list of career options. In each case, a variable has been translated into a specific measure or measures and alternate translations could have been used. Equally important, there is room for error both in the translation of a variable to a measure and in the measuring process itself. The remainder of this chapter discusses the measurement process and how error may occur.

Finally, the researcher included in the questionnaire an open-ended question regarding life experiences that led to choice of field of practice. In this last question, the researcher does not concretely translate a variable but asks the subjects to share experiences that may help her to develop a definition of the variable "life experiences affecting choice of field." Because this variable is not concrete, the researcher will have to start by developing a theoretical translation or definition before considering an operational definition. The fictional article provides several examples of operationally defined variables but includes no theoretical definitions. As we discuss some specific methods for collecting information about variables, we see examples of theoretical definitions that were in the articles found by the RN in the vignette (see Table 8–1 for the theoretical and operational definitions of those variables).

## METHODS FOR CONSTRUCTING THE MEANING OF VARIABLES IN QUALITATIVE RESEARCH

In qualitative research, the study methods used to collect data are intended to allow the researcher to construct a description of the meaning of the variable(s) under study. Remember that a qualitative approach assumes that truth is a moving target. The more we can know, feel, or understand about a variable of interest, the closer we will come to a full and complete meaning, but that meaning will always be context laden and, therefore, changing and evolving. A qualitative method for data collection, then, does not aim to measure specifically or make concrete a variable of interest. Rather, these data collection methods aim to expand our understanding about a variable or variables on as many levels as possible.

Qualitative methods of data collection depend on the participants' open sharing of their thoughts, feelings, and experiences verbally, visually, in writing, with music, and within life activities. Although it may not be surprising that participants can share through speaking and writing, other means of expression, such as music or cooking a meal, are probably less frequently considered but can be meaningful avenues for understanding a participant's experiences or feelings. Therefore, the data methods include interviews, journaling, participant observation, and art analysis. Interviews are probably the most frequently used methods for collecting data in qualitative research, with two broad categories of interviews used: unstructured interviews and group interviews.

**Unstructured interviews** involve asking questions in an informal and open fashion, without a previously established set of categories or assumed answers, to gain understanding about a phenomenon or variable of interest. Unstructured interviews in qualitative research assume that the product of the interview reflects the interactions among the interviewer, participant, and interview environment or setting. Depending on the type of qualitative study, the researcher may identify and purposely set aside or bracket his or her beliefs or expectations about the variable, or he or she may carefully document and incorporate his or her beliefs and perspectives into the data collection process. In any case, data collection using an unstructured interview includes not only the actual words of the participant but also notes about the participant's tone, expressions, and associated actions, and what is occurring in the setting. These notes are often called **field notes**, because they are a record of the researcher's observations about the overall setting and experience of the data collection process while in that setting or field itself. Field notes are used to enrich and build a data set that is thick and dense.

Unstructured interviews may take several forms, including in-depth interviews, oral histories, story telling, and life reviews. In all forms, the intent is to openly explore the understanding and experiences of the study participants. Unstructured interviews usually are tape-recorded or videotaped, then transcribed verbatim into a written form that will include notes on pauses; vocalizations that are not actual words, such as sighs; and even voice tone at times.

A related method of data collection is participant observation. In **participant observation**, the researcher intentionally imbeds himself or herself into the environment from which data will be collected and becomes a participant. From the perspective of active participation in the experiences and lives of those studied, the researcher/participant records observations, feelings, conversations, and experiences regarding the phenomenon of interest. The trajectory of death article states that data collection was "in-depth interviews with families supplemented by participant observation in the home. First each family member was interviewed individually; then the family was interviewed as a group" (Steel, 2000, p. 54). Thus, the researcher's data included both unstructured interviewing and her own observations as she spent time with the families in the study. Data from both sources helped the researcher gain an understanding of the experience of living with a child who is certain to die when the "how" and "when" of that death are unknown.

Group interviews also are used to collect data in qualitative research. **Group interviews** involve collection of data by interviewing more than one participant at a time. The data collected, then, is not just each individual participant's responses, but the responses that occur due to the interaction of the participants as they hear and respond to each other. Group interviews may take the form of focus groups, in which a preset topic is addressed in an open-ended fashion and the researcher keeps the focus of the group on that topic. Another form of group interview is brainstorming, in which no particular focus or direction is established and a group dialogues about a broad topic in an unstructured discussion. Group interviews may occur spontaneously in a setting where a researcher finds or facilitates two or more participants in naturally dialoging about a phenomenon of interest. For example, a researcher studying the experience of receiving government assistance and observing a group of women waiting for their food stamps might see several women talking about what it is like to shop with the stamps. The researcher might introduce himself or herself, obtain consent, and join the discussion, asking a few questions and listening to what the women have to say. In general, group interviews are rich in data and can be a relatively inexpensive method of data collection. However, use of group interviews may limit hearing and knowing unique individual perspectives or ideas, because groups limit some individual expression.

Use of journals is another approach that can be used to collect data in qualitative studies. In journaling, a researcher can ask participants to describe, in writing, their ongoing experiences with a phenomenon of interest. This type of data collection can provide continuous and evolving information from an individual perspective that cannot be collected in face-to-face interviews. However, it clearly depends on the participant's ability and willingness to write on a regular and detailed basis. The researcher also depends on the participant's own description of the setting and interactions related to an experience under study, because he or she is not present during the journaling. A more limited form of written data can be collected by directly asking participants to write a response or description about a phenomenon on the occasion of data collection. This approach is often called a free write. The fictional article about students' choices of fields of nursing used a limited version of written data collection by asking an open-ended question about students' experiences that had affected their choices of field in nursing. This can be considered to be a form of qualitative data collection, because it does not constrain or limit the responses that students can give and lends itself to providing data about the meaning of life experiences for future life choices.

A similar form of data collection involves the use of art forms, such as drawing or photography, which reflect the participant's perception and interpretation of certain experiences. When art is used, often an interview also is included so that the participant can share or interpret his or her art to the researcher. For example, homeless individuals might be given disposable cameras and asked to take photographs that reflect their experiences of being homeless. The researcher might then analyze the photographs for common subjects or common reflected moods.

Another form for data that are collected in qualitative research is documents and records. These types of data are used in historical research and may include personal and business letters, logs, contracts, accounts, and other written records from the past. These data are compiled and examined to create a clear picture of some past aspect. These types of data are particularly useful when the phenomenon of interest has evolved over time, such as the elimination of wearing nursing caps in the clinical setting.

In all these methods, the researcher is not collecting discrete, clearly defined, and limited information. Qualitative data are used to develop theoretical meaning by creating a verbal, a visual, or an auditory picture of a variable of interest. Although data collection in qualitative research is not structured and objectified, it is carefully planned and thought through, and it involves clearly identified methods for the overlapping processes of collecting, handling, and analyzing the data. We discuss how these methods are used to assure the rigor of a study later in this chapter.

## METHODS TO MEASURE VARIABLES IN QUANTITATIVE RESEARCH

In quantitative research, the methods used for data collection aim to measure clearly, specifically, and accurately the variables of interest. Earlier, we said that an operational definition of a variable is a description of how it will be measured and that a researcher doing a quantitative study almost always must decide how to measure the variable of interest, even when it is as concrete as a subject's gender. Remember, also, that the goal in quantitative research is to measure variables numerically so that they can be statistically described and analyzed. Therefore, the methods used for data collection in quantitative research include physiologic measurements, chemical laboratory tests, systematic observations, and written measures containing carefully defined questions, questionnaires, and/or scales.

Physiologic measurement is probably the most concrete type of data collection in quantitative research and may include anything from a simple measurement of blood pressure to the calculation of pulmonary function values. As was pointed out with the gender variable, physiologic measures still must be defined operationally, because most of them can be measured in several different fashions and with different levels of accuracy. A research study that examines a physiologic variable should report specifically how the physiologic parameter was measured so that you can evaluate the accuracy and appropriateness of that measure. Similarly, a study that includes a variable measured by a laboratory test should specify the actual test or procedure used to arrive at the study values. For example, if blood sugar was measured in a study, the report should indicate whether it used a capillary sample or a venous sample and what type of control and calibration was used to ensure consistency and accuracy.

A second method of measuring variables in quantitative research involves systematic observation of the variable of interest. Measurement by systematic observation differs from the observation data collection methods used in qualitative research, because it is structured and defined to ensure that each measurement is accurate and comparable to earlier or later measures. As a result, systematic observation does not try to collect as much detail and variation as possible but has a narrow focus on specific components of the variable under study. For example, in the fecal incontinence study, the researchers operationalized the variable fecal incontinence as the presence of uncontrolled release of stool and/or soiled clothing (Bliss, Johnson, Savik, Clabots, & Gerding, 2000). The variable is clearly defined, and the data collection focuses on the specific components of the definition. Therefore, data collectors were not interested in factors such as urinary incontinence, skin condition, type of bedpan, staffing ratio, or the subject's ability to use the call button. Data collectors were looking for and recording reports by the staff or the client of involuntary release of stool, and they counted the presence or absence of the defined components to give each subject a value of "yes" or "no" for the variable fecal incontinence.

A more detailed and complex example of measurement using observation in a quantitative study is provided in the report of the study of mothers of medically fragile infants. One of the variables in that study was parental competence. The authors theoretically define this relatively abstract variable as "the quality and effectiveness of parenting" (Miles et al., 1999, p. 132). They then operationally define parental competence as "a composite score that included four interview rating items, the amount of four mother–child interaction items from a naturalistic setting, and six subscale scores from the Home Observation for Measurement of the Environment (HOME)" (Miles et al., 1999, p. 132). Thus, scores on three different measures were combined to measure parental competence. The last of these three measures, the HOME, is further described in some detail to be a standardized instrument that uses semistructured interview responses and observations of mother–child relationship and of the kinds of play materials available to a child.

**Instrument** is used in research to refer to a device that specifies and objectifies the data collecting process. Instruments are usually written and may be given directly to the subject to collect data or may provide objective description of the collection of certain types of data. The HOME measure depends on observers noting certain specified and defined types of behaviors of the mother and the child, counting the presence or absence of those behaviors, and converting them into a final numeric score. When a researcher uses this type of observational measurement, the components that define the variable have been specified before data collection begins, and the study does not seek to expand the understanding of the components of that variable, as would a qualitative approach, but to count the extent to which they are present.

We have said that instruments are devices that define and objectify the data collection. The HOME instrument defines and objectifies the identification of children at risk for developmental delay. Many instruments that are used in nursing research collect data in a written form, provided directly by the subjects in the study. Instruments that collect data in writing are also called questionnaires or scales; in fact, these three words are sometimes used interchangeably. Instrument is the broadest term and, as we have said, can include interview questions, directed observations, or written collection of data. A **questionnaire** is an instrument used to collect specific written data, and a **scale** is a set of written questions or statements that, in combination, are intended to measure a specified variable. The questions or statements included on a scale are often called **items**. The language of research when discussing measurement of variables can get confusing, but understanding the basic meanings of some of these terms will allow you to better understand the meaning of a study for your clinical practice. Box 8–1 summarizes and gives an example of each of the frequently used terms in quantitative measurement.

The HOME instrument described in the maternal distress article also used the answers to semistructured questions. Semistructured questions are an example of data collection using specific planned questions. Telephone surveys often consist of semistructured questions, such as "how many hours of television do you watch per day?" or "how many members of the household eat breakfast daily?" Data collection using

---

**BOX 8-1    Definitions and Relationships Among an Instrument, Questionnaire, Scale, and Item**

*Instrument*–a device that specifies and objectifies the process of data collection
*Example:* Written instructions for a focused observation of behaviors indicating pain
↓

*Questionnaire*–An instrument that is completed by the study subjects
*Example:* Three-page written form that asks subjects about their personal characteristics, medications, past medical history, and pain
↓

*Scale*–a set of written questions or statements that measures a specified variable
*Example:* Three questions that ask the subjects to rate how often they experience pain in different situations
↓

*Item*–the individual question or statement that comprises a scale
*Example:* How often do you wake up in the night because of your pain?

| 0 | 1 | 2 | 3 |
|---|---|---|---|
| Never | Rarely | Occasionally | Frequently |

structured or defined questions establishes what data is wanted ahead of the collection. In contrast, unstructured questions seek to determine what data, experiences, or ideas are relevant and meaningful without previous narrowing of the definition or specification.

Many of the abstract concepts that we want to measure in nursing research are operationalized using written scales of one type or another. Because the concepts are abstract, it is not logical or reasonable that we could measure them with a single question. For example, suppose we want to measure the concept of "stress." One could simply ask subjects: "are you stressed—yes or no?" However, answers to this question alone will not capture levels of stress, negative versus positive stress, sense of managing or not managing stress, or the nature of the stresses. To collect a fuller and more complex measure of stress, one needs more than one simple question, hence the use of scales that consist of several statements or items related to the concept being measured.

The first step in developing a scale to measure an abstract concept is to identify items or questions that are relevant to the concept. Identification of items for a scale may be based on previous research about the concept, theory related to the concept, experts' knowledge regarding the concept, or individuals' experiences with the concept. Often, items for a scale are created based on several of the sources described. For example, a list of items to measure stress might first be developed based on a theory of stress and coping, then reviewed by experts in the field of stress and coping for suggestions, and, finally, reviewed or tested with small groups of individuals who are experiencing stress to see what they think about the items. The result might be five items such as those listed in Box 8–2. (Note—this is not an existing and established stress scale; it is simply intended to be an example.)

In addition to developing items that all are intended to address the same abstract concept or variable, scale development requires deciding how subjects will be asked to respond to the items. One type of response that is sometimes used asks subjects to respond whether each item is true or false. A second approach to responding to items is called a **Likert-type response scale**. A Likert-type response asks for a rating of the item on a continuum that is anchored at either end by opposite responses. For example, a Likert-type response scale that asks subjects to rate the frequency with which they experience what is described in each item that reflects stress from Box 8–2 might range from "always" at one end to "never" on the other end, as illustrated in Figure 8–1. Another example of a Likert-type response scale that could be used with the same items intended to measure stress could ask about frequency

---

**BOX  8-2  Sample Stress Measurement Items**

1. How often do you feel anxious?
2. How often do you have difficulty sleeping at night?
3. How often do you feel overwhelmed?
4. How often do you feel tired, even after a good night's sleep?
5. How often do you feel angry for no identifiable reason?

**FIGURE 8-1    Example of a Likert-type scale for stress.**

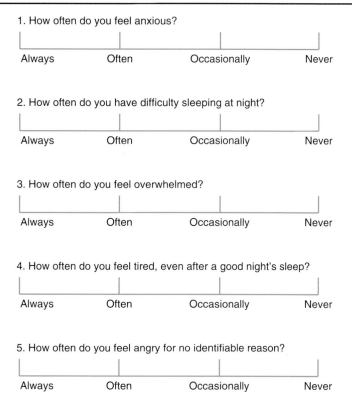

1. How often do you feel anxious?

| | | |
Always          Often          Occasionally          Never

2. How often do you have difficulty sleeping at night?

| | | |
Always          Often          Occasionally          Never

3. How often do you feel overwhelmed?

| | | |
Always          Often          Occasionally          Never

4. How often do you feel tired, even after a good night's sleep?

| | | |
Always          Often          Occasionally          Never

5. How often do you feel angry for no identifiable reason?

| | | |
Always          Often          Occasionally          Never

of experiencing what is described in the item with four options: 0 = never, 1 = once a week, 2 = two to three times a week, and 3 = daily. Likert-type scales may include from three to as many as eight or more choices, although the usual number of responses ranges from four to six. Notice that the answers to these questions are structured so that the subject cannot answer anything that he or she wishes, such as "once every other week" or "sometimes." Use of this scale to measure stress would result in a number between 0 and 15, which is a sum of the number for each item. The score on the scale could be considered to reflect the stress of the individual subject with subjects who answered "never" for all items, getting a score of 0, and subjects who answered "daily" for all items, getting a score of 15.

　　**Visual analog** is another response format that can be used in scales that differs from true/false, yes/no, and Likert-type scale responses. A visual analog consists of a straight line of a specific length that has extremes of responses at either end but does not have any other responses noted at points along the line. Subjects are asked to mark the line to indicate where they fall between the two extreme points. Often, the line is 100 mm, and the subject's response is scored from 1 to 100, depending on the placement of his or her mark. For example, a subject might be asked to rate the level of stress that different situations cause for him or her, ranging from no stress to extreme stress, as illustrated in Figure 8–2.

FIGURE 8-2    **Example of a Visual Analog scale.**

Rate your level of stress in each of the following situations by placing an "X" on the line below each situation. The left side of the line represents NO STRESS, and the far right side of the line represents EXTREME STRESS.

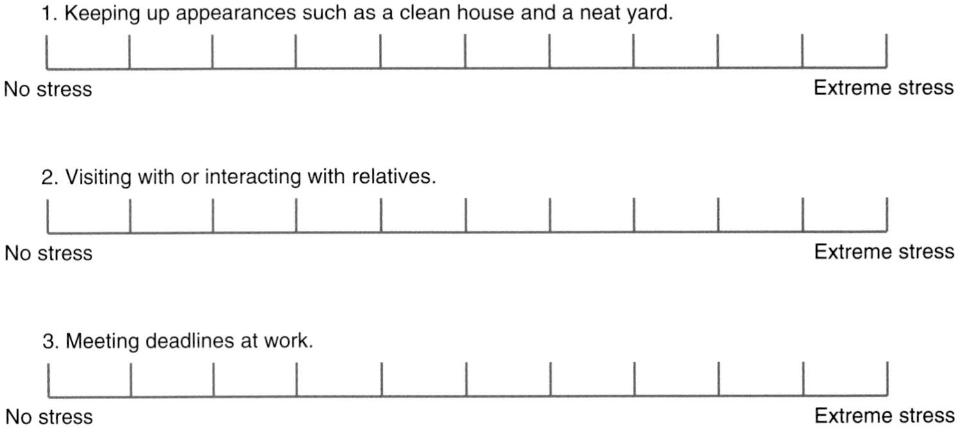

1. Keeping up appearances such as a clean house and a neat yard.

No stress                                                                                               Extreme stress

2. Visiting with or interacting with relatives.

No stress                                                                                               Extreme stress

3. Meeting deadlines at work.

No stress                                                                                               Extreme stress

The maternal distress study report describes the use of several scales, including the Maternal Identity Scale, the Parental Stressor Scale, and the Child Health Worry Scale (CHWS) (Miles et al., 1999). In each case, the authors tell us the theoretical definition of the variable that is measured by the scale, then tell us about the scale itself. Information about the scales usually includes the number of items, the general nature of the items, how subjects are asked to respond to the items, and how to interpret the numbers from the scale. For example, the CHWS is described as a scale to "assess the distress related to worry about the child's health" (Miles et al., 1999, p. 133). Because the CHWS is one of three measures used for the variable called maternal illness-related distress, we now have one part of the theoretical definition of that variable. The authors state that mothers were asked to rate their distress on five aspects of their child's illness. These aspects are reflected in items such as: (1) worry about the child's medical problem, (2) worry about whether the child will be normal, or (3) worry about whether the child might die or will always be sick. The response scale used a Likert-type format, ranging from a value of 1 for "no worry" to 5 for "very much worried." After reading this description of the measures used in the maternal distress and growth study, the RN in our vignette has a clearer idea about what was meant by maternal illness-related distress and how it was measured. This allows her to consider whether the measure is relevant to what she has observed in clinical practice.

In the previous two sections, we discussed methods to collect data and specific measurement approaches. We also have mentioned that, at times, error can occur in the methods or in the process of measurement. The potential for error occurs in both qualitative and quantitative methods of data collection. Understanding how error can occur in data collection is important so that you can consider what that potential error means for understanding and using research in clinical practice.

# ERRORS IN DATA COLLECTION IN QUALITATIVE RESEARCH

In qualitative research, error can be introduced into a study in two major ways. Problems can occur with the process of data collection, with the process of data analysis, or both. Because data collection and analysis are so closely linked in qualitative research, error that occurs in data collection is not easily separated from error that occurs in data analysis. When considering aspects of data collection and analysis that can create error, qualitative researchers aim to ensure the rigor of the data collection process and the associated data analysis process. **Rigor** is both a strict process of data collection and analysis and a term that reflects the overall quality of that process in qualitative research. Rigor is reflected in the consistency of data analysis and interpretation, the trustworthiness of the data collected, the transferability of the themes, and the credibility of the data. Qualitative researchers use several tools and processes to guarantee that each of these aspects of rigor is ensured.

## Trustworthiness

**Trustworthiness** refers to the honesty of the data collected from or about the participants (Lincoln & Guba, 1985). To collect trustworthy data, the researcher must have a meaningful relationship with the participants, which may require time to develop. Participants also must want to share information so that they can communicate their feelings, insights, and experiences without feeling pressured or wanting to censor what they share (Lincoln & Guba, 1985). For example, the parents who participated in the trajectory of certain death study were not likely to share their experiences and perceptions honestly and openly unless they believed that the researcher had a real interest in their perceptions and an acceptance of them and their life experiences. Participants do not develop such openness without first getting to know the researcher, at least to some extent. The researcher in the trajectory article used hospital and hospice staff to make the introductions that were the beginning of the relationships with the researcher. In this manner, the trust and relationship already developed with that staff was used to initiate a relationship. The researcher then went to the families' homes, thus using a setting that was safe to the participants. Each of these strategies was carefully thought through aspects of the data collection process, implemented to ensure trustworthiness.

Trustworthiness of data collection may also be supported by using a consistent protocol in data collection. Use of a protocol may seem contradictory to the open-ended nature of most qualitative data collection methods. However, a protocol can provide a broad framework for data collection and ensure a similar setting and interaction, without structuring the data collected. The trajectory of certain death article describes a protocol when the author states that she first interviewed each family member individually and then the family as a whole and that the ill children were not included in the interviews.

## Confirmability

A second aspect of ensuring rigor in qualitative data collection is **confirmability**—that is, the consistency and repeatability of the decision making about the process of data collection and data analysis (Lincoln & Guba, 1985). One approach taken to ensure confirmability of data in qualitative research is developing and maintaining an audit trail. An **audit trail** is an ongoing documentation regarding the researcher's decisions about both the data analysis and the collection processes. The documentation included in the audit trail may include field notes about the process of data collection, theoretical notes about the working hypotheses or developing ideas during the analysis, or methods notes regarding approaches to categorizing or organizing the data. The audit trail can be used both to assist the researcher in being consistent and to demonstrate the presence of consistency when sharing the data.

Qualitative researchers use computer software programs, such as NU.DIST and N.VIVO, to help them to organize and analyze their data. These programs do not perform the thinking and conceptualizing that is at the heart of qualitative data analysis, but they can be used to examine the data efficiently and organize it around themes and dimensions as they are identified in the data. As the researcher begins to identify a data theme, different units of language or observations can be categorized under this theme. As new themes arise, the data can be reorganized consistently by the software. In addition, a record of the evolving decisions about themes and the classification of data are maintained, ensuring that the researcher is consistent in the analysis of all the data and assisting the qualitative researcher in maintaining an audit trail.

Taking a simple example, suppose that the researcher for the choice of field study reported in the fictional article had broken down the students' written answers describing experiences that contributed to their choices of field into units that were the individual sentences and then stored them within a computer program. The researcher might decide that whenever students described some kind of experience with fiction about health care, such as a novel or television series, that this reflected a theme. The researcher now must explore the data to decide what are and are not examples of experiences with fiction about health care. For example, novels, plays, movies, and television series may all clearly fit into the theme of fiction, but are advertisements that depict health care also part of this category? As she decides and tells the program that references to television, radio, literature, film, and theatre all reflect exposure to media, the computer will find and place into a category sentences with those references. When the researcher later adds some additional data from another class of students, she might decide that identification with selected actors or actresses is a separate theme from the broader media exposure. The computer can be told to reorganize the data, looking for references to particular actors or actresses, but it will also retain the information about how the original category was formed. This provides the researcher with an ongoing record of decisions and decreases the possibility of the researcher defining or describing a category inconsistently from one time to another.

### Transferability

A third aspect of rigor in a qualitative study is the transferability of the concepts, themes, or dimensions identified. **Transferability** refers to the extent to which the findings of a study are confirmed by or are applicable to a different group or in a different setting from where the data was collected (Lincoln & Guba, 1985). Transferability is different from generalizability, because the focus is not on predicting specific outcomes in a general population. Rather, the focus is on confirming that what was meaningful in one specific setting or with one specific group is also meaningful and accurate in a different setting or group. One of the methods used to ensure transferability is to describe themes that have been identified in one sample to a group of similar participants who did not contribute to the initial data collection to determine if the second group agrees with the themes. This procedure is sometimes called external checks. Transferability also can be ensured if the researcher actively seeks sources of data that contradict the ideas that are emerging from the data. If disconfirming data are found, they can be used to modify or reinterpret the total body of data to develop more comprehensive and credible findings. Findings that reflect the breadth of experiences or ideas will then be more easily transferred or related to different groups.

## Credibility

Credibility, the fourth aspect of rigor of concern to qualitative researchers, overlaps with transferability and trustworthiness. **Credibility** refers to the confidence that the researcher and user of the research can have in the truth of the findings of the study. Lincoln and Guba (1985) suggest that the credibility of qualitative data can be supported by a researcher performing several actions, including seeking feedback from participants regarding evolving findings and interpretations and seeking participants whose perceptions differ from those already included in the study. The former activity is often referred to as member checks. **Member checks** means that the data and the findings from data analysis are brought back to the original participants to seek their input concerning the accuracy, completeness, and interpretation of the data. Steele, in the trajectory study, indicates that "during the following year, the evolving analysis was shared with the families" (2000, p. 54), thus telling us that the interpretation of the data was reviewed and confirmed as correct by the participants.

Credibility also is ensured through processes that guarantee trustworthiness and transferability, such as spending time with the participants and maintaining thorough, phenomenon-focused observations. It can be further ensured through the use of triangulation. **Triangulation** is the process of using more than one approach or source to include different views or to look at the phenomenon from different angles (Lincoln & Guba, 1985). Triangulation focuses on the data, seeking different types of sources of information regarding a phenomenon, or it can focus on the use of more than one investigator, the use of several theories, or the use of numerous methods in the study (Denzin, 1989). The trajectory study could be considered to have used triangulation by including data from interviews, observation, and groups. Specifically, the author collected data through individual interviews and family group interviews, as well as through her own observations. When multiple sources of data all lead to the same conclusions, the credibility of those findings is increased.

Table 8–2 summarizes the aspects of rigor that we have discussed. As we read and consider using results from qualitative research in practice, we must consider the rigor of the data collection methods and analysis. The greater the rigor in the study, the more we can be confident that the findings are meaningful truths that we can use to understand our patients. What helps us to be confident in the rigor of a study includes the use of processes to ensure the trustworthiness of the data, such as

| TABLE 8-2 | Aspects of Rigor | |
|---|---|---|
| **Aspect** | **Definition** | **Methods** |
| Trustworthiness | The honesty of the data collected from and about participants | Establishment of ongoing or meaningful interactions Use of a protocol |
| Confirmability | The consistent repeatable nature of the data collection and analysis | Use of computer software to organize and analyze data Audit trails |
| Transferability | The extent to which findings relate to other settings or groups | External checks Seeking disconfirming cases or outlyiers |
| Credibility | The confidence in the truth of the findings | Triangulation Member checks |

the researcher establishing meaningful interactions and maintaining ongoing contact with participants. That the data are confirmable can be indicated by the researcher stating that an audit trail was maintained or that selected software was used to assist in data analysis. Use of approaches, such as external checks and searching for participants who differ or have dissenting views, can help to ensure us of the transferability of the data. The credibility of the data can be supported by member checks and triangulation.

## ERRORS IN DATA COLLECTION IN QUANTITATIVE RESEARCH

In quantitative research, the data analysis process usually is separated from the data collection process. There also are two general areas in which error can occur in quantitative data collection: in the quality of the measures used to collect data and in the implementation of those measures or the data collection process itself. These two areas are not entirely discrete and do overlap. We start by talking about the quality of the measures used to collect quantitative data.

### The Quality of Measures—Reliability and Validity

Accuracy and consistency in measurement are at the heart of successful quantitative research. As an intelligent reader and user of research, you must ask yourself two questions about any measure used in a quantitative study: how consistently does the instrument, questionnaire, or procedure measure what it measures, and does the instrument, questionnaire, or procedure measure what it is supposed to measure. The

# CORE CONCEPT

*Consistent measurement is reliable measurement. Accurate or correct measurement is valid measurement.*

first question addresses the reliability of a measure, and the second question addresses its validity.

**Reliability** means that a measure can be relied on consistently to give the same result if the aspect being measured has not changed. Consider, for example, measuring the gender of a sample: if three independent observers each record the gender of 1000 adults as they individually walk into a room, there will be a quite high level of consistency in the final count of the numbers of men and women in the sample. However, if even five or six of the sample are androgynous in their appearance, there may be some small differences in the final counts provided by the three observers. We have already said that this leads to some small error in the measure. If we changed our sample to 1000 diapered infants all dressed in white, we would expect much more inconsistency in the final totals, because gender identification of infants by observation is much more difficult to do consistently. If, instead, three laboratories conducted genetic testing of each of the 1000 infants, there should be no differences in the final totals for boy and girls (assuming no laboratory error). Thus, the data collection on gender (particularly for infants) using the method of observation is less reliable than the data collection on gender using the method of genetic testing.

The reliability of a measure becomes more difficult to ensure as the measurement process becomes more complicated, because complexity allows for more opportunities for error through inconsistency. Several approaches are taken to ensure or examine the reliability of measurement in quantitative research, depending on the type of measurement being used. When data are being collected by observation, a researcher often trains the observers and then tests them with different cases, until all the observers agree on their observations the majority of the time.

The maternal distress study provides a good example of this when it describes the use of the HOME scale. The authors tell us that the "HOME was administered by three observers who were trained by an experienced HOME tester until they had a minimum interrater reliability of 95%" (Miles et al., 1999, p. 132).

In other words, the observers practiced making the observations needed to obtain a score on the HOME scale until they each reached the same score at least 95% of the time. The authors also tell us that "the interrater reliabilities for the data collectors averaged 97%" (Miles et al., 1999, p. 132). **Interrater reliability** is present when two or more independent data collectors agree in the results of their data collection process. In the case of the HOME scale when the three independent observers collected data from the families in the study, they agreed an average of 97% of the time. By providing this information, the authors help the RN in our vignette to know that this complicated procedure to get a measurement of parental competence was used consistently across the different families. That consistency in use decreases the chances that any differences between families were due to inconsistent measurement rather than real differences. Assurances of reliability of a measure allow us to be comfortable that little error occurred in the measurement because of inconsistent use of the scale or instrument.

When a measure of a variable in a study is a written questionnaire or scale, two other types of approaches can be taken to ensure that the measure is reliable. The first is to test the measure before it is used in the study by having individuals complete the questionnaire or scale at two or more time points that are close enough together that we would not expect the "real" answers to have changed. This kind of reliability is called **test-retest reliability**; what we hope for is consistency in the answers in the different time points. If a scale or questionnaire is confusing or does not have a lot of meaning for a subject, his or her responses from one time to another are likely to differ. That means that the scores from that measure will not be consistent and differences found may occur because of a lack of reliability of the measure rather than actual differences. For example, one would expect that nursing students' choices of field of practice would not change much during a week. If the author of the fictional article had administered her questionnaire to the students twice, a week apart, and found big differences in choice, we would believe that the questionnaire was not measuring this variable consistently. That inconsistency would then shed significant doubt on the findings of the study, because we could not be sure that the study truly measured choice of field.

A second way that reliability is often measured for quantitative measures is by calculating a statistic called an alpha coefficient. This statistic reflects a computation of how closely the answers to different questions or items within a scale are related and is, therefore, often called the **internal consistency reliability** coefficient. Internal consistency reliability is the extent to which responses to a scale are similar and related. Remember that we said that many abstract concepts in nursing and other fields are measured using scales consisting of several items or questions that all relate to the same aspect being studied. If, in fact, all the items or questions address the same aspect or variable, we would expect a consistent pattern in how subjects respond to or answer the items.

Let's go back to the five items that we are pretending were developed to measure stress (see Box 8–2). We would expect that a highly stressed person would indicate that most of the experiences listed were happening regularly. If, instead, we found that subjects indicated that one or two of the items were occurring regularly but that others were not occurring at all, there would be a low internal consistency among the items. Alpha coefficients, often called Chronbach's alpha after the statistician who developed the test, can range from 0 to 1.0, with a value of 0 indicating that there are absolutely no relationships among the responses to the different items in a scale, and a value of 1.0 meaning that the answers to the items were all completely connected or related to each other. In general, researchers hope for an alpha coefficient of greater than 0.7, indicating a relatively strong relationship or connection among the responses to the different items on any particular scale.

Many quantitative studies that use scales to measure variables report internal consistency reliability coefficients or alpha coefficients to let the reader know how internally consistent that measure was. For example, the RN in our vignette reads that the "Cronbach's alpha was .71 at hospital enrollment and .90 and .85 at 12 and

16 months" (Miles et al., 1999, p. 133) for the CHWS. This tells her that the CHWS, which we previously learned consisted of five items, was answered relatively consistently throughout the study but that there was more internal consistency at the second use than either initially at the hospital or at 16 months.

To summarize, the reliability of a measure reflects how definite we can be that the measure will yield the same data consistently if the actual or "real" variable stays the same. When quantitative data are collected using observation, the rate of agreement, or interrater agreement, tells us how consistent the observational measure was. Test-retest reliability can tell us if a measure stays consistent over time when the aspect measured has not changed. Internal consistency reliability or a Cronbach's alpha coefficient is a statistic that tells us how consistently subjects responded to a set of items or questions. In all three cases, the goal in quantitative research is to use measures that will most consistently measure the variables of interest.

**Validity** is the second aspect of measurement that must be considered when deciding on use of research in clinical practice. Validity reflects how accurately the measure yields information about the true or real variable being studied. A measure is valid if it measures correctly and accurately what it is intended to measure. The validity of a measure becomes more of an issue the more abstract the variable to be measured; with a concrete variable such as gender, validity of a measure is not a great concern. We are generally confident that gender self-report will yield a true measure of gender. However, let's look at another demographic variable that may seem as concrete: the variable of race. To measure this variable, researchers might ask subjects to indicate their race by checking one category from a list that looks like the one in Box 8–3. On initial inspection, we might assume that this list is clear and should yield valid results. However, although the use of the term "native American" to represent those individuals who represent the indigenous peoples of the Americas is considered politically correct, it also can be interpreted to mean "born in America." If many subjects interpret it this way, then the measure will yield inaccurate information about race.

The issue of validity of a measure becomes much more complex in scales used to measure variables such as depression, stress, efficacy, motivation, or coping. Scales or written instruments that are developed to measure abstract concepts such as these must find a way to describe or ask about factors that are specific to the concept and clear enough to avoid confusion with other concepts. Three types of validity are sometimes described within reports of research: content validity, criterion-related validity, and construct validity.

---

**BOX 8-3    Potentially Invalid Forced Choice Race Item**

Please check the item below that best describes you.

| | | | |
|---|---|---|---|
| _____ | Black | _____ | Latino/Latina |
| _____ | White–non-Hispanic | _____ | Asian–not Pacific Islander |
| _____ | Native American | _____ | Pacific Islander |

The simplest of the three, and the one that is most easy for a reader of research to assess, is content validity. **Content validity** asks whether the items or questions on a scale are comprehensive and appropriately reflect the concept that they are supposed to measure. Put simply, the question becomes: is the *content* of the scale complete and appropriate? Researchers who have to develop their own measure of a concept will try to establish the content validity of the measure by asking a group of experts to review the items on the scale for completeness and appropriateness. If researchers are using a measure that has only been used a few times in other research, they may describe what type of assessment was made of the measure when it was developed to ensure content validity. As a user of research, you can assess what is called the face validity of a measure, which is simply one person's (perhaps not an expert's) interpretation of content validity. Face validity is a judgment of how clearly the items on a scale reflect the concept they are intended to measure.

If we consider the face validity of the items listed in Box 8–2 that were proposed to measure stress, we might begin to question them. In fact, the items listed in that box generally reflect the symptoms that we expect to see when someone is experiencing depression rather than stress. Although depression and stress may be related, we do not necessarily expect everyone who is experiencing significant negative stress to also be depressed. Therefore, the face validity of these items must be questioned. In all likelihood, if a panel of stress experts reviewed these items, they would decide that the items were not valid items for a stress scale.

The RN in our vignette can make some of her own judgments about the face validity of most of the scales used in the maternal distress study, because the authors give the reader information about the content of the items on several of the scales. In the example of the CHWS, the five items are described as:

> the degree to which they worry about the child's medical problem; about whether the child will be normal, might die, or will always be sick; and about when the parent will be able to take the baby home (Miles et al., 1999, p. 133).

The RN can think about her experience with parents of sick children and decide whether these five ideas are inclusive of the major worries of parents and are clearly related to the concept of worry. In thinking about this, the RN is making her own judgment about the face validity of the scale; if she decides that it is not valid, she may then decide the that results of the study connected with this variable are questionable for use in practice.

The second type of validity that may be described in a research report is criterion-related validity. **Criterion-related validity** is the extent to which the results of one measure match those of another measure that is also supposed to reflect the variable under study. The question asked with this type of validity is: do the results from the scale relate to a known criterion relevant to the variable? If a researcher were trying to test the criterion-related validity of the five-item "stress" scale in Box 8–2, subjects might be asked to answer those five items and then to rate their stress level on a scale from 1 to 100. If scores from responses on the five items closely matched ratings of stress on the 100-point scale, they might be considered to provide some evidence for the criterion-related validity of the 5-item scale. The criterion used in this example is a direct self-rating of stress level, and the example is one of a test for concurrent criterion-related validity. That is, the test looked for a relationship between two measures concurrently, or at the same time.

A second type of criterion-related validity looks for a relationship between the scale being tested and some measure that should be closely related that occurs in the future. This type of validity is called predictive validity. An example of predictive validity for a scale called the Mental Development Index (MDI) is provided by the authors of the maternal distress study when they tell us that "in very low birthweight, premature infants, the 12-month MDI had a correlation of .48 with preschool year IQ . . ." (Miles et al., 1999, p. 133). This tells us that this scale that is supposed to measure mental development in infants predicted intelligence quotient when the children were preschool age. The authors provide this information to let the reader of the study know that the measure that they chose to use had already been shown to have predictive criterion-related validity in earlier research; this tells us that we can be more confident that the MDI scores found in the maternal distress study did reflect the mental development of the children in the study.

The last type of validity that is sometimes discussed in a report of research is construct validity. **Construct validity** is the broadest type of validity and can encompass both content and criterion-related validity, because it is the extent to which a scale or an instrument measures what it is supposed to measure. The construct validity of a scale or an instrument is supported with time if results using the measure support theory about how the construct (variable) being measured is supposed to behave. This may include predictive validity and concurrent validity but also will include other less direct predictions that arise from theory. Several approaches can be taken to measure the construct validity of a scale or an instrument, including use of statistical procedures, such as factor analysis or structural equation modeling, comparison of results from the measure to closely related and vastly differing constructs, and the development of hypotheses that are then tested to provide support for the scale. In all cases, the goal is to build evidence that the construct, or abstract variable, is being measured by the scale.

There is a relationship between the validity and reliability of measures: a scale can be reliable but not valid. However, a scale cannot be valid and not also be reliable. A scale may consistently measure something (reliability) but not the something it is supposed to measure (validity). However, if a scale measures what it is supposed to measure (validity), then it will inherently also be consistent (reliable). For example, we have suggested that the five items in Box 8–2 have questionable validity as a measure of stress, but it is possible that subjects might answer those five questions consistently, giving us reliable data about something—just not about stress.

One last note about reliability and validity is related to data collection from sources such as medical records. In nursing research, using medical records to collect certain types of data is quite common. However, some unique issues surrounding this data must be considered. As all nurses know, we can be confident that whatever is documented on a record has a high likelihood of having occurred. Therefore, if we are collecting data about pain level and we find notations regarding the patient's pain complaints, we can be sure they are accurate. However, we cannot be as confident that the absence of a notation about pain means that the patient did not have pain. If a great deal happened during a particular shift and a patient's pain was not exceptional in some way, it is possible that the pain was not charted. Thus, the reliability of certain types of data from medical records—that is, the consistency with which the kinds of data are documented—must be considered when choosing to use medical records to measure study variables. This is not to say that records are unreliable, only that there is inconsistency in the documentation of certain care aspects in records.

The different types of reliability and validity that must be considered when understanding quantitative studies are summarized in Table 8–3. Although reliability focuses on the consistency of a measure, validity focuses on the accuracy or correctness of a measure. Three types of validity are considered by researchers. Content validity refers to the extent to which the scale or instrument is comprehensive and addresses the concept or variable of interest. Criterion-related validity can be either concurrent or predictive and refers to how closely the results on the measure in question relate to results on other measures of the same concept in the present or future. Construct validity refers to the overall ability of the scale to measure what it is supposed to measure and is established only after the repeated use of a measure yields results that reflect the theoretical expectations for the concept being measured. An instrument of measurement can be reliable but not valid. However, if a measure has been shown to be valid, then it will be reliable.

### Error in Implementation of Quantitative Data Collection

We said that error can be introduced into the measurement of variables in quantitative research because of problems with either the quality of the measure or the process of implementing the measure. Although reliability and validity speak to the quality of a measure, even a reliable and valid measure can be implemented incorrectly and lead to error. Implementation of data collection requires careful and detailed planning to ensure that the process is consistent and does not invalidate the measures. For example, a researcher could be using a reliable and valid measure of blood sugars, but subjects may fail to understand the dietary restrictions of fasting before samples are collected, thus introducing errors into the data. A procedure that confirms true fasting status would ensure that the measure yielded meaningful data. Another example of an implementation error occurs when a written scale that may have been shown previously to be reliable and valid is administered with incorrect directions or the subjects are prompted in a way that sways their responses to a measure. Pointing out that the financial support for an agency depends on positive reviews before asking subjects to complete a satisfaction survey is an obvious example.

The order in which subjects are asked to complete questionnaires also can affect their responses. For example, if subjects are asked to complete a scale that asks several questions about symptoms of depression and then are asked to rate their level of overall depression, the scale likely will have increased their awareness of how depressed they really are, thus affecting their total depression ratings. In addition, different timing and environments affect data collection. For example, asking nursing students about their choices of field when they have just completed an exciting clinical rotation in the emergency room could lead to more of them selecting the emergency room than would have selected it if they had been asked some time after that rotation.

| TABLE 8-3 | Aspects of Reliability and Validity | |
|---|---|---|
| **Aspect** | **Definition** | **Methods** |
| ***Reliability—how consistent is the measure?*** | | |
| Interrater reliability | Agreement between two or more independent data collectors about the results of their data collection process | Carefully structured instruments Practice until a high level of agreement is reached |
| Test–retest reliability | Consistency in answers on tests when we would not expect the real answers to have changed | Repeated administration of measures or tests to calculate consistency in responses |
| Internal consistency reliability | The extent to which responses to a scale are similar and related | Calculation of a Cronbach's alpha coefficient |
| ***Validity—how accurate is the measure?*** | | |
| Content validity | The comprehensiveness and appropriateness of the measure to the concept it is intended to measure | Expert panel review Face validity |
| Criterion-related validity | The extent to which results of one measure match those of another measure that examines the same concept | Concurrent validity Predictive validity |
| Construct validity | The extent to which a scale or instrument measures what it is supposed to measure | Content and criterion-related validity Hypothesis testing Statistical procedures such as factor analysis |

Other types of error that can occur in the measurement process include sloppy handling of data, resulting in a loss of some of it. Failure to keep careful records can lead to missed opportunities for repeat measures, because subjects' addresses or telephone numbers are misplaced or not accurately recorded. This is a problem particularly in longitudinal studies, such as the maternal distress study, in which subjects are asked to complete measures at five different time points.

Finally, the implementation of data collection can introduce error by arbitrarily changing a measure through translating it to another language or administering it in a format other than that which was intended. Measures that are reliable and valid have been successfully translated into other languages, but this requires a careful translation process and then translating the measure back into the original language by independent translators to ensure that the meanings of items on a scale remain intact when the language changes. In the TB-screening article discussed in several earlier chapters (Poss, 2000), the author gives us detailed information about the process used to translate the measures for that study into Spanish. By giving this information, the author assures us that the measures retained the basic validity and reliability that had been established for the English versions. An issue similar to translation to another language exists when a measure that was developed to be read *by* a subject is instead read *to* a subject. The subject is then hearing the words rather then seeing them, and this can definitely affect his or her understanding and potential response to the items.

In summary, measurement in quantitative research must be carefully planned and controlled. The variables to be measured must be clearly defined. If the variables are abstract, we should expect to see both a theoretical definition and an operational definition, so that we can judge both the meaning of the variable and how well that meaning was translated into data through measurement. Errors in measurement can be present because of problems with the measure itself or incorrect implementation of the measure.

The measurement language in both qualitative and quantitative research can be complex and confusing. Overall, the important points are that data collection must be trustworthy, confirmable, and consistent, as well as transferable, credible, and accurate. Both the process and the actual measures in data collection must be considered as we decide how to use the results of research in practice. To decide how measurement in a study has affected results and conclusions, we must receive complete and clear information about the measures. This leads us to consider what might be some common problems with written reports of data collection.

## COMMON ERRORS IN WRITTEN REPORTS OF DATA COLLECTION METHODS

Probably the most common error that occurs in written reports of research studies is provision of incomplete information. This was not a problem with either of the articles read by the RN in our vignette, because both reports provided a great detail about the data collection process. In contrast, the fictional article does leave several gaps in the information provided about the collection of the data. For example, the author does not give us a clear theoretical or operational definition of the dependent variable in this study—choice of field. Theoretically, "choice" could be defined as what students would really like to do if all options were open to them or it could be defined as what students expect to do, given current openings and other aspects of their personal situations. The results section of this report does give us some idea about how "field of choice" was operationally defined, because those categories that were elected by the students are listed. We know that the students were not permitted to write in their choice but were given a list of nursing career options from which to select. However, the author does not tell us what was included in the original list of options, so we do not know if the final categories reported in Table 1 included all the possible options or if there were options that were not selected or were collapsed into one of the reported categories. In other words, we are not clear about the operational definition for the dependent variable either. This lack of clear information jeopardizes the usefulness of the research for practice, because it becomes difficult to be comfortable with conclusions based on measurement that we do not understand or believe was consistent or accurate.

A second common error with written reports of data collection is a failure to organize clearly the information in a manner that makes it understandable. Although the maternal distress article provides a wealth of information about the measures used in the study, the information is not easily understood in the winding narrative format in which it is presented. The information summarized in Table 1 would have been helpful to have at the beginning of the data collection section of this report, with the various specific measures listed below each variable. Having the variables clearly organized and defined in a table format would have been helpful. For example, such a table might have indicated that the variable "Maternal competence" was measured using (Miles et al., 1999, p. 132):

1. four interview rating items,
2. the amount of four mother–child interaction items from the naturalistic observations, and
3. six subscale scores from the HOME (numbers inserted by author).

A third error that occasionally occurs in written reports of data collection methods is a failure to reference the source of measures used in a study. Although the practicing nurse may not choose to do so often, the option of reading other studies that previously used a measure that was used in the new study should be available. Referencing reports of previous studies that indicated the reliability and validity of a measure is particularly important, because it gives the reader the option to learn more about that specific measure and increases one's confidence in the quality of the measure.

## CONNECTING DATA COLLECTION METHODS TO SAMPLING, RESULTS, AND DISCUSSION/CONCLUSION

At the beginning of this chapter, we said that the RN needed to understand how the study variables were measured to understand the meaning of the results of the studies about aspects of family functioning with severely ill children. One thing that may have become clear to the RN as she learned more about research methods is that sampling and data collection methods are linked in both quantitative and qualitative research. Particularly in qualitative studies, data collection and analysis drive the sampling, because additional participants often are sought purposely to focus on aspects of the phenomenon that are emerging from the data. We also discussed trustworthiness and the use of both member and group checks. These aspects of rigor in data collection require sampling strategies that ensure a trusting and open relationship with the data collector. Further, a researcher can ask the right questions about a phenomenon but fail to gain access to the right groups to answer those questions; so, as we read about data collection, we must consider the sampling process as well.

In quantitative research, sampling is most connected to data collection in follow-up for repeated measures with time. However, the data collection process also can be affected by the nature of the sample or vice versa. For example, a study of homeless patients that uses measures written in English that have no established Spanish version may exclude a group of Spanish-speaking subjects. Another problem in data collection that is closely related to sampling is the educational level assumed in the measures. A complex written scale that uses language aimed at a high school reading level may become unreliable when used with subjects who have a lower education level. Thus, sampling and data collection can be closely linked in quantitative research as well as in qualitative research.

Throughout this chapter, we have stressed that if variables are not clearly defined or are not consistently and accurately measured, the results of the study must be questioned. Similarly, if rigor is not maintained through both data collection and analysis, the results of qualitative research are jeopardized: the results of a study are only as good as the data that went into those results. Therefore, understanding how data were collected and recognizing how potential sources of error in the data collection were addressed is closely linked to our ability to accept the results of a study. This, in turn, clearly affects our willingness to accept and adopt the conclusions of a study.

A last link between data collection and the rest of the research process is the link between data collection and the section of a research report that speaks to limitations of a study. Despite the best plans and efforts, problems do arise with data collection. These may be mentioned in the write-up of the data collection itself, but the implications of those problems for the conclusions of a study are often addressed when the author discusses limitations. For example, the maternal distress study found some surprising results regarding depression and distress. The authors for this study comment on the effects of measurement on their findings in the discussion sections of their article by stating:

> *Measuring only depressive symptoms as a measure of distress may not capture other aspects of distress that are important. In addition, while the measure of growth was assessed as objectively as possible by the research team based on their extensive observations of and interviews with the mothers over time, there still likely was some bias in the ratings. It is recommended that future studies use additional measures of distress such as measures of anxiety and mood disturbance, and also use a valid and reliable self-report measure of growth in order to assess the mother's own perspective about her developmental impact* (Miles et al., 1999, p. 138).

Thus, the conclusions of a study are directly linked back to the measurement process.

## PUBLISHED REPORTS—WOULD YOU USE THESE STUDIES IN CLINICAL PRACTICE?

At the beginning of this chapter, the RN was concerned about how to help S.G.'s parents and how to avert a problem between the nursing staff and S.G.'s parents concerning his care. After considering the data collection methods in the trajectory of certain death article, the RN is comfortable that the experiences described in that article are credible and transferable to S.G.'s parents' experiences. The researcher developed a trusting relationship with the families, used several methods to triangulate the data, used member checks to ensure credibility, and systematically analyzed the data to generate the dimensions described in the findings of the study, thus ensuring confirmability. The RN is comfortable that the results of this study will help her to understand the crisis S.G.'s parents are probably facing falling off their plateau with S.G. However, the RN is not sure why the researcher chose to use a method called grounded theory for collection of the data or why children with NLTI were specifically targeted for data collection. To answer these questions she must read the section of the report that describes the research design.

After reading about the data collection methods used in the maternal distress study, the RN was sure that great effort went into measuring several abstract and complex variables. She recognizes that each variable has been carefully defined, both theoretically and operationally, and that the reliability of the different measures is discussed. Validity of the measures is not discussed as completely as reliability was, and the study itself is complex because of both many measures and many points of measurement. The RN wonders why so many variables were included in this study and why the study was carried out over so many time points. She believes that the findings have given her some insight into how she might take a more active role in working with S.G.'s parents, as well as S.G. himself. However, she would like to understand better the design of this study and what this type of design may mean for the applicability of the results to practice.

## OUT-OF-CLASS EXERCISE:

### Free Write

The next chapter continues to address the question of why a study included the people it did and why the study was done the way it was by talking about research designs. Before reading that chapter, consider the question of whether being in nursing school affects the students' well-being. If you were going to conduct a study to address this question, how would you go about it? What do you think would be the best way to conduct a study to answer this question, and what do you think would be the most realistic approach? Are they the same or different, and why? Think about this, then write, in as much detail as possible, your ideas about how to conduct a study to determine if and how being a nursing student affects well-being. Wherever you can, write your rationale for conducting the study in the manner on which you have decided. After you have completed this assignment, you will be ready to move on to read about research designs in Chapter 9.

## References

Bliss, D. Z., Johnson, S., Savik, K., Clabots, C. R., & Gerding, D. N. (2000). Fecal incontinence in hospitalized patients who are acutely ill. *Nursing Research, 49*(2), 101–108.

Denzin, N. K. (1989). *Interpretive interactionism.* Newbury Park, CA: Sage Publications.

Lincoln, Y. S., & Guba, E. G. (1985). *Naturalistic inquiry.* Beverly Hills, CA: Sage Publications.

Miles, M. S., Holditch-Davis, D., Burchinal, P., & Nelson, D. (1999). Distress and growth outcomes in mothers of medically fragile infants. *Nursing Research, 48*(3), 128–140.

Poss, J. E. (2000). Factors associated with participation by Mexican migrant farmworkers in a tuberculosis screening program. *Nursing Research, 49*(1), 20–28.

Steele, R. G. (2000). Trajectory of certain death at an unknown time: Children with neurodegenerative life-threatening illnesses. *Canadian Journal of Nursing Research, 32*(3), 49–67.

## Resources

Campbell, D. T., & Russo, M. J. (2001). *Social measurement.* Thousand Oaks, CA: Sage Publications.

Denzin, N. K., & Lincoln, Y. S. (Eds.). (1998). *Collecting and interpreting qualitative materials.* Thousand Oaks, CA: Sage Publications.

LoBiondo-Wood, G., & Haber, J. (1998). In *Nursing research: Methods, critical appraisal, and utilization* (4th ed.). St. Louis: Mosby.

Locke, L. F., Silverman, S. J., & Spirduso, W. W. (1998). Reading and understanding research. Thousand Oaks, CA: Sage Publications.

Polit, D. F., & Hungler, B. P. (1999). *Nursing research: Principles and methods* (6th ed.). Philadelphia: Lippincott.

**LEARNING OUTCOME:**

*THE STUDENT WILL* interpret the strengths and weaknesses of research designs in relation to sampling, data collection methods, and the meaning of the results and conclusions.

# Research Designs: Planning the Study

## *How Were Those People Studied—Why Was the Study Done That Way?*

**KEY TERMS**

Clinical trials
Comparison group
Control group
Correlational
Descriptive
Ethnography
Experimental design
Experimenter effects
External validity
Grounded theory

Hawthorne effect
Historical
History
Instrumentation
Internal validity
Longitudinal
Maturation
Measurement effects
Mixed methods
Model testing

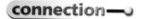

For additional activities go to
http://connection.lww.com/go/macnee.

| | |
|---|---|
| Mortality | Reactivity effects |
| Multifactorial | Repeated measures |
| Novelty effects | Research design |
| Phenomenology | Retrospective |
| Pretest-posttest | Selection bias |
| Prospective | Testing |
| Quasi-experimental | |

## CLINICAL CASE

Z.B., a 72-year-old man, was admitted to the coronary care unit (CCU) with acute congestive heart failure secondary to ischemic cardiomyopathy. A review of his medical history indicates that Z.B. was enrolled in a special exercise training program after his last CCU admission 6 months ago, with the goal of improving his daily functioning and prognosis. At discharge from his last admission, Z.B. had an ejection fraction of 38%, but on this admission, the ejection fraction has decreased to only 28%.

The RN assigned to care for Z.B. is a recent graduate who has just completed his orientation period to the CCU. He wonders how Z.B.'s exercise program may have contributed (positively or negatively) to the current health crisis. The RN also is concerned about implementing even simple daily care activities, such as turning Z.B. to make his bed or bathing him, given the decline in his cardiac functioning as indicated by the low ejection fraction. The charge nurse tells the RN that she recently read a nursing study regarding the effects of position change on $SvO_2$ (mixed venous oxygen

saturation) in critically ill patients with a low ejection fraction. According to the charge nurse, the study findings indicate that changing the positions of these critically ill patients generally is safe. The RN decides to find and read this article and to search for additional information about the effects of movement and exercise on cardiac functioning. He finds the article, entitled "Effect of positioning on $SvO_2$ in the critically ill patient with a low ejection fraction" (Gawlinski & Dracup, 1998). He also finds an online article that is a synthesis of current research about exercise and heart failure, entitled "Exercise in heart failure: A synthesis of current research" (Adams & Bennett, 2000). Both articles are available at the Connection Web site and in Appendix A. Read them before you continue with this chapter, so that the examples discussed in the chapter will help you.

We also will return to many of the articles used in the earlier chapters, so you may want to review those. All the articles used as examples are available in full text at the Connection Web site and in Appendix A.

## RESEARCH DESIGNS: WHY ARE THEY IMPORTANT?

As we have considered how to interpret and use research findings in nursing practice, we have been moving from the end of research reports toward the beginning of those reports. We have learned that the conclusions of a report usually do not provide enough information to allow us to fully understand the findings. The usefulness of the study results depends on the sample and the methods used to collect data. We have learned also that various approaches to sampling and data collection have different strengths and weaknesses. Thus, we need to better understand the overall purpose and nature of research designs, because research designs direct the sampling and data collection processes. This chapter discusses research designs to help explain why a study is planned and implemented using any particular research design and how different research designs affect approaches to sampling and data collection, which, in turn, influence the study results and conclusions.

The RN in the clinical case notes that the study of the effects of positioning used an experimental design, but he is not sure why. He also notes that one critique of the many exercise studies described in the synthesis article about heart failure is that there have been too few randomized longitudinal studies. The RN knows that much of nursing research is not experimental and wonders how important experimental design is to the usefulness of research results for practice. He also wonders why more research is not randomized or experimental if that is the "best" type of design to use.

A **research design** is the overall plan for acquiring new knowledge or confirming existing knowledge. In Chapter 1, we said that research is characterized by a systematic approach to gathering information to answer questions, which is in contrast to those approaches that use intuition, seek expert advice, or follow tradition. The research design is the plan for that systematic approach, conducted in a way that ensures the answer(s) found will be as meaningful and accurate as possible. The research design identifies how subjects will be recruited and incorporated into the study, what will happen during the study, including timing of any treatments and measures, and when the study will end. A research design is selected with two broad purposes: (1) to plan an approach that will best answer the research question and (2) to ensure the rigor and validity of the results. We will discuss each of these purposes in general terms, and then we will look at specific approaches to research design.

## Answering the Research Question

The first purpose in selecting a research design is to plan a systematic collection of information that will answer the research question of interest. Two considerations are important: (1) the fit of the design to the research question and (2) the functionality of the design for the purpose of the study. *Fit* refers to how well the design matches the question of interest. It is in considering fit that we begin to address the question the RN in our vignette has asked about why all research is not experimental. In the simplest terms, not all research questions can be answered through experiments, because experimental designs answer questions that require a lot of knowledge. For example, simply setting up an experiment would not answer a research question regarding the characteristics of student nurses who select nonacute settings for their first practice after graduation. Why? Because an experiment assumes that we know some factors that we want to manipulate to see if and how they affect an outcome. If we do not know what factors are influencing the outcome of interest (in this example, choice of practice after graduation), we have nothing to manipulate!

Research questions can be broadly categorized as questions that seek to describe or understand, questions that seek to connect or relate, and questions that seek to predict or study the effects of manipulation (see Box 9-1). Generally, if we

BOX **9-1**   General Types of Research Questions

- Questions that describe
- Questions that connect or link factors or concepts
- Questions that predict or examine effects of manipulation

do not have adequate knowledge about a phenomenon of interest to nursing, we have to start by describing and understanding it. Once we have some idea of the meaning of the selected aspects of the phenomenon, we can ask questions about connections or relationships among those aspects. Only after we know something about the connections and relationships can we begin to ask questions that seek to predict or manipulate aspects of the phenomenon.

For example, the effect of positioning study uses an experimental design to test how oxygen delivery ($DO_2$) and oxygen consumption ($VO_2$) predict $S\bar{v}O_2$. To ask this question, there already had to be answers to the questions: (1) what physiologic factors affect a patient's overall cardiac output? and (2) is there a relationship between physiologic factors, such as $DO_2$, $VO_2$, position, ejection fraction, and $S\bar{v}O_2$ and cardiac output? The answers are that as oxygen demand and $VO_2$ increase, $DO_2$ must increase and usually does through increased cardiac output. In patients with cardiac failure reflected in low ejection fractions, however, the ventricles may not meet the need for increased output. Oxygen deprivation may develop, as reflected in lowered venous oxygen saturation ($S\bar{v}O_2$). Thus, we know that $VO_2$, $DO_2$, and $S\bar{v}O_2$ are related. Having this knowledge allows us to ask that third type of question: how do the $DO_2$ and $VO_2$ factors predict $S\bar{v}O_2$? An experimental design fits this third type of research question.

A research design must fit the type of question asked to provide appropriate and effective answers. A research design intended to answer questions about prediction will not be useful or appropriate for questions that seek to describe. Similarly, a design meant to allow meaningful description would not answer research questions that seek to predict. The fit of a design to a research question depends on the function of the design. In other words, different research designs serve different functions and, therefore, are particularly suited to specific types of research questions.

The functions of specific research designs can be broadly categorized, just as types of questions can:

1. Designs for describing or understanding
2. Designs for connecting or relating
3. Designs for manipulation and prediction

## CORE CONCEPT

*The type of research question being asked affects the type of research design that will and can be used.*

Two other important considerations are designs that include timing or time as a factor in the study and designs that seek to control or not to control. Although several other factors differentiate types of research designs, the framework we will use for understanding how research designs influence the meaningfulness of research for practice focuses on three factors: (1) the overall function of the design, (2) how time or timing is incorporated into the design, and (3) whether the design seeks to control or not control study factors. Figure 9–1 depicts these three broad factors and how they relate. We will discuss specific designs that fit into each category later in the chapter.

In summary, when deciding upon a research design, a researcher must consider several factors, including the functions of a design and the fit of those functions to the purpose of the research. Research designs differ in terms of the type of questions they can answer, whether they include time as a factor, and whether they focus on control within the study. The fit and functionality of a research design significantly influence whether the study can answer the research question of interest.

**FIGURE 9-1**    **Three broad factors that affect research design and associated terms.**

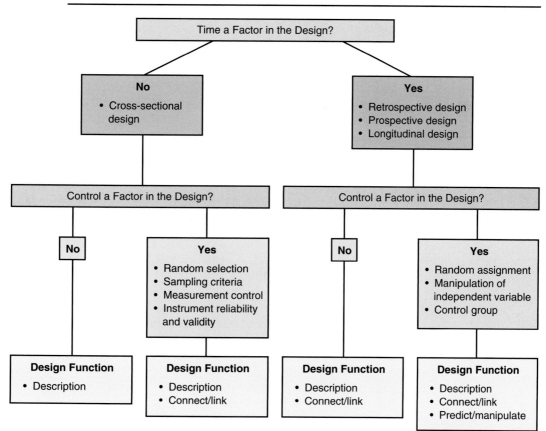

### Ensuring Rigor and Validity

**QUALITATIVE**

In addition to examining function and fit to answer the research question, the research design has as a purpose to ensure the rigor and validity of a study. In Chapter 8, we discussed both rigor and validity in the context of specific strategies for data collection and measurement. The terms rigor and validity also are used in a broader sense to refer to the overall study. In Chapter 8, we said that rigor is both a strict process of data collection and analysis and a term that reflects the overall quality of that process in qualitative research. It is in the broader sense of overall quality that we consider rigor when discussing study design. Study designs in qualitative research usually are nonspecific and flexible and often are described as "emerging" to indicate that the design evolves as the study progresses. Nevertheless, the overall design still must have functions that fit the research question and provide the foundation that ensures the overall rigor of the study.

**QUANTITATIVE**

Like the term rigor, the term validity is used in research to refer both to specific ways that measures can correctly and accurately reflect their intended variable and to the accuracy of the overall results. Although use of the word validity in reference to measurement and to design may be confusing, remember that the word validity always has the same general meaning: accuracy or correctness. Content validity, criterion-related validity, and construct validity all refer to aspects of the accuracy of a measure. Validity of a study refers to its overall accuracy.

Study designs in quantitative research provide the foundation that ensures overall validity. Two types of validity are mentioned frequently when discussing research design. The first type, called **internal validity**, is the extent to which we can be sure of the accuracy or correctness of the findings of the study. Thus, internal validity of a study refers to how accurate the results are within the study itself or internally. The second type, called **external validity**, is the extent to which the results of a study can be applied to other groups or situations. In other words, external validity refers to how accurately the study provides knowledge that can be applied outside of or external to the study itself. Figure 9–2 summarizes and illustrates the relationships among measurement validity, internal validity of a study, and external validity of a study.

Research designs can affect both internal and external validity, and these two types are related in many research designs. Generalizability, discussed in Chapter 6, is a big aspect of external validity, because it refers to the ability to infer that findings for a particular sample can be applied to the entire population. External validity also includes the extent to which the findings from a study in one setting can be applied to other similar settings. Logically, if a study lacks internal validity, it automatically lacks external validity: if the results were not accurate within the study, they clearly will not be accurate in other samples or settings. Similarly, if a study lacks measurement validity, it will lack internal validity. However, a study can have measurement validity and not have internal validity, or it can have correct findings and thus be internally valid but not externally valid. That is, the findings of a study may be real and correct to the specific sample and setting of the study but not applicable to the general population or to other settings. This relationship is illus-

**FIGURE 9-2** **The relationships among measurement validity, internal validity, and external validity.**

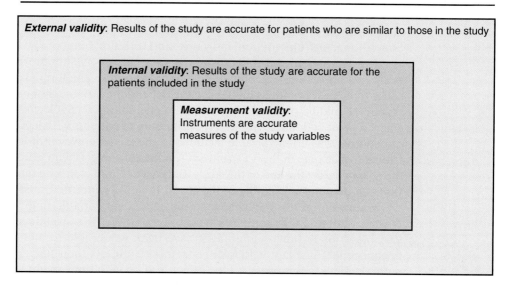

trated in Figure 9–2 by the nesting of the three boxes representing the three types of validity.

Several aspects of study design can potentially lead to problems with internal and external validity. These potential problems are referred to as threats to validity, because they threaten the accuracy of internal findings or the ability to apply the findings to other samples or settings. The threats to internal and external validity often discussed in research literature are listed in Table 9–1.

**TABLE 9-1** **Threats to Internal and External Validity**

| Internal Validity—accuracy of findings within the study | External Validity—accuracy of findings to settings and samples outside of study |
| --- | --- |
| History | Reactivity effects (Hawthorne effect) |
| Maturation | Measurement effects |
| Testing | Novelty effects |
| Instrumentation | Experimenter effects |
| Mortality | |
| Selection bias | |

### *Threats to Internal Validity*

Threats to internal validity are potential problems that can affect the accuracy or correctness of findings within a study. They include problems of history, maturation, testing, instrumentation, mortality, and selection bias.

The threat referred to as **history** is some factor outside those examined in a study that affects the outcome or dependent variable. The term history is used, because some past event has influenced the dependent variable. For example, suppose that in the middle of the study of effect of positioning on $S\bar{v}O_2$ the unit switched to a new type of bed that facilitated repositioning of patients with less effort. The type of bed used was not a variable included in the study; however, it would likely contribute to a change in the $VO_2$ and $S\bar{v}O_2$ values of subjects who were repositioned in the new beds. By the end of the study, the past event of changing types of beds could threaten the internal validity of the study. It would be termed "history."

**Maturation** refers to a change in the dependent variable simply because of the passage of time. In the synthesis article, some studies that examined the dependent variable of daily functioning might have been vulnerable to maturation, because people generally adapt with time to factors that affect their functioning. Thus, the natural adaptation process, a type of maturation with time, might lead to increased daily functioning, regardless of whether the subjects participated in an exercise program. Those studies with a design that did not include a control group would be vulnerable to maturation. We talk more about the role of control groups shortly.

The threat called **testing** refers to changes in a dependent variable that result because it is being measured or because of the measure itself. For example, the mere presence of a nurse taking measurements and recording values might increase a patient's anxiety, changing his or her heart rate and thus $S\bar{v}O_2$ level. Another possible example is a study in which a pretest of depression might make a subject more aware of how bad he or she feels, thus increasing his or her depression. A related threat to internal validity, called **instrumentation**, refers to changing the measures used in a study from one time to another. Instrumentation was not a problem in the study of effect of positioning. If the researchers had changed the protocol for measurement of a variable such as cardiac output, however, the results at the different time points or between different subjects would not be comparable, compromising the results. For example, suppose that the number of injections was changed from three to four or that the timing of the injection in the respiratory cycle changed midway through the study. The change in the measurement might lead to different results; thus, values using the first method would not be directly comparable to values from the revised method.

The last types of threats to internal validity frequently considered when selecting a research design are called mortality and selection bias. We have examined both of these threats in Chapter 6 during the discussion of potential problems with sampling, although we did not use the actual terms mortality and selection bias. **Mortality** refers to the loss of subjects from a study because of a consistent factor related to the dependent variable. Occasionally, the loss of subjects is from death. At other times, mortality refers to subjects withdrawing from a study. The authors of the effects of positioning article do not indicate that any subjects in the study were excluded or lost. Nevertheless, if even 2 or 3 of the 42 critical subjects for this study

**BOX  9-2  Summary of Threats to Internal Validity**

Internal validity is threatened because some *outside factor* **(history)** or *time* **(maturation)** affects the dependent variable, because the *measurement process* itself **(testing)** or *changes* in a manner **(instrumen-** **tation)** affect results for the dependent variable, or because the sampling process is biased *by loss of subjects* **(mortality)** or *selection of subjects* **(selection bias)**.

had died or been dropped from the study, we would have to wonder whether some factor directly related to $S\bar{v}O_2$ led to their death or being dropped and how that factor then affected the accuracy of the findings.

**Selection bias** refers to subjects having unique characteristics that, in some manner, relate to the dependent variable, raising a question whether the findings from the study resulted from the independent variable or the unique characteristics of the sample. Several studies reviewed in the synthesis article used random assignment to a control and to an experimental group, thus avoiding the threat of selection bias. Remember, we examined random assignment in Chapter 6 and learned that when we randomly assign subjects, any possible systematic bias in a sample has an equal chance of being present in the subjects in either group. This negates the potential threat of selection bias when comparing two groups.

Suppose that the effects of positioning study had not used random assignment to the position order but simply varied the order on a regular basis. Further suppose that some of the patients required an additional piece of equipment by the bedside, such as a suction machine, that made it more logical to change a patient's position from supine to left lateral and then to right lateral. As a result, the researchers might have inadvertently introduced selection bias into their study by always selecting the patients who needed the suction machine at the bedside to receive the turning from supine to left and then right. The bias would occur because the health problem that required use of suction might also affect the $S\bar{v}O_2$ during position changes, thus confounding any differences that might occur solely because of the order of position change.

### Threats to External Validity

Threats to external validity are potential problems in a study that affect the accuracy of the results for samples and settings other than those of the study itself. As we said earlier, threats to internal and external validity are related, and, in fact, overlap exists in the language used to describe the different threats. Because we are

## CORE  CONCEPT

*Studies with problems in internal validity automatically will have problems in external validity. Having internal validity, however, does not guarantee that the study will have external validity.*

discussing being able to apply the results of a study to other samples and settings, research literature often refers to threats to external validity as the **effects** of a threat to validity. Several effects are considered when selecting a research study design to ensure external validity. They include the effects of reactivity, measurement, experimenter, and/or novelty.

**Reactivity effects** refer to the responses of subjects to being studied. Threats to internal validity, such as testing, may cause reactivity, such as the example we used earlier of heart rate changing because the nurse was recording values from the monitors. However, reactivity also can occur in a broader sense simply because subjects know they are being studied. For example, the maternal distress study (Miles, Holditch-Davis, Burchinal, & Nelson, 1999) presented in Chapter 8 depended on observing a mother and child for several measures throughout the study. Clearly, the subjects were aware that they were being observed closely, and, although they may not have known what specific aspects of their behavior were being observed, the mere fact of being observed likely changed their behavior somewhat. If being observed, in fact, greatly affected the maternal behavior, the results of that study would differ in settings where behavior was not being observed. This then would be considered a threat to external validity. Another term sometimes used to describe reactivity is the **Hawthorne effect**. This name came from a study at the Hawthorne Electric Plant in which productivity of workers improved simply because they were being studied, no matter what intervention was applied. Reactivity and the Hawthorne effect are the same concept.

**Measurement effects** are changes in the results of a study resulting from the various data collection procedures. This effect sounds similar to instrumentation and testing (threats to internal validity). Remember that any threat to internal validity automatically affects external validity negatively, and overlaps between internal and external validity can get confusing. Just as there are other forms of reactivity effects besides those inherent in threats to internal validity, there are other forms of measurement effects that are not threats to internal validity.

For example, suppose that the placement of a fiber-optic pulmonary artery catheter alone increased $S\bar{v}O_2$ (as far as the author knows, this is not so but is simply used as an example). If the fiber-optic pulmonary artery catheter affected $S\bar{v}O_2$, then the results of the effects of positioning study would be accurate or internally valid, but they would not apply to patients who did not have such a catheter. If fiber-optic pulmonary artery catheters increased $S\bar{v}O_2$, then the measurement used in the study would not have compromised the results of the study itself, because all subjects had the catheter in place. The external validity of that study may be affected, however, because not all patients with low ejection fractions necessarily would have such a catheter.

The last two effects for us to consider are called novelty effects and experimenter effects. Both involve uncontrolled or unmeasured effects from being in a study. **Novelty effects** occur when the knowledge that what is being done is new and under study somehow affects the outcome, either favorably or unfavorably. Once the independent variable is used outside the context of a study, the enthusiasm or doubts that affected the results are no longer present, so that the results are no longer accurate in a setting that is not known to be a study. For example, using a self-help intervention for smoking cessation might be associated with success in quitting smoking in a study, leading the researchers to conclude that the self-help intervention was effective. However, in fact, it was the novelty of the intervention and the subjects' knowledge that it was a new approach that actually led to their success in quitting, and, when the intervention is later used in a clinical setting without a study being implemented, the success rate decreases.

**Experimenter effects** occur when some characteristic of the researcher or data collector influences the study results. For example, subjects may answer the questions the way they believe a researcher wants them to answer, so that results change when subjects are not responding to cues from the researcher.

No matter which threat affects external validity, it reflects some problem with the environment or the research process that may make the results of the study less valid or accurate for other samples or settings. The names of the different effects and threats are intended to reflect the threat or effect, but they can be confusing. What is most important for the RN in our vignette and you to know is that research designs are selected not only for their function and fit to the research question, but also to do the best possible job of ensuring the rigor and validity of the study. To review, rigor refers to the overall quality of a qualitative study, internal validity refers to the accuracy of the overall results within a quantitative study, and external validity refers to the accuracy of the overall results of a quantitative study in relation to settings and samples that are different or external to that study. Different research designs have different strengths and weaknesses in relation to rigor and validity. The next two sections of this chapter describe some of these specific designs considering their functions, timing, and efforts at control.

## QUALITATIVE RESEARCH DESIGNS

Figure 9–3 places qualitative designs within the framework of the broad factors of function, time, and control. As has been said throughout this book, the goal of qualitative research is to gain knowledge that informs our practice broadly and holistically, understanding that all knowing is evolving and contextual. That means that a design or method for a qualitative study will not focus on controlling factors to isolate specific aspects of a phenomenon. Rather, the methods focus on acquiring the richest possible data—that is, data with the greatest complexity and variety. Therefore, the designs intentionally seek to avoid external control over setting and factors.

In this chapter, we said that there are three broad types of research questions: those that seek to describe and understand, those that seek to connect or relate, and those that seek to predict or manipulate. Qualitative research questions seek to describe, understand, and connect or relate, but they do not seek to predict or manipulate. The three broad functions of qualitative research designs are to increase understanding, to promote participation/immersion, and to link ideas and concepts. Designs that function to facilitate understanding answer descriptive questions. Designs that seek to promote participation/immersion answer questions of both description and connection. Designs that seek to link ideas and concepts answer questions of connection or relationship. We will discuss four general types of designs or methods for qualitative research. Within each general method are variations of-

**FIGURE 9-3**    **Three broad factors that affect research design, with associated terms and associated qualitative designs.**

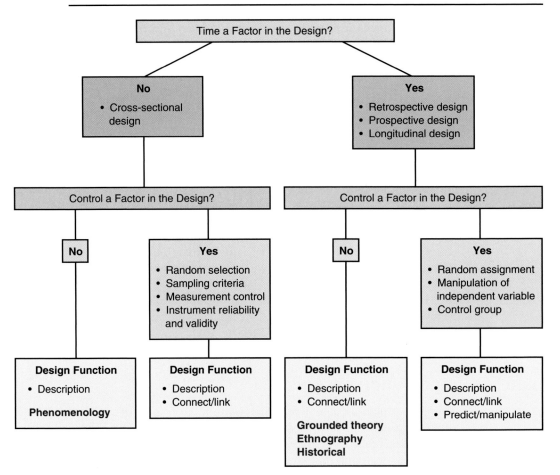

ten associated with the names of the methodologists who developed it. Some reports of qualitative studies use these specific names, rather than the more general method name. It is beyond the scope of this book to describe these variations, but Table 9–2 lists some names frequently connected with each of the four general methods.

## Phenomenology

**Phenomenology**, or the phenomenologic method, is a qualitative method used to discover and develop understanding of experiences as perceived by those living the experience. As with all qualitative studies, the method seeks to avoid external control by going as directly as possible to those who have lived or are living the experience being studied. The method assumes that lived experiences can be interpreted or understood by distilling their essence. The study of satisfaction with care for homeless individuals (McCabe, Macnee, & Anderson, 2001) used phenomenologic

| TABLE 9-2 | Common Names of Methodologists Associated With the Major Qualitative Methods |
|-----------|------------------------------------------------------------------------------|
| **Major method** | **Specific Methodologists** |
| Phenomenology | Parse<br>van Kaam<br>Colaizzi<br>Giorgi<br>Paterson and Zderad<br>Munhall and Boyd<br>van Manen |
| Grounded theory | Glasser and Strauss<br>Strauss and Corbin<br>Stern |
| Ethnography | Goodenough (ethnoscience)<br>Geertz (ethnographic algorithms)<br>Sanday (ethnobehavior)<br>Leininger (ethnonursing) |
| History | Bullough<br>Hamilton |

methods to identify the essence of what satisfactory health care means to a homeless person. It may be helpful to go back and read the methods section of that research report for an example of a study using phenomenology.

There are several variations on the phenomenologic method (Spiegelberg, 1976; van Kaam, 1966; Giorgi, 1971; Colaizzi, 1973), but, in general, the method includes identifying the people who are living or have lived the experience of interest and seeking, usually through unstructured interviewing, their perceptions. As data are collected, the researcher uses the processes of intuiting, analyzing, and describing to discover essential themes in the experience of the phenomenon (Parse, 2001). Skilled interviewing is needed to promote the most open, rich sharing of experiences as participants lived and perceived them. As presented in Chapter 4, phenomenology uses a spiraling process of data collection and analysis, and detailed field notes of observations during data collection augment the richness and fullness of data. Time is not necessarily a major factor in phenomenologic methods, except as the participants in the study experience it. In fact, the method supports seeking participants who are both currently experiencing the phenomenon of interest and have already experienced it to get a breadth of perceptions of experiences. Neither length of time for collecting data nor number of participants is defined before the study starts in phenomenologic methods. Rather, data are collected until all information is redundant of previously col-

lected data–until saturation occurs. Sampling in phenomenology is always a convenience sample, because only those who have had the experience of interest are sought,
and neither limits nor criteria are placed on who can be a participant, other than the
ability to communicate about and having lived the experience. Depending upon the
specific phenomenologic method used, the researcher often starts by identifying his or
her own perceptions or expectations about the phenomenon to be studied and then
attempts to consciously bracket them—hold them separate—so that they will not
color either the data collection or the analysis process (Spiegelberg, 1976).

In the satisfaction with care study (McCabe et al., 2001), the authors describe
going to various settings, including a soup kitchen and shelters, to interview homeless people. The authors all worked with homeless clients, giving them insight into
the experience of homelessness. The interviews consisted of only three unstructured
questions: What was homelessness like for the participants? What did health mean
to them? What had been good and bad experiences with health care? The duration
of each interview and the overall study were not established ahead of time. The
number of participants reflected the point of data saturation. The sample is described as purposive, because people who were homeless and had experiences with
health care were sought for the study. No effort was made, however, to control factors such as gender, race, age, or length of time homeless. This study highlights the
major characteristics of the phenomenologic method.

## Ethnography

The second method commonly used in qualitative research is the ethnographic
method or **ethnography** (Spradley, 1979). A closely related method that was developed by Leininger (1991) within nursing is called ethnonursing. This method originated in the discipline of anthropology, and its purpose is for the researcher to
participate or to immerse himself or herself in a culture to describe a phenomenon
or phenomena within the context of that culture. Ethnography and ethnonursing assume that culture exists, even though it is not visible, and that the only way to know
a culture is to get both an insider's view and an outsider's perspective. The insider's
view is sometimes called an emic perspective. The study of Mexican American family survival (Niska, 2001) from Chapter 4 used an ethnographic method to understand family survival within the Mexican American culture. Reviewing that study
report will give you an example of this method.

Again, controlling the environment or aspects of the study is not part of this qualitative method. The researcher tries to become part of the culture studied to acquire
an insider's understanding that he or she can then translate into a common language
understood by those outside the culture (Spradley, 1979). Because cultures are, by
nature, complex, ethnographic methods take time, and the concept of time itself may
be studied within the culture, but there is no set use of time within the method itself.
That means that there is no structured plan concerning when data are collected or
when the study ends. In general, data are collected as they happen and as opportunities present themselves, although the researcher may seek specific opportunities to
interact within the culture. The researcher collects and analyzes data simultaneously,
so that he or she immediately uses knowledge gained to guide additional data collection. Therefore, there is no structured format for the collection of data.

In the family survival article (Niska, 2001), the author tells us that she lived within the research area with Mexican American families not in the study. She gives this information to indicate her immersion within the culture that she was studying. The general purpose of this research was to characterize family goals of survival, continuity, and growth from the perspective of Mexican American parents, recognizing this as a unique cultural community. Some other aspects of ethnographic methods are less obvious in this particular article, because the author does not directly talk about cultural aspects in Mexican American families. The entire study, however, reflects the unique culture of Mexican American families. In addition to studies with recognized cultural groups, ethnographic methods frequently are used in nursing to describe unique subcultures, such as adolescent drug users, people living in homeless shelters, and people residing in halfway houses.

## Grounded Theory

**Grounded theory** is the third qualitative method commonly used in nursing research (Glaser & Strauss, 1967). The function of grounded theory is to study interactions to understand and to recognize links between ideas and concepts or, in other words, to develop theory. The term "grounded" refers to the idea that the theory developed is based upon or grounded in participants' reality rather than on theoretical speculation. Grounded theory is best used to study social processes and structures, hence the focus on links and interactions among ideas or categories. The article about trajectory of certain death (Steele, 2000) from Chapter 8 used a grounded theory method and provides a good example of this method.

Grounded theory methods often incorporate time into the study, because the focus usually is on processes or change. The method itself, however, does not specify any particular timing to the data collection and analysis process. Sampling in grounded theory usually will be purposive—that is, purposely seeking participants experiencing the process or changes under study (Strauss & Corbin, 1994). Data collection in grounded theory can include interviews and careful observation of interactions and processes. As with all qualitative methods, grounded theory has as a goal avoiding placing limits or external controls on the processes being studied, because the function of the method is to ground theory in natural reality.

In the trajectory of certain death article (Steele, 2000), the author comments that the grounded theory method was particularly appropriate to her research question because she was interested in studying families, and grounded theory focuses on social processes, such as those within families. The author also tells us that she used both interviews and observation to collect data and that she shared results of analysis with the families and used them as the basis for second interviews to develop the theory. The results describe social processes over time, such as "navigating uncharted territory," demonstrating that the function of the method is to describe processes and linkages.

## Historical

The last general qualitative method sometimes used in nursing research is called the **historical** research method. Its function is to answer questions about links in the past to understand the present or to plan the future. Historical research methods require the researcher to define a phenomenon in a manner that can be clearly delineated so that data sources can be identified. For example, a phenomenon that might lend itself to historical research is to understand the process of nurse practitioners' legitimization as health care providers. Nurse practitioner legitimization, however, is too undefined to be approached using the historical method, because it is not clear what time period or data sources would be relevant. The phenomenon of credentialing of nurse practitioners as a vehicle to legitimization of the role, on the other hand, defines a focus for data sources, as well as a time period, because the development of credentialing occurred throughout a definable number of years. Data sources in this example would target the development and implementation of the process of credentialing nurse practitioners and how that process related to perceptions of the legitimacy of the role of nurse practitioners.

Data sources in historical research may include records, videotapes, photographs, and interviews with people involved in the phenomenon, or review of published reports. As with the other qualitative methods discussed, the researcher tries to acquire as broad a sample of data sources as possible. Unlike the other methods, in the historical method, a focus of data collection includes evaluation of data sources for their reliability. For example, an editorial in the *Journal of the American Medical Association* regarding the process of nurse practitioner credentialing might reflect a bias that makes the description of the process questionable. That same editorial, however, might be a reliable data source about the professional climate in which credentialing developed. A researcher using the historical method would evaluate the data source and consider this potential bias when deciding how to use it.

We have not had a research study that used the historical method as an example in this text. An example of research using that method is an article on the use of side rails in American hospitals (Brush & Capezuti, 2001). You can find this article on the connection Web site and in Appendix C.

We have now discussed four different methods used in qualitative research, the functions of which vary. Phenomenologic methods provide in-depth data about a particular life experience and, therefore, are particularly useful in answering descriptive questions. Ethnographic methods provide immersion and active participation in a particular culture or subculture and are useful in answering both descriptive and connection/linkage questions. Grounded theory methods provide data about social interactions, which can be built into a theory based on reality. Grounded theory methods are particularly useful in answering questions about interactions or links among social processes. Historical methods provide data about past processes to gain insight about the present and future. They answer questions about links/connections. All the qualitative methods we have examined specifically attempt to avoid introducing external control into the study design because all are interested in gathering data that are as complex and rich as the real world. Nevertheless, all four methods entail a systematic process for sampling, data acquisition, and data analysis. Strict criteria for timing are not part of any of the methods, but time is an inherent component of the historical method, is often a part of the culture studied using ethnography, and is usually an aspect of interactional processes reported in grounded theory studies.

Throughout this section discussing qualitative design, the word "methods" has been used more frequently then the word "design." That is because design suggests a more formalized and standardized plan than is often present within qualitative methods. Qualitative research designs are consciously and intently unstructured and flexible to reflect the unpredictable and complex nature of phenomena as they occur in life. As we will see in the next section that discusses quantitative designs, the word design is more appropriate in quantitative research, because quantitative methods seek to standardize and to formalize the process of sampling, data collection, and data analysis.

## QUANTITATIVE RESEARCH DESIGNS

We will once again use the three broad factors of function, time, and control to categorize quantitative designs (Figure 9–4). The language used to describe quantitative designs can be confusing initially, because terms are used in different

**FIGURE 9-4** **Three broad factors that affect research design and associated terms and quantitative designs.**

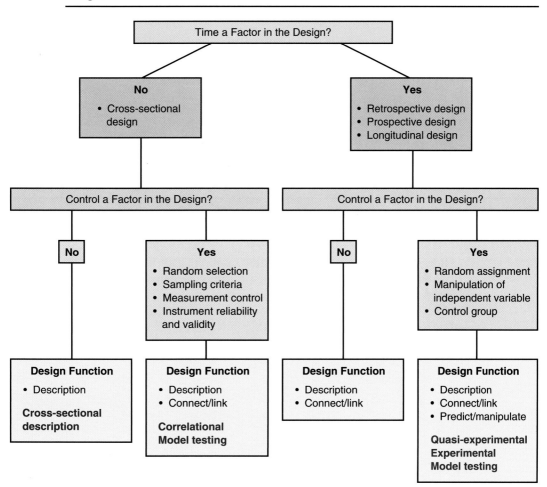

combinations to define different methods. Rather than start with the functions of different designs, we start by discussing the language used to address time and control when discussing quantitative research design.

### Time

Whereas time is a factor to study or to incorporate into the fabric of a method in qualitative research, time is a specific factor that defines different research designs in quantitative research. Quantitative designs are described as either **retrospective** or **prospective**. Retrospective designs are designs in which data are collected about past events or factors. Prospective designs are designs in which data are collected about events or variables as they occur, moving forward in time. In addition to considering whether data are collected moving backward or forward in time, designs are described in terms of point of time of measurement. Research designs are **cross-sectional** if they collect data all at one point in time. Research designs are called **longitudinal** if they collect data at different time points. Therefore, a prospective study automatically is longitudinal as well. A cross-sectional study, however, does not have to be retrospective.

Consider a study of patient satisfaction with care. A retrospective and cross-sectional study would collect data from patients at some point after they visit a clinic, perhaps 1 or 2 weeks later, and ask them to recall their level of satisfaction during their visit. Data are collected at one time point looking at past experience. A study of patient satisfaction that surveys patients as they leave a clinic also would be cross-sectional, because data are collected at only one time point for each subject. However, it would not be retrospective, because it is not going back in time; data are being collected about present variables. A prospective longitudinal patient satisfaction study might collect data before a visit to a clinic, immediately after the visit, and 1 week later, looking for changes in selected variables over time. At each measurement point, the question might be "How satisfied are you right now with the clinic care?" Thus, data are not being collected about past experiences or perceptions, even when they are collected 1 week after the visit.

From this example, it should be clear that it is a combination of factors that define research designs in quantitative research. This idea is important to grasp.

Terms used to describe the use of time in quantitative research designs include those we have discussed and another important term: repeated measures. **Repeated measures** mean just what the words say–a design using repeated measures repeats the same measurements at several points in time. When you see the term repeated measures, it suggests that a variable or variables were measured more than just two

---

## CORE CONCEPT

*The labels for quantitative research designs usually are combinations of words or terms that define the design in terms of function, use of time, and use of approaches to provide control.*

or three times, and you can expect that the analysis of the study examines the pattern of change in the variable over time.

A longitudinal prospective study may or may not have repeated measures. We have reviewed several longitudinal studies throughout this book, but only some of them included repeated measures. For example, the fecal incontinence study (Bliss, Johnson, Savik, Clabots, & Gerding, 2000) in Chapter 2 was longitudinal and used repeated measures, because the same data about the same variables were collected in the same way regularly over time. This included data about number of stools, consistency of stools, and rectal swabs for culture. In contrast, the longitudinal prospective study of maternal distress and growth from Chapter 8 (Miles et al., 1999) repeated only 6 of the 12 measures used in the study. Variables such as depression were measured at two of the five time points in the study, but the variable parental stress was measured only at one time point. Although some measures were used more than once, the maternal distress and growth study would not be considered a design using repeated measures.

## Control

In addition to differences in how they consider the factor of time, quantitative research designs differ in the amount of control of extraneous factors that they attempt to impose on a study. Remember that quantitative research seeks to clearly define and to measure specific variables. To do so, research designs seek to ensure that outside factors not specifically defined and measured in the study are not allowed to affect what is included in the study. Outside or extraneous factors not considered and measured within a quantitative study are sources of error. In Chapter 8, we discussed error in measurement in relation to measurement reliability and validity. We are now considering error in a broader manner, just as we examined validity of an entire study previously in the chapter. Designs in quantitative research seek to ensure the internal and external validity of the study by minimizing error. They do so by imposing different controls on the sampling, data collection, and analysis.

The areas within which research designs seek to create or to impose control include the sampling process and the measurement process. Control in the sampling process can be imposed by establishing criteria for inclusion or exclusion that attempt to prevent some outside difference among subjects from confusing the findings of the study. Another method of control in the sampling process is the use of random sampling, by which the entire population is enumerated and all have an equal chance of being asked to be in the study. A third way to create control in the sampling process is random assignment, because all subjects have an equal chance of being included in any particular group in the study. Thus, any differences in the subjects will likely be distributed equally within different groups that will be compared. We reviewed each of these approaches to control in Chapter 6. Quantitative research designs partly reflect and define the sampling approach that a study will take.

Control within the data collection process can be imposed by ensuring the validity and reliability of the measures or by ensuring that the measurement process itself is consistent, avoiding instrumentation threats. Control in measurement also can be imposed by creating comparison group(s), so that either exposure to the factors studied is manipulated in a controlled fashion or the timing of the measurement process is manipulated around a factor of interest. Studies designs that include a **comparison group** create control by comparing subjects in two groups who differ in an independent variable of interest. Inclusion of a comparison group eliminates such threats to internal validity as history and maturation, because both groups experience the same history or process of maturation. A design using a comparison group attempts to ensure that two groups are as similar as possible on most factors that could affect the dependent variable of interest and assume that they differ clearly in an independent variable. Therefore, such designs hope to isolate the influence of that independent variable on the dependent variable of interest. Study designs that include a **control group** create a greater level of control by manipulating the independent variable of interest so that the control group is not exposed to it, whereas the experimental group is. Again, a dependent variable is examined for differences to see if the factor manipulated affected that dependent variable.

## Functions of Quantitative Research Designs

Having considered the factors of time and control, we now discuss specific quantitative designs considering these two factors, as well as overall function. Quantitative research designs vary in the level of control that they impose from limited in descriptive and correlational studies to more control in quasi-experimental studies to the most control in true experimental designs.

### Descriptive Designs and Correlational Studies

**Descriptive** designs function to portray as accurately as possible some phenomenon of interest. **Correlational** studies use a descriptive design to describe as accurately as possible interrelationships among variables. Researchers generally consider studies that look at correlations to be a subtype of descriptive designs and refer to them as "studies" rather than the broader term "design." Clearly, descriptive designs are used to answer research questions that seek to describe. Correlational studies are used to answer research questions that seek to link or connect. Both types focus on exerting control through the quality of the measurement—that is, by using reliable and valid measures as discussed in Chapter 8—and through sampling criteria or procedures. Descriptive and correlational studies may impose control by establishing certain criteria for inclusion or exclusion from the study. Remember, this also can be called purposive sampling or use of a convenience sample. Both types of design can impose even greater control over extraneous factors by using randomly selected samples.

Descriptive and correlational designs can be longitudinal or cross-sectional, and they can be retrospective or prospective. Decisions about how time is a factor are based on the nature of the question, the potential sample, and the measures. Some phenomena, such as growth or productivity, clearly entail a time element that would make it logical for a researcher to use a longitudinal design. As we discussed in Chapter 6, however, finding, following, and maintaining subjects over time can be difficult and costly, so some studies may use a single cross-sectional design to avoid problems of following subjects over time. Certainly, some measures can be repeated easily, whereas others cannot, because they measure stable concepts unlikely to change or because the measurement process is too intrusive to repeat often. For example, the concept of an individual's sense of coherence is a stable sense of the world and oneself within the world and, although a researcher may be interested in measuring this as a variable in a study, it would not be helpful to measure it more than once, because it will remain stable. An example of an intrusive measure might be a bone marrow analysis. It could be that data from weekly bone marrow tests would be ideal in evaluating a new cancer drug. However, this test is too intrusive and painful to repeat at that kind of interval.

A special type of correlational study is a design for **model testing**. A model is the symbolic framework for a theory or part of a theory. In Chapter 2, we discussed Lazarus's Theory of Stress, also shown as a model in Figure 9–5. A design testing such a model identifies measures for each concept and examines how the concepts relate. A study testing Lazarus's theory would identify ways to measure the variables of personal beliefs and resources, event, primary appraisal, secondary appraisal, and stress. Then the study would statistically analyze relationships among the results of these measurements of the variables to see if the relationships found were of the type and direction predicted by the model.

Often designs for model testing are longitudinal, so that some parts of the model are measured at one time point and other aspects are measured at a second, later time point. This allows researchers to propose causal relationships between concepts in the model. Therefore, model testing designs often attempt to answer questions that predict as well as relate.

An example of a study that used a model testing design is the study of factors associated with tuberculosis (TB) screening discussed in Chapters 4 and 5 (Poss, 2000). In that study, the model is a combination of two theories and is shown in Figure 1 in the article (Poss, 2000, p. 21). Data were collected at three time points: before screening, at the time of screening, and when screening results were read. For example, measures of intention to get a purified protein derivative (PPD) before screening were measured and then tested for their statistical relationship with behavior at a later time point, thus examining how much intention to do a health behavior may actually predict actions related to that behavior. A model that is tested in research predicts certain relationships. The model testing design allows the researcher to see if, indeed, those relationships were present in a particular setting and sample.

**FIGURE 9-5    Schematic model of Lazarus's Theory of Stress.**

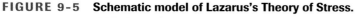

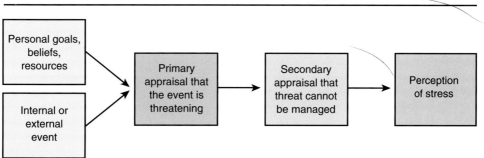

In summary, descriptive designs function to portray a phenomenon of interest and may be retrospective, prospective, cross-sectional, or longitudinal. They also may impose varying levels of control through sampling strategies, such as purposive samples or random sampling. Correlational designs function to describe or to identify interrelationships among factors of interest; they also may be retrospective, prospective, cross-sectional, or longitudinal. Because correlational designs describe relationships, occasionally you will see them called "descriptive correlational designs." Correlational designs may use the same range of sampling strategies used in descriptive designs. Model testing designs are a special type of correlational design that usually incorporate time in some manner, either through longitudinal data collection or through use of measures that combine retrospective and concurrent data collection.

### Quasi-Experimental and Experimental Research Designs

Quasi-experimental and experimental research designs function to answer questions involving prediction and the effects of manipulation. Quasi-experimental designs differ from experimental designs primarily in the amount of control that they impose. Both types include control of an independent variable, but a true **experimental design** always includes a control group and random assignment to groups. Remember, a control group is a group of subjects who do not receive an intervention, so that the control group can be compared to those who do receive the intervention.

When researchers discuss quasi-experimental and experimental designs, they often use a set of symbols to diagram the particular form of design used. When they do this, they use the symbol "O" to indicate occasion of observation or measurement, with a subscript number designating the time point of the observation. They use the letter "X" to denote the intervention, meaning the independent variable, and they use "R" to denote that subjects were randomly assigned to groups. Figure 9–6 is an example of this type of diagram. It translates to mean that two groups were formed using random assignment (R). Each group had measurements taken ($O_1$), one group received the intervention (X), and both groups had a second measurement taken ($O_2$). This design includes manipulation of the independent variable, random assignment, and a control group; therefore, it is experimental. Because it includes an observation both before and after the intervention, the type of design in Figure 9-6 is called a **pretest-posttest** experimental design.

Although most experimental and quasi-experimental designs are longitudinal, it is possible for an experiment to be implemented at only one time point. Figure 9–7 shows how a single-time-point experimental design would look. Because experi-

---

**BOX  9-3  Components of Experimental Designs**

- Manipulation of the independent variable
- Random assignment of subjects to groups
- A control group

**FIGURE 9-6**    **Schematic of pretest–posttest experimental design.**

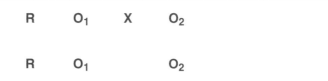

$$R \qquad O_1 \qquad X \qquad O_2$$

$$R \qquad O_1 \qquad\qquad O_2$$

mental designs always involve manipulation of an independent variable, they are never retrospective. Finally, a term sometimes associated with experimental design is **multifactorial**, which refers to several independent variables being manipulated in a study. The examples we have considered have all had a single independent variable; however, some studies control and manipulate two or more independent variables.

A **quasi-experimental** design lacks both a control group and random assignment. It may not include two groups at all. Instead, it may involve a series of observations, followed by an intervention and then another series of observations (Figure 9–8). In this case, there is manipulation of the independent variable but no control group. The threats to internal validity in this type of design include instrumentation and testing, as well as selection bias and mortality. There also are quasi-experimental designs that have two groups of subjects, but the groups are nonequivalent, because subjects are not randomly assigned to each group. Such a design is referred to as a nonequivalent control group pretest-posttest quasi-experimental design, and it entails observations of two groups, followed by one group receiving the intervention and then a second set of observations. Because both groups receive the same measurement, this quasi-experimental design is less threatened by instrumentation and testing but still is threatened by selection bias and mortality. Thus, a rather long name for a design tells us a great deal about how the research study was implemented.

The effect of positioning study that the RN in our vignette found is described as "an experimental two-group repeated-measures design" (Gawlinski & Dracup, 1998, p. 293). In reading the article, we learn that there were two groups of patients and that patients were randomly assigned to the groups. The independent variable (the variable manipulated in this study) was the order in which the subjects' positions were changed. We said that to be experimental, a design must include manipulation of an independent variable, a control group, and random assignment. There is no real control group in the effect of positioning study. Both groups receive positioning changes, but they differ in the order of the changes. This design stretches the definition of experimental. It is considered experimental because two groups were randomly assigned and subjects served as their own controls, with their $S\bar{v}O_2$ values after being turned compared with their values before being turned. The use of the

**FIGURE 9-7**    **Schematic of an experimental design with only one point of measurement.**

$$R \qquad X \qquad O_1$$

$$R \qquad\qquad O_1$$

**FIGURE 9-8**    **Schematic of repeated measures quasi-experimental design.**

$$O_1 \quad O_2 \quad O_3 \quad O_4 \quad X \quad O_5 \quad O_6 \quad O_7 \quad O_8$$

term experimental for this study demonstrates just how complex the language of research design can become.

The other phrase used to describe the design in the study of effect of position change is "repeated measures." We have already said that this phrase means that multiple measures of the same variable were taken over time. In the effect of positioning article, measures were taken before turning, immediately upon turning, and every minute for 5 minutes, then at 15 and 25 minutes, for a total of eight $S\bar{v}O_2$ measures. This is a good example of the frequency of measures you would expect if a design is said to use "repeated measures."

The article discussed in Chapter 3 that evaluated the effects of three types of HIV risk-reduction programs (Nyamathi, Flaskerud, Leake, Dixon, & Lu, 2001) is an example of a study that used a quasi-experimental design. That study had three interventions and used random assignment of the interventions to shelters rather than random assignment of individual subjects to the interventions. We discussed in Chapter 3 the possibility that selected shelters housed women with common characteristics, which may have created significant differences in the groups that received the intervention. Therefore, the lack of true random assignment to the intervention groups and the lack of a control group make this study quasi-experimental.

In summary, the language used to describe quantitative research designs reflects their function, such as descriptive, correlational, or experimental. Other language used to describe designs reflects how time is a component, such as retrospective, cross-sectional, or longitudinal. Finally, the language of designs reflects the level of control imposed in the study, with experimental designs imposing the greatest control over extraneous variables. We have reviewed several of the studies used throughout this book as examples of various designs. To provide familiar examples of several research designs, Table 9–3 categorizes each of the 10 studies in this text according to type of research design used.

## HOW CAN ONE GET THE WRONG DESIGN FOR THE RIGHT QUESTION?

Let us return to the question our RN in the vignette was considering about why all studies are not experimental. We have already addressed one part of the answer to that question: the research question must ask about prediction or the effects of manipulation before an experimental design will fit. For a question to seek to examine effects of manipulation or to predict, we must have certain baseline knowledge already in place. The other reason that experimental designs are not the right design for every question involves the strengths and weaknesses of the design itself. Experimental designs are strong on control; therefore, they have the fewest threats to internal validity. That same control, however, makes experiments dissimilar from the "real" world of patient care, where variety and complexity are the rule. Therefore, generally the results of a study using an experimental design are accurate, and we can trust highly that the findings are correct. However, the findings may not be

**TABLE 9-3  Categorization of Research Designs of the Ten Articles Used in This Text**

| Chapter and Reference | Research Design |
|---|---|
| Chapter 1: Lipman, T. H., Hayman, L. L., Favian, C. V., DiFazio, D. A., Hale, P. M., Goldsmith, B. M., et al. (2000). Risk factors for cardiovascular disease in children with type I diabetes. *Nursing Research, 49*(3), 160–166. | Descriptive, mixed longitudinal |
| Chapter 2: Bliss, Z. B., Johnson, S., Savik, K., Clabots, C. R., & Gerding, D. N. (2000). Fecal incontinence in hospitalized patients who are acutely ill. *Nursing Research, 49*(2), 101–108. | Prospective, longitudinal, repeated measures |
| Chapter 3: McCabe, S., Macnee, C. L., & Anderson, M. K. (2001). Homeless patients' experience of satisfaction with care. *Archives of Psychiatric Nursing, XV*(2), 78–85. | Phenomenology |
| Chapter 3: Nyamathi, A., Flaskerud, J. H., Leake, B., Dixon, E. L., & Lu, A. (2001). Evaluating the impact of peer, nurse case-managed, and standard HIV risk-reduction programs on psychosocial and health-promoting behavioral outcomes among homeless women. *Research in Nursing and Health, 24*, 410–422. | Quasi-experimental |
| Chapters 4–5: Niska, K. J. (2001). Mexican American family survival, continuity, and growth: The parental perspective. *Nursing Science Quarterly, 14*(4), 322–329. | Ethnography |
| Chapters 4–5: Poss, J. E. (2000). Factors associated with participation by Mexican migrant farmworkers in a tuberculosis screening program. *Nursing Research, 49*(1), 20–28. | Correlational Model Testing |
| Chapter 8: Steele, R. G. (2000). Trajectory of certain death at an unknown time: Children with neurodegenerative life-threatening illnesses. *Canadian Journal of Nursing Research, 32*(3), 49–67. | Grounded theory |
| Chapter 8: Miles, M. S., Holditch-Davis, D., Burchinal, P., & Nelson, D. (1999). Distress and growth outcomes in mothers of medically fragile infants. *Nursing Research, 48*(3), 129–140. | Longitudinal, multivariate |
| Chapter 9: Adams, C. D., & Bennett, S. (2000). Exercise in heart failure: A synthesis of current research. *The Online Journal of Knowledge Synthesis for Nursing, 7*(5). | Systematic review |
| Chapter 9: Gawlinski, A., & Dracup, K. (1998). Effect of positioning on $S\bar{v}O_2$ in the critically ill patient with a low ejection fraction. *Nursing Research, 47*(5), 293–299. | Experimental |

easily applied or generalized to clinical practice, where many of the factors controlled in the experiment will not be controlled.

For example, subjects in the effect of positioning article had to receive a two-dimensional echocardiograph or radionuclide ventriculography to confirm that their ejection fraction was lower than 30%. They also needed a fiber-optic pulmonary artery catheter in place, and they could not have a diagnosis of septic shock. The availability of technology to confirm ejection fraction reflects a certain level of hospital and, in most cases, a certain level of insurance coverage. Thus, uninsured patients and those from rural settings without access to tertiary care centers were probably underrepresented or not represented in this study. Yet, being uninsured or living in a rural setting are factors that may affect physiologic functioning and resilience. The very controls that ensured that the patients did have low ejection fractions and allowed the measurement of $S\bar{v}O_2$ without unnecessary intrusion also may limit the generalizability of the study. In reality, the controls exerted in this particular study probably do not greatly influence the utility of the results for more general practice; however, this example gives you an idea of why the aspects that provide control in a design also may limit the clinical usefulness of the results.

Quasi-experimental studies lose some of the internal validity of an experimental design but often gain some applicability to real life. Often, a quasi-experimental design is selected to answer a research question when implementing a true experimental design is not feasible. For example, the researchers studying HIV-prevention programs would have faced great difficulty randomly assigning homeless women to different programs, because homeless people generally do not follow schedules or have circumstances that would enable them to attend programs not located conveniently. If the researchers had tried to implement several different programs in one shelter (randomly assigning the women in the shelter to a program), it is likely that the women would have shared activities from the different programs, causing the programs to blur and making it impossible to isolate the effects of one compared to the other. Had the researchers been testing HIV-prevention programs with high school students, they might have more easily randomly assigned subjects and created a true experiment. Nevertheless, results with high school students would not be easy to apply to the different lives and experiences of homeless women. Therefore, the very control possible with high school students would preclude the study being as useful for homeless women.

As we move to descriptive and correlational designs, control decreases even further, because the researcher no longer controls the independent variable. Selection criteria or random selection, however, can still provide some control. In addition, measurement reliability and validity increase our confidence about the accuracy of the factors being studied. Because descriptive and correlational designs still impose control through sampling and measurement, however, the richness and diversity of real-life clinical situations is limited. Phenomenologic, ethnographic, and grounded theory designs impose the least control over the process of research and, therefore, capture the greatest detail and depth of real experiences. Yet, they can become so subjective or conceptual that the results also may be difficult to apply to real practice. Qualitative designs are not intended to develop knowledge about predictions; however, we often seek knowledge that will allow us to predict in nursing.

Therefore, the answer to the question, "How can one get the wrong design for the right question?" involves feasibility in terms of who or what is being studied, what measures are available, and what is already known about the problem or phenomenon. A study of the process of tobacco addiction cannot ethically manipulate the variable of exposure to tobacco, so it will, by necessity, be nonexperimental. A study of drug efficacy requires careful control of as many extraneous factors as possible, lending itself to experimental design. However, withholding drug treatment in some cases may be unethical, leading to the use of quasi-experimental design. Studies of subjective experiences, such as pain, grief, or satisfaction, require understanding best acquired through seeking the insights of those who have experienced or are experiencing the phenomenon, lending themselves to qualitative designs. Yet, a researcher may not be skilled in qualitative methods and so may choose a cross-sectional descriptive design instead.

What should be evident at this point is that study design shapes the approach taken to sampling, measurement, and data analysis. Understanding the basic language of design will allow you to understand many of the decisions made by the researcher(s) regarding the study, clarifying the approaches taken to acquiring subjects or participants and to the data collection itself. Recognizing that the terms used in quantitative design are combined differently to specify the function, control, and time factor in a design will help you to better understand the types of designs described in published research.

In addition to terms that reflect the function of and the use of control and time in a design, some designs are described as **mixed methods**. Mixed method refers to some combination of methods in relation to function, time, or control. The first study we discussed in Chapter 1 about risk factors in children with type 1 diabetes states that the study method was "mixed-longitudinal" (Lipman et al., 2000). In fact, the study collected retrospective data when it asked parents to complete a questionnaire about family history, their children's activity, and smoking behavior. This is an example of collecting data about how things were, thinking back in time. In addition, this study collected data concurrently about Tanner stage, cholesterol, blood pressure, and $HgA_1$. The authors call the study longitudinal, because it linked data from the past about activity, history, and smoking with data from the present about blood pressure, cholesterol, and $HgA_1$.

Another use of the term mixed method is to refer to a combination of qualitative and quantitative methods. The fictional article about nursing students' choices of clinical practice used a somewhat mixed method, because it included data collection using a pen-and-paper quantifiable questionnaire and a written open-ended question that was analyzed using methods associated with qualitative research. As nursing research develops, more and more researchers are recognizing the value of both qualitative and quantitative methods to more fully answer questions of interest to nursing. This has led to increased use of a combination of qualitative and quantitative designs in single studies.

Before beginning this chapter, you were asked to consider how you might best conduct a study of the effects of nursing school attendance on well-being. Now that we have examined various research designs and some of the advantages and disadvantages to each, let us consider what would be some choices you would need to make if you were going to conduct such a study.

First, you could approach a study of the effects of nursing school attendance on well-being from a qualitative perspective or a quantitative perspective. The decision would depend partly on what is already known, such as what is known about influences on well-being in college students, how nursing programs differ from other undergraduate programs, and whether nursing students differ from other undergraduate students in some important ways that might affect well-being. If little is known about any of these factors, a qualitative study of the lived experiences of nursing students in terms of sense of well-being while in school might be the research design to use. If little is known about well-being and nursing students, a researcher might implement a grounded theory design to examine interactions that affect well-being.

A researcher also might decide to do a descriptive correlational study measuring well-being and other factors that would logically be relevant, such as general health, age, family commitments, work schedule, and grade point average, to see how they relate. If implementing a quantitative study, the researcher could decide to do measurements only at one time point and perhaps include students just entering school, those halfway through school, and those preparing to graduate. Such a study would be cross-sectional. To address problems with internal validity, the researcher would need to consider how comparable students in the three different classes were in factors that affect well-being other than nursing school attendance.

Alternately, a researcher might decide to do a longitudinal study following a group of nursing students from the time they enter school to graduation. This type of study would take much time and many resources; it also would be open to such threats to internal validity as mortality, testing, and instrumentation. The question of effects of nursing school attendance and well-being probably does not lend itself to or fit with either quasi-experimental or experimental designs, unless something already has been shown to be a factor that could be manipulated to try to change well-being.

This example demonstrates why studies addressing approximately the same question may use different research designs. As an intelligent user of nursing research, you do not have to decide what type of design to use, but it is helpful for you to understand some considerations that go into selecting a design, as well as the meaning and strengths and weaknesses of different research designs.

## COMMON ERRORS IN PUBLISHED REPORTS OF RESEARCH DESIGNS

As you read published studies, such as those the RN found in our vignette, there may be problems with the information about the study design. One possible problem is a lack of detail about the design, leaving the reader uncertain concerning the methods used. In some cases, the only thing we are told is that a particular method or design was used. This happens more in published reports of qualitative studies than in reports of quantitative studies. This may occur partly because qualitative methods were less well known or used in nursing for some years. A written report of a study design should not simply tell the reader the label for the design; it also should describe enough of the actual process of the research study to assure the reader that the design was implemented appropriately.

For example, a study that states it uses phenomenologic methods also should tell you enough about the subjects to assure you that they were rich and appropriate sources of data and generally both how data were collected and analyzed. A study that tells you it used an experimental design also should provide specific information about the random assignment process, creation of the control group, and manipulation of the intervention.

As with measurement in research, a study design can be complex. Nevertheless, it is the responsibility of the author(s) to communicate in writing all the essential aspects of the design so that the reader can intelligently read and understand the study. The use of a timeline often helps readers to understand a study design, particularly if it is longitudinal. The other aspect that occasionally is lacking in published reports is a rationale for the choice of research design. We have discussed that a researcher has to make several decisions when selecting a research design. Occasionally, the rationales for decisions, such as not including a control group, can help the reader to understand better the problems of the study and how those may affect usefulness for clinical practice.

## PUBLISHED REPORTS—DID DESIGN AFFECT YOUR CONCLUSION?

The RN in our vignette is trying to understand how Z.B.'s exercise program might have influenced current health status, and how concerned he must be about turning Z.B. for activities, such as bed making and bathing. We have discussed the exercise synthesis article only briefly. It is an example of an evidence-based study or synthesis to address a clinical question. The design for a literature synthesis could be called descriptive, because the study samples research studies to reach conclusions about what is known with regard to a particular research question. A literature synthesis describes the current state of our knowledge based on existing research findings. What makes the synthesis article especially appropriate as an example when we are examining research design is that most evidence-based studies focus on research in the form of clinical trials and use as a gold standard those studies that used true experimental designs. **Clinical trials** refer to studies that test the effectiveness of a clinical treatment, and some researchers would say that a clinical trial must be a true experiment. For many problems in clinical practice, however, there have been only a few true experimental studies, so it is not uncommon to see clinical trials defined more broadly, as in the exercise synthesis article.

The questions that must be asked about research synthesis studies are: (1) is the research question appropriate for an evidence-based approach? and (2) was the evidence included in the synthesis appropriate? Considering the question for the synthesis article, the RN concludes that an evidence-based approach is probably one appropriate approach to addressing the question of the role of exercise in heart failure. The fit is good partly because it is a question that lends itself to quantitative studies that can be more readily synthesized than qualitative studies. The fit also is good because several studies already have examined the question.

In the synthesis article about exercise in patients with heart failure, the RN finds that Table 1 (Adams & Bennett, 2000, p. 3) lists the design/patient selection used in each of the studies included in the review. The presence or absence of randomization and a control group is noted in every case, suggesting that the reviewer believes that these aspects of design are important for studies looking at the effects of exercise. Given that the question being asked is one of prediction—how does exercise predict function?—it makes sense that the best design might be experimental. One can speculate, however, that there is a reason many of the studies reviewed did not randomize. Withholding an exercise program by randomly assigning some patients with heart failure to a group that would not receive the exercise program might be considered unethical. It also is likely that some studies focused on simply evaluating the effects of a program—that is, relating the exercise to function after the program, rather than seeking to predict. In that case, the question asked in the study might have best fit the descriptive correlational or quasi-experimental design that was used.

When the RN considers whether the evidence included in the synthesis was appropriate, he recognizes that the emphasis on quasi-experimental and experimental designs means that the evidence is likely to be relatively accurate and not too vulnerable to threats to internal validity. He also recognizes that, with the exception of one study, the samples were relatively small, several studies were limited to men, and interventions tested were diverse, making comparison of the studies difficult.

Nevertheless, given the nature of the question and the evidence from the studies, the RN concludes that Z.B.'s exercise program probably should not have precipitated his worsening condition and may, in fact, improve his prognosis at this point. The RN wonders why so many different exercise training programs were tested instead of just one or two. He will need to read the beginning of several of the research articles themselves to better understand the background that led to different researchers selecting different approaches to exercise training.

The RN's understanding of the strengths and weaknesses of an experimental design also help him to interpret better the effect of positioning study. In particular, the RN notes that the intervention that was the basis for the experiment, the variation in order of position change, did not significantly affect $S\bar{v}O_2$ level. After that result, the researchers analyzed the data with all the subjects in one group, looking at the subjects' own baseline values for $S\bar{v}O_2$ to see how positioning changed them and how $DO_2$ and $VO_2$ were related to $S\bar{v}O_2$. Once the two randomly assigned groups became one group for the analysis of the contributions of $DO_2$ and $VO_2$ to $S\bar{v}O_2$ changes, the effects of randomization were no longer relevant. That then raises questions about selection bias in this study. Nevertheless, the results that indicate that patients with low ejection fractions recovered quickly from position changes, despite an initial 8.5% to 11.3% decrease in $S\bar{v}O_2$, reassure the RN that basic daily care, such as bathing and bed making, will be safe with Z.B. The results also suggest the importance of giving Z.B. an opportunity to recover from each change before making the next change. That is something the charge nurse did not mention to the RN, so he is glad he chose to read the study itself. The RN wonders why the researchers were so concerned about the order of position change. To answer that question, he will have to read the beginning of the article that describes the background for the study and the research problem.

Clearly then, the type of research design used in a study affects the usefulness and meaningfulness of the results for clinical practice. The language of research design is complex and confusing at times, because several terms are used in different ways in different contexts. Nevertheless, it is possible to acquire a good general understanding of the meaning of most of the terms, so that this important aspect of a research study can be understood and interpreted as related to the applicability of the study to clinical practice.

## OUT-OF-CLASS EXERCISE

### How to Set the Stage for a Study

At the end of Chapter 8, you were asked to develop some ideas for a research design to study the effects of nursing school attendance on well-being. We have discussed in this chapter some possible designs you may have considered and the need to have a better idea of what is already known before you can necessarily settle on a design. Chapter 10 discusses the background and statement of the research problem sections of research reports. It is this first part of a research report that provides the rationale for a study as well as information about previous research. Before reading Chapter 10, take a piece of paper and write one or two paragraphs that describe why a study of nursing students' well-being and the effect of attendance in nursing school are important to warrant a research study. If you were going to conduct such a study, what would you need to describe at the beginning to set the stage? After you have written your case for studying the nursing students' well-being, you are ready to begin Chapter 10.

## References

Adams, C. D., & Bennett, S. (2000). Exercise in heart failure: A synthesis of current research. *The Online Journal of Knowledge Synthesis for Nursing, 7*(5).

Bliss, Z. B., Johnson, S., Savik, K., Clabots, C. R., & Gerding, D. N. (2000). Fecal incontinence in hospitalized patients who are acutely ill. *Nursing Research, 49*(2), 101–108.

Brush, B. L. & Capezuti, E. (2001). Historical analysis of siderail use in American hospitals. *Journal of Nursing Scholarship, 33*(4), 381–385.

Colaizzi, P. F. (1973). *Reflection and research in psychology: A phenomenological study of learning.* Dubuque, IA: Kendall/Hunt.

Gawlinski, A., & Dracup, K. (1998). Effect of positioning on S$\bar{\text{v}}$O$_2$ in the critically ill patient with a low ejection fraction. *Nursing Research, 47*(5), 293–299.

Giorgi, A. (1971). Phenomenology and experimental psychology: II. In A. Giorgi, W. Fischer, & R. von Eckartsberg (Eds.), *Duquesne studies in phenomenological psychology* (Vol I). Pittsburgh, PA: Duquesne University Press.

Glaser, B. G., & Strauss, A. L. (1967). *The discovery of grounded theory: Strategies for qualitative research.* New York: Aldine.

Leininger, M. (1991). *Culture care diversity and universality: A theory of nursing.* New York: National League for Nursing Press.

Lipman T. H., Hayman, L. L., Favian, C. V., DiFazio, D. A., Hale, P. M., Goldsmith, B. M., et al. (2000). Risk factors for cardiovascular disease in children with type 1 diabetes. *Nursing Research, 49*(3), 160–166.

McCabe, S., Macnee, C. L., & Anderson, M. K. (2001). Homeless patients' experience of satisfaction with care. *Archives of Psychiatric Nursing, XV*(2), 78–85.

Miles, M. S., Holditch-Davis, D., Burchinal, P., & Nelson, D. (1999). Distress and growth outcomes in mothers of medically fragile infants. *Nursing Research, 48*(3), 129–140.

Niska, K. J. (2001). Mexican American family survival, continuity, and growth: The parental perspective. *Nursing Science Quarterly, 14*(4), 322–329.

Nyamathi, A., Flaskerud, J. H., Leake, B., Dixon, E. L., & Lu, A. (2001). Evaluating the impact of peer, nurse case-managed, and standard HIV risk-reduction programs on psychosocial and health-promoting behavioral outcomes among homeless women. *Research in Nursing and Health, 24,* 410–422.

Parse, R. R. (2001). Qualitative inquiry: *The path of sciencing.* Sudbury, MA: Jones and Bartlett Publishers and National League for Nursing Press.

Poss, J. E. (2000). Factors associated with participation by Mexican migrant farmworkers in a tuberculosis screening program. *Nursing Research, 49*(1), 20–28.

Spiegelberg, H. (1976). *The phenomenological movement* (Vols. I and II). The Hague: Martinus Nijhoff.

Spradley, J. P. (1979). *The ethnographic interview.* New York: Holt, Rinehart & Winston.

Steele, R. G. (2000). Trajectory of certain death at an unknown time: Children with neurodegenerative life-threatening illnesses. *Canadian Journal of Nursing Research, 32*(3), 49–67.

Strauss, A., & Corbin, J. (1994). Grounded theory methodology: An overview. In N. K. Denzin & Y. S. Lincoln (Eds.), *Handbook of qualitative research* (pp. 273–285). Thousand Oaks, CA: Sage.

van Kaam, A. L. (1966). Application of the phenomenological method. In A. L. van Kaam (Ed.), *Existential foundations of psychology.* Pittsburgh, PA: Duquesne University Press.

## Resources

Denzin, N. K., & Lincoln, Y. S. (Eds.). (1998). *Collecting and interpreting qualitative materials.* Thousand Oaks, CA: Sage Publications.

LoBiondo-Wood, G., & Haber, J. (1998). *Nursing research: Methods, critical appraisal, and utilization* (4th ed.). St. Louis: Mosby.

Pedhazur, E. J., & Schmelkin, L. P. (1991). *Measurement, design, and analysis: An integrated approach.* Hillsdale, N.J.: Lawrence Erlbaum Associates Inc.

Polit, D. F., & Hungler, B. P. (1999). *Nursing research: Principles and methods* (6th ed.). Philadelphia: Lippincott.

CHAPTER

10

# Background and the Research Problem

## *Why Ask That Question? What Do We Already Know?*

SOURCES OF PROBLEMS FOR RESEARCH

BACKGROUND SECTION OF RESEARCH REPORTS

LITERATURE REVIEW SECTIONS OF RESEARCH REPORTS

  Directional and Nondirectional Hypotheses

  Null and Research Hypotheses

LINKING THE LITERATURE REVIEW TO THE STUDY DESIGN

PUBLISHED REPORTS—HAS THE CASE BEEN MADE FOR THE RESEARCH STUDY?

COMMON ERRORS IN REPORTS OF THE BACKGROUND AND LITERATURE REVIEW

**KEY TERMS**

Conceptual framework
Deductive knowledge
Directional hypothesis
Inductive knowledge
Literature review
Nondirectional hypothesis
Peer review
Primary sources

Research hypothesis
Research purpose
Research problem
Research questions
Secondary source
Specific aims
Statement of purpose
Theoretical framework
Theory

**connection—**

For additional activities go to
http://connection.lww.com/go/macnee.

## CLINICAL CASE

The RN works in a large primary care clinic in a rural county in the south. The clinic is staffed by several family physicians, a pediatrician, an obstetrician, a certified nurse midwife, and two family nurse practitioners. The RN manages the patient flow in the clinic, supervises two medical assistants, and provides professional nursing care to clients seen in the clinic, including such procedures as nebulizer treatments, diagnostic tests (such as electrocardiograms [ECGs]), and health education. The clinic sees a high volume of patients, because it is the only source of health care for most of the county. At the weekly staff meeting, the obstetrician and the nurse midwife propose that the clinic participate in a large epidemiologic study of risk factors in pregnancy that is being implemented jointly by the colleges of medicine, nursing, and public health at the state university. The study is being implemented in several clinics and settings throughout the state. Participation requires that the entire staff receive a half-day training session in the study protocol. Much of the study data would be collected through a questionnaire and through repeated measurement of selected physical and laboratory parameters throughout patients' pregnancies. Most of the work will be performed by the RN and the medical assistants, who will track any subjects enrolled in the study, ensure that all forms are completed in a timely fashion, and record the relevant physical finding on a special log. The benefits of participation are that the patients themselves would receive numerous tests free of charge and all results from the study pertaining to the clinics' patients will be given to the staff to use in planning future care. The staff is generally supportive of participating in this study but asks the RN to decide whether the additional effort required of her and her assistants is reasonable, given the contribution that the study may or may not make to future practice. To better understand the study, the RN asks to see the research proposal for the study to review the background and rationale for the study.

## SOURCES OF PROBLEMS FOR RESEARCH

We started this book by discussing knowledge and knowing and why research is an important source of knowledge. This led us to recognize the need to understand and intelligently use research in nursing practice. As we moved through discussions of the different sections of most reports of research, we ended each chapter with a "why" question: Why did the researcher come to that conclusion? Why did the researcher use those patients and those measures? Why did the researcher plan the study in that way? We are now ready to discuss the beginning of research reports, in which the most important "why" question of all is asked: Why do this study? This is the most important "why" question because if there is no good rationale or basis for a research problem, then the rest of the study and report becomes trivial.

A **research problem** is a knowledge gap that warrants filling and can be addressed through systematic study. Research problems are derived from several sources, but the two general sources of research problems are those derived from practice and those derived from theory. Figure 10–1 illustrates how research, practice, and theory can be viewed as one large braid, because they wind together to develop knowledge.

FIGURE 10-1    **The woven, or braided, relationships between practice, research, and theory.**

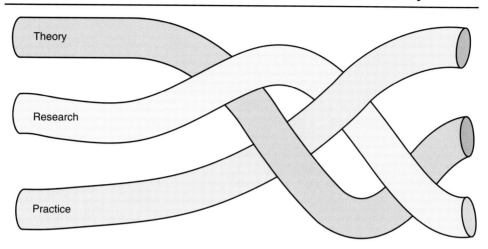

We have focused on research questions that directly relate to practice, and practice is one of the major sources for identification of gaps in knowledge that must be researched. Nursing practice is broad and is a rich source of questions and problems for which we currently do not have answers. Examples of some of the questions that must be answered include:

- What are the best ways to support physiologic functioning in acutely ill patients?
- How can we facilitate individual and family growth through the stress of health crises?
- How can we assist patients in making major adjustments associated with chronic illness?
- How can we facilitate and promote positive healthy living, and what makes for a positive and healthy balanced life?
- What allows some people to adapt or cope with illness when some cannot?
- What makes some people more vulnerable to health and illness problems?
- How can we facilitate individuals and families during the transition from life to death?

These questions are all broad and cannot be directly tested in a research study, but they do demonstrate the diversity of research areas that arise from nursing practice. Research problems derived from practice may be based on experiences in the practice arena, may be problems derived from mandated evaluation or accrediting requirements, or may reflect social issues as they affect practice.

Theory is another source of research problems. A **theory** can be defined as an abstract explanation describing how different factors or phenomena relate. In Chapter 8, we discussed theoretical definitions of variables, saying that a theoretical definition describes a variable conceptually rather than concretely. It is the conceptual or abstract nature of the ideas that, by definition, make something theoretical.

Lazarus's Theory of Stress, used in several previous examples, provides an abstract explanation for how individuals and their environments interact to lead to stress (see Figure 9–5). Nursing theories that you have studied in other courses provide an abstract explanation of how nursing, persons, environment, and health all interrelate. Any theory can be a source of research problems, because theory and research are closely intertwined: theory is based on and guides research, whereas research tests theory to generate new knowledge.

In general, knowledge can be developed inductively or deductively. **Inductive knowledge** is developed by pulling observations and facts generated through research together to generate theory. That theory is then used to suggest further observations that might be expected and that are then used to refine the theory. **Deductive knowledge** is developed by proposing a theory regarding a phenomenon of interest, breaking down the parts of the theory, and seeking observations and facts to support the abstract relationships proposed in that theory. Observations that support or refute a theory's predictions of relationships are used to revise or refine the theory, which then undergoes further testing. In nursing, many of the observations for either inductive or deductive knowledge development arise from research studies, as well as from practice, hence, the intertwining relationships among practice, research, and theory that are illustrated in Figure 10–1.

Although practice and theory are the major sources of research problems, much more is required to develop a specific research problem than just identifying a broad question from either source. In the background section of a research report, we should be able to follow the trail of thinking that has led from a relatively general research problem to a specific research purpose.

The first sections of most research reports are labeled "Background," "Introduction," "Problem," "Theoretical Framework," "Literature Review," or some combination of these. In all cases, these first sections of a research report should: (1) provide the broad context or rationale for the problem, (2) define the problem, and (3) summarize what is already known about the problem. These three purposes are not always discrete and distinct, because one purpose also may relate to another purpose. Therefore, information about what is known about a problem also may help to define it, or the context or rationale for a problem also may include what is or is not known about it. However, after reading the introductory sections of a research report, we should have a general understanding of these three purposes. The purposes of context and definition are often discussed in the introduction or background section of a research report, whereas a section titled "Literature Review" often specifically describes the current state of knowledge about a problem. Our discussion will follow this division.

## BACKGROUND SECTION OF RESEARCH REPORTS

To provide a context for a research problem, most study reports start with a broad and general description of a health concern derived from theory or practice. This broad description of the concern can be based on national health statistics; a description of the costs of an important health problem; the goals or agenda of an organization that supports health, such as the American Nurses Association (ANA);

or an emerging health crisis. For example, the beginning of the report of the study about risk factors of children with type 1 diabetes (Lipman et al., 2000) states that type 1 diabetes is a major disease that causes morbidity and mortality, particularly affecting the cardiovascular system. It goes on to point out that we know several of the risk factors that predict diseases of the cardiovascular system. The exercise in heart failure synthesis (Adams & Bennett, 2000) starts by pointing out that exercise intolerance is a major limit for those who have heart failure, affecting their functioning and their quality of life. It further states that pharmacologic treatment is only partly successful in improving exercise tolerance. In both of these research reports, the authors set the stage by providing the context for the specific problem they are going to study.

Providing the context for a specific research problem also often establishes the relevancy of the problem for health care in general and, possibly, nursing specifically. That diabetes is a major health problem that affects many people and has significant health consequences gives us a clear idea of why a study aimed at health problems in diabetics is important. However, it does not directly connect the problem to nursing. Some research reports include a subsection at the beginning of the report that specifically addresses the relationship between the research problem and nursing. More often, the potential nursing implications of the problem are addressed indirectly as the research problem is framed and refined.

The background section of a research proposal differs from a published research report in the quantity and depth of information that is included, with research proposals usually having longer and more extensive background sections. However, the purposes of the background sections are similar. Therefore, the RN in our vignette needs the same kind of understanding when she reads the research proposal that she would need to read and understand a published research report. The RN in our vignette knows that health behaviors and risk factors during pregnancy affect birth outcomes, but she is surprised to discover in the background of the research proposal that her state has one of the highest rates of low-birth-weight and premature births. She also is surprised to learn that there are differences in rates of low-birth-weight and premature births between rural and urban counties in her state. Both of these pieces of information provide her with a beginning understanding about the purpose of the study to which she is being asked to contribute.

In addition to setting a broad context for a research problem that may also define the clinical relevancy of that problem, the background section of a report should narrow and refine the research problem. General problems, such as low birth weight and differences in vulnerability in rural and urban settings, are not specific enough to be easily examined using research. Even with qualitative research methods, a specific phenomenon, an aspect of a cultural group, or social interaction must be refined and delineated as the focus of the study to guide data collection and analysis.

Research problems are usually refined either through reference to existing literature about the problem or through theoretical frameworks. Existing literature used to refine a research problem may include scholarly papers, research studies, or clinical case studies. The focus of the literature when refining the research problem is on the aspects of the problem that have been recognized, what is known about these aspects, and how they may relate. Although the background section refers to existing literature, that literature will be relatively general and address the overall research problem. Often, a background section is followed by a literature review section, in which the literature referenced is usually more focused on the particular research problem than the literature in the background section. The literature used in the background usually differs from the more extensive literature review, because the former is relatively general and addresses the overall research problem. The literature review section of a research report usually addresses the research problem after it has been refined. The background and literature review sections of a research report, then, might fit together to develop a story. The background gives us the general scene and characters, perhaps including the relationships among the characters, and it ends by presenting a specific conflict or problem among selected characters. The literature review continues the story and gives us a much more complete description of the central characters specifically relevant to that problem.

Another approach that may be used to refine a research problem, either by itself or in combination with literature, is application of a theory, theoretical framework, or conceptual framework to the research problem. A **theoretical framework** is an underlying structure that describes how abstract aspects of the research problem interrelate based on developed theories. A **conceptual framework** also is an underlying structure, but it comprises concepts and the relationships among the concepts. We have said that a theory is an abstract explanation describing how different factors or phenomena relate. In the purest sense, these three different terms have different meanings, but understanding those meanings is not essential to intelligently use research, because they all describe proposed relationships among abstract concepts.

We must be clear that we are not talking about theoretical definitions of specific variables at this point. The word "theory" does refer to something that is abstract, so theoretical definitions of variables are abstract definitions of specific variables to be studied. And, theoretical definitions of variables may derive from a specific theory or a specific framework. However, before we can focus on specific variables, we must have refined the research problem to a point that it can be systematically studied. Therefore, in the background section of a report, we expect that a broad and general concern, such as cardiovascular disease in young individuals with type 1 diabetes, will be narrowed to a specific research purpose. The **research purpose** is a clear statement of factors that are going to be studied to shed knowledge on the research problem. The factors to be studied may also be referred to as the variables to be studied. In general, we expect the research purpose to identify the major variables in a study.

In Chapters 4 and 5, we discussed a study of factors associated with participation in tuberculosis (TB)-screening programs by Mexican migrant farm workers

---

### C ORE  C ONCEPT

*Theory, theoretical frameworks, and conceptual frameworks all provide a description of the proposed relationships among abstract components that are aspects of the research problem of interest.*

(Poss, 2000). That study used a conceptual framework that was a combination of two well-established theories, the Health Belief Model and the Theory of Reasoned Action. The author chose these theories because they both describe how abstract factors interrelate to lead to a health behavior. The use of these theories is logical, because the research problem of interest is decreasing the incidence of undetected TB, and the way that is accomplished is through the health behavior of TB screening. The author decided to combine these two well-known theories and presents her own conceptual framework in a figure in the introduction to the study. According to this framework, several factors contribute to an individual's intention to carry out a health-related behavior:

1. An individual's beliefs about a behavior that is related to a health problem (behavioral beliefs) affects his or her attitude about that behavior (attitude), which, in turn, affects his or her intention to do a behavior related to a health problem (intention).
2. An individual's experiences related to the behavior (cues to action), beliefs about his or her vulnerability to the health problem (susceptibility), and beliefs about the seriousness of the health problem (severity) all affect an individual's intention to do a behavior related to the problem (intention).
3. The normative beliefs about health and health behavior that surround an individual affect his or her individual norm about health and health behavior (subjective norm) and, in turn, affect his or her intention to do a health behavior (intention).

The intention to do a health-related behavior, then, predicts whether the individual carries out the behavior. Notice that this conceptual framework breaks down health behavior into nine components, each of which can be defined and measured. It also leads to a specific purpose for this study, to:

> *analyze the relationship between variables (susceptibility, severity, barriers, benefits, cues to action, normative beliefs, subjective norm, attitude, and intention) from the Health Belief Model (HBM) and the Theory of Reasoned Action (TRA) and participation by Mexican migrant farmworkers in a tuberculosis screening program* (Poss, 2000, p. 20).

Thus, the general research problem of TB infection in migrant farm workers and the importance of effective screening programs for TB in this population has been refined to a specific research purpose based on a combination of two theories about health behavior.

Similarly, the study of risk factors for cardiovascular disease in children with type 1 diabetes (Lipman et al., 2000) used the epidemiologic framework that organizes risks according to "agent," "host," and "environment" and applied it to the general research problem. This guided the researchers in identifying 12 factors that would contribute to cardiovascular disease (CVD) that they could examine and describe in this at-risk population.

In contrast, the fecal incontinence study (Bliss, Johnson, Savik, Clabots & Gerding, 2000) used literature to refine the research problem into a specific research purpose. These authors cite scholarly work showing that studies conducted on fecal incontinence in long-term care settings indicate that diarrhea or liquid stools exacerbate fecal incontinence. Nosocomial infections, particularly with *Clostridium difficile,* also can cause nosocomial diarrhea. Tube feeding, receipt of antibiotics or sorbitol-containing medications, and selected patient characteristics all have been associated with *C. difficile* infection. This background literature brings the researchers to the specific purpose of their study:

> *to determine the extent and severity of fecal incontinence in hospitalized patients who are acutely ill, and to examine the relationship among fecal incontinence and stool consistency, diarrhea,* C. difficile-*associated diarrhea, tube feeding, and diarrhea during tube feeding* (Bliss et al., 2000, p. 102).

In this research report, the background section first provides the context of the problem of cost and significance, then uses literature to refine the problem to a specific research purpose.

Another example of using literature to refine a research problem into a research purpose is found in the homeless patients' satisfaction with care study (McCabe, Macnee, & Anderson, 2001). The authors of this study provide the context for the problem by establishing the extent of homelessness and the problem of homeless individuals following up on health care. They then refine the problem by discussing the role of patient satisfaction in follow-up for health care in White middle-class populations and use this literature to identify the purpose for this study, which is to "address. . .what constitutes satisfaction with primary health care for homeless clients" (McCabe et al., 2001, p. 79).

In addition to the term "research purpose," some research reports may refer to **specific aims**, **research question**(s), or research objective(s). For example, the reports of the fecal incontinence study (Bliss et al., 2000) and the TB-screening study (Poss, 2000) use the term "research purpose," whereas the study of risk factors in children with type 1 diabetes (Lipman et al., 2000) and the study of effects of positioning (Gawlinski & Dracup, 1998) use the term "objectives" and the study evaluating HIV programs (Nyamathi, Flaskerud, Leake, Dixon, & Lu, 2001) refers to the research question. All these terms mean essentially the same thing: they refer to a statement of the specific variables that will be studied.

Often, the research purpose (or question, specific aim, or objective) also will include language that defines the type of question being asked in the research—whether the question is descriptive, relational, or predictive. The research purpose for the TB-screening study uses the phrase "analyze the relationships," thus clearly identifying that it is asking a question about relationships or connections. The fecal incontinence study also uses the word "relationship," as well as the words "to determine," indicating a descriptive component to the study objective as well. The risk

---

# CORE CONCEPT

*The terms research purpose, research question, study, or specific aim(s) or research objective(s) all refer to the statement of the variables to be studied that are related to the broad research problem.*

factors in children who are in the diabetic study also uses the word "determine," indicating that the type of question asked is descriptive.

In our vignette, the RN finds that the proposed research has used a modified version of the Health Belief Model to identify factors that may affect health-related behaviors of women who are pregnant. The purpose of the study is to test factors from this modified model (perceived barriers, benefits, self-efficacy, and social support) with the spectrum of health-related behaviors associated with pregnancy, including smoking, alcohol use, prenatal care, exercise, and nutrition. Although the proposed research described in this chapter is fictional, a similar study that resulted in several publications was implemented in the past (Aaronson & Macnee, 1989a; Aaronson & Macnee, 1989b).

In summary, the background section of a research report has two major purposes: to establish the context for the research problem and to refine that problem to a specific research purpose. The section of the report that we are referring to as background may simply be the beginning of the report without any title, may be titled "Introduction," or may be titled "Background." Information that provides the broad context for the research problem may include issues from either practice or theory and may reflect societal concerns, health care policy changes, or major health concerns. Refining the research problem may be accomplished using literature, theory, or both. In either case, the goal is to move from the general problem to a specific purpose or question that identifies the variables to be included in the study and often the type of question being asked.

## LITERATURE REVIEW SECTIONS OF RESEARCH REPORTS

We said earlier that the use of literature to refine the research problem is not necessarily the same as the formal literature review. A **literature review** is a synthesis of the literature that describes what is known or has been studied regarding the particular research question or purpose.

Much of the literature review consists of a synthesis of existing published research, but some scholarly and theoretical work that is not actual research also may be included in the review. The literature review is more than a listing or summary of relevant research; it entails the combination of several elements or studies to provide a different or new focus on the research problem. For example, the literature review—titled "Relevant Literature"—in the TB-screening study has a sentence that describes the types of behaviors that have been examined using the Health

> ## CORE CONCEPT
> *The literature review is guided by the variables that have been identified in the research purpose and aims to give the reader an overview of what is known about those variables, how those variables have been studied in the past, and with whom they have been studied.*

Belief Model. The new perspective created in this sentence is the identification of the breadth and variety of behaviors that have been examined. Each of the 15 studies cited in this single sentence examined one particular behavior. A recitation of all of them would have been monotonous and useless. However, it is useful for the reader to know that behaviors such as immunization programs, breast cancer screening, colon cancer screening, genetic disease screening, hypertension screening, and general health examinations have all been studied using the Health Belief Model.

The RN in our vignette can expect that the literature review in the research proposal will help her to understand and evaluate several aspects of the proposed study. Specifically, the literature review should tell her the state of the science regarding the variables to be studied. Included within that review should be information about how the variables have been studied and in what circumstances or with whom they have been studied. Box 10–1 summarizes the purposes for these reviews.

To assure us that the literature review reflects the state of the science, the author must include current or recent studies. Usually, we expect that most of the literature cited in a literature review has been published within 5 years of the date of the study or the publication of the report. However, sometimes little research has been conducted on selected variables, there has been a gap in time since the problem was addressed, or some important or classic studies may have been done more than 5 years ago. In these cases, we may appropriately see literature cited that was published more than 5 years ago. We care about how current the literature cited is because we want to know that the researcher is building on the most current knowledge related to the problem of interest.

Another way of ensuring that a study, either proposed or reported, is based on current knowledge is its use of primary sources. **Primary sources** are the sources of information as originally written. To be accurate and current, it is important that the researcher has read and synthesized the actual research reports or scholarly papers that are relevant to the study. A **secondary source** is someone else's description or interpretation of a primary source. For example, Poss (2000) states in her literature review that "Champion (1985) used the HBM [Health Belief Model] to study breast self-examination (BSE) frequency in women. Stepwise multiple regression revealed that 26% of the variance in BSE was accounted for by all the HBM variables tested together" (Poss, 2000, p. 21). This is an example of using a primary source, because Poss has read Champion's study and is reporting on it. However, suppose the authors of the proposal being reviewed by the RN in our vignette read the article by Poss about TB screening and then stated in her literature that "Champion (1985) found that 26% of variance in breast self-exam was explained by the variables in the

**BOX 10-1**  **Specific Purposes of the Literature Review**

- Description of what is known about the variables for the study
- Description of how the variables have been studied in the past
- Description of with whom the variables have been studied

Health Belief Model" (Poss, 2000). In this case, they would be citing a secondary source: she has not read the Champion study itself, only Poss's description of it.

One problem with secondary sources is the potential for inadvertent error or distortion of the findings of a study. Think about the childhood game of telephone, in which 6 or 7 children sit in a circle and one person starts a message around the circle by whispering it into the ear of the person next to him or her. That person then whispers the message that he or she heard into the next person's ear. As we all know, by the time the message gets around the circle, it is likely to have changed significantly from what was originally stated. The same problem can occur with reports of research or other scholarly work. The greater the number of times that the work is interpreted beyond the original, the greater the possibility that the actual results will be distorted or changed.

The second reason that we expect a researcher to use primary sources is that we expect the researcher to do some discriminating in terms of the quality of the sources used to support his or her current research study. If we depend on Poss's two sentences about Champion's study, we are also depending on Poss's judgment about the quality of that study related to her TB-screening study. Once we read the report of the Champion study itself, we might decide that it is not relevant to the proposed study of health behaviors in pregnant women.

In addition to the use of current and primary sources, the RN in the vignette should expect to see literature that has been published in referred or peer-reviewed journals. We mentioned in Chapter 1 that the quality of information acquired on the World Wide Web must be carefully evaluated, because anyone can create a Web site and claim to be an authority on a subject. Similarly, there is variety in the quality of published literature. A standard that ensures that a published report has been carefully scrutinized to ensure the quality is the use of peer review. **Peer review** means that the manuscript for the published report has been read and critiqued by two or more peers before it was accepted for publication. "Refereed" is another term that means that there was critical review of manuscripts before they were accepted for publication. Manuscripts that are peer reviewed are intentionally sent to individuals who have expertise in the manuscript's topic. Therefore, the reviewers' comments are likely to reflect current and well-established knowledge. Not all sources of reports on research are peer reviewed or refereed. You can find out whether a particular publication is refereed by checking the author's guidelines for a journal, often available on a Web site or in the journal itself.

All of the studies used as examples in this text are from peer-reviewed journals. However, not all of the citations listed when you do a search using search programs such as CINAHL will be from peer-reviewed publications. As an intelligent user of research for clinical practice, you should consider not only the content of the research study but also the type of publication. When you read research published in refereed journals, you know that the published report has been reviewed by several individuals with expertise in the research area, giving you some assurance about the quality of the study before you read it.

Part of what assures us of the quality of a literature review and, therefore, the knowledge on which the study was based, is that the literature cited was from refereed publications. Therefore, the RN in our vignette will read the literature review in the proposal, expecting that recent literature, from primary sources and peer-reviewed journals, will give her information about what is known about the variables in the study and how and with whom they have been studied.

The satisfaction with care among homeless research report (McCabe et al., 2001) provides a good example of a review of the literature. The article was published in 2001. If we look at the literature cited, we see a range of publication dates from 1983 to 1997. Most of the literature was published after 1993, and, when we look at the 1983 citation, we see that it relates to "recognized" measure of satisfaction, suggesting that this is an example of a "classic" or an important element related to the topic. Further, the references cited are all studies published in major nursing journals that are peer reviewed.

The literature review content gives us background about what satisfaction means conceptually and how it has been measured in the past. The synthesis of the literature includes information about what has been a potential problem in existing research: the lack of variability in studies with less educated or disadvantaged populations. This way, the authors address the variable of satisfaction that is central to the purpose of the study. The other factor that is important to consider in this literature review is the population that has been studied in the past. Homeless individuals have not been included in previous satisfaction studies, so the literature review describes what is known about the homeless population in terms of their health and their use of health care. The authors' synthesis of this literature focuses on the unique nature of the concerns of those who are homeless. The authors set the stage for a qualitative study that seeks to understand the unique experiences of this population.

In contrast to the report of the study about satisfaction with care, the literature review in the TB-screening article focuses on research that tested the two theories that are the basis for the conceptual framework for that study. Again, most of the literature is current, although some is older, because both theories were originally developed some time ago. The publications are all from peer-reviewed journals. The author gives us a description of the research that has been completed in the past with each model, pointing out how successful the models and the different factors within the models were in predicting health behavior. In the process, the author offers the reader a better theoretical understanding of the variables included in the study, as well as information about who has been included in studies and how studies have been implemented.

As the RN in our vignette reads the literature review of the research proposal for a study of factors affecting pregnancy outcomes, she gains an increased understanding about the variables to be studied. The proposal cites literature that indicates how important exercise, smoking, alcohol intake, nutrition, and prenatal care are to birth outcomes. The review also points out that many pregnancy outcome studies have been retrospective and that a longitudinal multi-measures study is needed to understand better the relative effect of these different behaviors on pregnancy outcomes. Finally, the literature review addresses known differences between rural and urban populations and presents a case for a study that relates pregnancy behaviors to pregnancy outcomes while comparing rural and urban samples. At the end of the literature review, the RN reads that the purpose of the study is:

> *To describe and compare the patterns of health related behaviors including smoking, alcohol use, use of prenatal care, exercise and nutrition among women in rural and urban settings, and to test the relationship among these behaviors and the outcomes of low birth weight and premature birth.*

Therefore, the literature review should provide focused information about the specific variable(s) to be examined in a study. The literature review should provide some understanding of what is known about the variables, how they have been studied in the past, and with whom they have been studied. This should logically support the design and methods for the research study reported. Returning to our earlier analogy, by the time the literature review is completed, the major plot and subplots for the story should be clear. For those plots to make sense, we must understand the characters and their past "relationships" or stories.

After the literature review, some research reports include detailed research questions or hypotheses. Not all reports do so, because not all research studies have detailed questions or hypotheses. In particular, we do not expect detailed questions or hypotheses in a study using a qualitative approach, because the emphasis should be on understanding the whole of an experience or a phenomenon, rather then breaking it down and studying its discrete parts. We also do not expect detailed research questions or hypotheses from quantitative studies whose purpose is general description. However, studies that test theory and predictions from theory or attempt to test the effect of manipulation usually have focused detailed research questions or hypotheses.

The language of research can be confusing at this point. We said earlier that a research purpose may also be called a research question and that it will specify the factor(s) or variable(s) to be examined in a study and the general type of question being asked. Now we are talking about "detailed" research questions. Another way to think about these questions is as subquestions to the general question or purpose of the study. For example, in Chapter 8 we discussed a study of maternal distress and growth (Miles, Holditch-Davis, Burchinal, & Nelson, 1999). This study states:

> *The purpose of this study was to examine the extent to which attributes of the mother, the mother's level of parental role attainment with the child, characteristics of the child's illness, and maternal illness-related distress influence adjustment in mothers caring for medically fragile infants (Miles et al., 1999, p. 130).*

This sentence clearly lists the variables to be examined in the study and suggests that the study is looking at prediction. In the next paragraph, the authors give specific research questions, which include:

> *(a) How do attributes of the mother, the level of maternal role attainment with the child, characteristics of the child's illness, and maternal illness-related distress influence maternal distress (depressive symptoms) at the infants' hospital discard and at 12 months of age? And (b) How do attributes of the mother, the level of maternal role attainment with the child, characteristics of the child's illness and maternal illness-related distress affect maternal growth (positive or negative developmental impact) at 6 and 16 months of age? (Miles et al., 1999, p. 130)*

Notice that these questions break down the larger research purpose into two more detailed and specific questions. The questions not only include the specific variables of interest in the study but also the specific relationship to be tested and the timeframe for that testing. As an intelligent reader and user of research, what is important for you to understand is that most reports of research studies start with a general problem, move to a more refined research purpose or question, and then, if appropriate, develop specific measurable questions or hypotheses, as illustrated in Figure 10–2. The research problem, purpose, and question are descriptions of the knowledge sought by the study that differ in their depth and specificity, but content from one may overlap with another at times. They also may differ in the actual terms used, such as the research purpose being called a specific aim or the research questions being written as objectives. However, a research report should include at least two, and often three, levels of depth and specificity of statements about the knowledge being sought in the study. These levels are differentiated by the specificity of the statements, with the problem being general, the purpose stating the variables for the study, and the questions or hypotheses stating specific measurable predictions or relationships.

In Chapter 5, we defined a hypothesis as a prediction regarding the relationships or effects of selected factors on other factors. We now know that the factors in a study are called variables. A research question and a **research hypothesis** are often opposite sides of the same coin, because they both state predictions about relationships among variables. A research question puts the predictions in the form of a question, whereas a hypothesis puts the predictions in the form of a statement. There are two types of research hypotheses and questions: those that are directional and those that are nondirectional.

## Directional and Nondirectional Hypotheses

A hypothesis may predict whether there will be a relationship between two variables, or it may state the nature of the relationship between them. When we speak about the nature of a relationship, we are referring to whether the relationship is

**FIGURE 10-2**   **Levels of development of the statements of the knowledge sought by the study.**

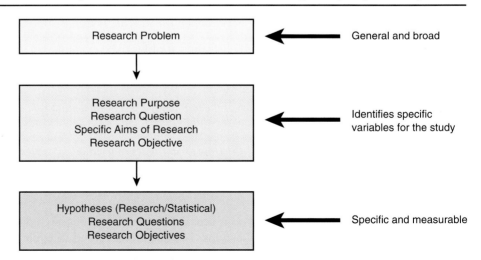

positive or negative; another word for this is the direction of the relationship. We also talked about negative and positive relationships in Chapter 6 when we discussed correlations. A positive relationship exists between two variables if one increases as the other increases and vice versa. A negative relationship exists if one variable increases as the other variable decreases. Figure 10–3 illustrates a positive relationship between sun exposure and number of freckles and a negative relationship between hours of work and ability to concentrate. A **directional hypothesis** predicts that two variables will be related and predicts the direction of that relationship. A **nondirectional hypothesis** predicts that two variables will be related but does not predict the direction of that relationship.

Research questions can be directional and nondirectional as well. If a researcher asks, "Is there a relationship between sun exposure and number of freckles?" this would be a nondirectional question. If a researcher asks, "Do the number of freckles increase as the amount of sun exposure increases?" this would be a directional research question. Whether a hypothesis or research question is directional or not depends on the current level of knowledge about the variables of interest or the extent to which theory has been developed about the variables. A well-developed theory proposes not only relationships among factors but also the direction of those relationships. Therefore, a study using such a theory would be more likely to have directional hypotheses.

If we look at the report of the TB-screening study with Mexican migrant farm workers (Poss, 2000) we find that the author had five specific hypotheses. This is logical, because the TB-screening study is testing a theoretical model that is based on two well-developed theories, making predictions possible. All of the hypotheses in this study were directional, predicting selected positive relationships among the various variables within the framework. Another example of a directional research question can be found in the study comparing HIV risk-reduction programs (Nyamathi, Flaskerud, Leake, Dixon, and Lu, 2001) that we discussed in Chapter 3. This study ends the literature review by asking "whether three cognitive-behavioral HIV risk-reduction programs would have a positive effect on substance use, sexual risk behaviors, and cognitive and psychological resources of homeless women and their intimate partners at 6 months and whether the effectiveness would vary by type of program" (Nyamathi et al., 2001, p. 412).

**FIGURE 10-3** **Graphs depicting positive and negative relationships among variables.**

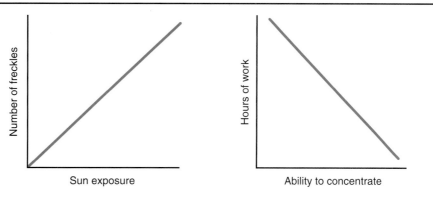

### Null and Research Hypotheses

In addition to hypotheses being directional or nondirectional, there are two forms for hypotheses: the null and the research forms. We described research and null hypotheses in Chapter 5. The research hypothesis predicts relationships or differences in variables, whereas the null hypothesis states that there will be no relationship or differences among variables. Remember that the null hypothesis is developed for statistical purposes and represents the assumption made in inferential statistics that most relationships or differences that may be found in any particular sample might have occurred by chance alone. Only when a difference or relationship among variables found in a sample is so large that it would only occur by chance in fewer than 5% of samples can the null hypothesis or statistical hypothesis be rejected. Usually when a study has a null hypothesis an alternate hypothesis also is stated, and that alternate hypothesis will predict both a relationship and a direction to that relationship. The idea of a "null" form is not applied to research questions, only to predictions in the form of statements.

Because we did not have any examples of use of a null hypothesis in the studies that we have read for the previous chapters, let's assume that the authors of the proposal about studying pregnancy behaviors to predict pregnancy outcomes did use statistical hypotheses. Let's suppose that the purpose of the study our RN found was "To describe and compare the patterns of health-related behaviors, including smoking, alcohol use, use of prenatal care, exercise, and nutrition among women in rural and urban settings and to test the relationship among these behaviors and the outcomes of low-birth-weight and premature birth." Two sets of possible hypotheses are stated:

$H_0$: There will be no differences in the pattern of tobacco use among pregnant women from urban and rural settings.

$H_1$: Women from rural settings will use tobacco more when pregnant than will women from urban settings.

$H_0$: Timing and regularity of use of prenatal care will not be related to birth weight among rural and urban samples.

$H_1$: Earlier and more regular use of prenatal care will decrease the incidence of low-birth-weight infants in both the rural and urban samples.

The symbol $H_0$ represents the null hypothesis, and $H_1$ represents the alternate hypothesis. You can see that the null hypothesis is a neutral or negative prediction, written primarily to support the assumptions of inferential statistics. A study that is using research hypotheses without null hypotheses also may use the symbol of an uppercase "H," but they will be numbered consecutively as $H_1$, $H_2$, $H_3$, and so on. A researcher should only include hypotheses at the beginning of a study if there is some basis for the predictions, from either previous research or theory, and the literature review should include the information from theory or research that supports the hypotheses.

## LINKING THE LITERATURE REVIEW TO THE STUDY DESIGN

When we first discussed the literature review, we said that it should give us an overview of what is known about the study variables, how they have been previously studied, and with whom they have been studied. We have discussed the quality of the literature review and mentioned that the research questions or hypotheses are specific predictions that should be supported by the literature review. The final aspect of the literature review that is important is the support it should provide for the study design.

The literature review should provide a synthesis of what is known but also should synthesize the approaches that have been taken to develop knowledge in this area. In this way, a literature review not only synthesizes but also critiques existing research about a problem. A true critique identifies strengths and weaknesses, and this is what we should expect to see in the literature review section of a research report. The strengths and weaknesses of previous research should serve as the basis for the study currently being described. The researcher should tell us at the beginning of the report how the results of this study would fit within the overall structure of knowledge about the problem. For example, the satisfaction with care study with homeless (McCabe et al., 2001) identifies in the literature review that homeless individuals differ from those who are not homeless in their perspective and behavior and that there have been no studies of satisfaction with primary care among homeless. This information supports a qualitative design, because it identifies that we lack knowledge about the unique experiences of homeless individuals. The authors also state that the results of this study are intended to be used to develop and measure satisfaction with care among homeless.

Similarly, Poss (2000) tells us in the literature review that, although TB screening has been studied, TB-screening behaviors among Mexican migrant farm workers have not. She also tells us that there are some well-tested theories about health behaviors, such as TB screening. These well-developed theories serve as the basis for her study, because she uses these theories to identify variables that may predict TB screening among Mexican migrant farm workers. A literature review may specifically address problems in study design from previous research or limitations of past samples. The literature review also may synthesize and critique the existing literature without directly addressing design and sampling issues. However, in either case, one of the purposes of the literature review is to identify the rationale for the design used in the study. Like a well-written story, each section or chapter should build a foundation for the next section or chapter. Choices of research design should be based upon approaches taken in the past, with the goal of improving on or expanding on previous knowledge.

In summary, the background and literature review sections of a research report set the stage for the remainder of the study. The background gives the broad context for the research problem and an overview of factors relevant to that problem. This overview may present an abstract set of concepts and their relationships to one another called a theory, conceptual framework, or theoretical framework. The background usually ends with a statement of a research purpose or questions that specify the variables to be studied. The literature review starts with the purpose and describes the current state of the science in relation to the study variables. To do so, the literature review must be current and use mostly primary sources from peer-reviewed journals. The literature review should include what is known about the variables and how and with whom they have been studied. It establishes the basis for the design of the study and may end in specific research questions or hypotheses.

## PUBLISHED REPORTS—HAS THE CASE BEEN MADE FOR THE RESEARCH STUDY?

We ended the last chapter with the RN wondering why the researchers in the effect of positioning study (Gawlinski & Dracup, 1998) were so concerned about position change. If we examine the literature review for this study, we find that several studies in the past have examined the effect of position on oxygenation. The authors' critique of these past studies is that they have used small samples, that the studies have not been done with patients who have low cardiac output, and that randomization of position change has not been used, introducing the possibility of a systematic bias in previous studies. The information about findings from previous studies and the limitations of previous studies set the stage for the authors' study, using random assignment to order of position change in a study of patients with low cardiac output.

After reading the background and literature review sections of the research proposal to study behavioral factors affecting pregnancy outcomes, the RN in the vignette for this chapter has a great deal more information with which to make her decision about participating in that study. She understands the general problem that the study is attempting to address and the specific research purpose. She also understands why the particular variables of smoking, alcohol, exercise, prenatal care, and nutrition were selected for study. She also has a clearer idea about previous research and how the design of this study will fill an important gap in knowledge. She decides that participation in the study will require extra work but that the study will make a valuable contribution to the care of future patients, so the work is acceptable.

At the end of Chapter 9, you were asked to make a case for why a study of nursing students' well-being should be implemented. After reading this chapter, you should have a clearer idea about how you might have developed that rationale and why it can be an important part of a research report. The background and literature review set the stage for the rest of the research report by giving us a general setting for the study in terms of the problem; the specific purpose of the study, including the study variables; and an understanding of how this study will fit with current theory and research-based knowledge.

## COMMON ERRORS IN REPORTS OF THE BACKGROUND AND LITERATURE REVIEW

One of the first errors that may occur in the background and literature review sections of a research report is a failure to develop a consistent link between the research problem, the research purpose, and any specific hypotheses or questions. The fictional article that describes the study of nursing students' choices of practice after graduation gives a good example of a background that does not directly link the problem, purpose, and research questions. The introduction to that report discusses the general problem of the nursing shortage and the need for workforce planning. It then states that, in addition to the sheer number of students, we must consider choice of practice in workforce planning, indicating that specific sites for practice will have greater needs for nurses in the future. International differences are mentioned, but there is no further mention of international aspects through the rest of the report. The next section, titled "Background," continues with the thread that students who will choose the most severe shortage sites should be targeted for recruitment to schools of nursing and concludes with a research purpose to "examine the relationships among nursing students' demographic characteristics and their choices for practice following graduation." At this point, the connections become weak. After the research purpose, the author lists three specific questions, the first of which addresses specific demographic variables (age, gender, race, and marital status), but the second and third of which introduce new variables that have not been mentioned at any point in the preceding section: students' well-being and students' experiences that relate to their choices of practice. This is like a fiction author dropping an entirely new character into the middle of a story without connecting that character to anything or anyone in the previous part of the story.

The example in the fictional article is somewhat extreme, and what makes it an even poorer example is that no literature review is included. Consequently, we have no idea of what research has been done with students and choice of practice, how it has been conducted, or with what types of students. Published research reports vary in the consistency and links that they draw between the research problem, purpose, and specific measurable questions. If, as an intelligent reader of research, you finish the background and literature review section and still do not know what is going to be studied and why, one explanation may be that connections between the problem, purpose, and research questions have not been clearly or consistently identified in this section of the report.

A second problem that can occur in published research reports is a failure to provide the information needed to fulfill the important purposes for these sections of the report. For example, a literature review may provide a thoughtful synthesis of what is known about the variables of interest in the study but may fail to connect it to the purpose of the study being reported. This may leave us uncertain concerning the basis for the researcher's selection of research design and approach to measurement or how the study will fit with current knowledge.

Another problem that can occur in literature reviews is a failure to adequately reference statements. If the author of a research report makes a statement about the variables of interest that reflects knowledge that is not common and does not provide a reference, then we are left wondering how much we can trust the statement. We must wonder whether the statement is simply the opinion of the researcher, some stray fact that was found on the World Wide Web, or a well-documented research-based piece of knowledge. Occasionally, the number of references imbedded in a sentence in a literature review can almost be distracting from the meaning of the sentence, but those references assure us that the information is well founded and accurate.

The last potential problems with background and literature review sections of research reports are those we have discussed: the use of secondary sources and the use of out-of-date references. The point of these beginning sections of a research report is to give us a clear and accurate picture of the state of knowledge about the research problem and to develop a coherent set of connections between that knowledge and the specific research purpose and questions. Secondary sources and references that are all more than 5 years older than the date of the study or publication of that study do not give us much confidence that the study will fit well with current levels of knowledge.

## OUT-OF-CLASS EXERCISE

### Pulling It All Together

We have now completed the second section of this book. We have looked at the entire research report, starting with the conclusions and moving forward to the background and literature review. As we discussed the sections of a research report, we also focused on selected aspects of the research process. The last two chapters of this book return to the traditional approach to discussing research: starting at the beginning of a study or report and moving to the end. We discuss how the research process is related to the published research report and to the nursing process itself. We also examine the history of nursing research and how evidence-based practice and quality improvement relate to the research process. To prepare you for the last two chapters in the book and to help you pull together the different sections of a research report, write an abstract that describes a research problem addressed by the in-class exercise. Decide on one question that you think could have been answered by that study. Then, in approximately 250 words (one page, double-spaced) write an abstract that includes: (1) background, (2) objective or purpose, (3) methods, (4) results, and (5) conclusions. If you have had the opportunity, you may be able to use real results generated in your class. If not, make up the results. The point of the exercise is to write a concise description of a research study using the specific language of research. Go back and read some of the abstracts of the research reports that we have used in this book, or find some published research of interest to you to serve as examples of what your abstract should look like. Remember that abstracts are organized differently in different journals, but for this exercise, try to use the five headings listed in this paragraph.

If you did not have an in-class study, you may want to take the fictional article and think of another question that might be addressed, given the variables in that study, or at least rewrite the abstract for that study using the headings listed in the previous paragraph. After you have completed this exercise, you are ready to move on to Chapter 11.

## References

Aaronson, L. S., & Macnee, C. L. (1989a). The relationships between weight gain and nutrition in pregnancy. *Nursing Research, 38*(4), 223–227.

Aaronson, L. S., & Macnee, C. L. (1989b). Tobacco, alcohol, caffeine use during pregnancy. *Journal of Obstetrical and Gynecological Nursing, 18*(4), 279–287.

Adams, C. D., & Bennett, S. (2000). Exercise in heart failure: A synthesis of current research. *The Online Journal of Knowledge Synthesis for Nursing, 7*(5).

Bliss, Z. B., Johnson, S., Savik, K., Clabots, C. R., & Gerding, D. N. (2000). Fecal incontinence in hospitalized patients who are acutely ill. *Nursing Research, 49*(2), 101–108.

Gawlinski, A., & Dracup, K. (1998). Effect of positioning on $SvO_2$ in the critically ill patient with a low ejection fraction. *Nursing Research, 47*(5), 293–299.

McCabe, S., Macnee, C. L., & Anderson, M. K. (2001). Homeless patients' experience of satisfaction with care. *Archives of Psychiatric Nursing, XV*(2), 78–85.

Miles, M. S., Holditch-Davis, D., Burchinal, P., & Nelson, D. (1999). Distress and growth outcomes in mothers of medically fragile infants. *Nursing Research, 48*(3), 129–140.

Nyamathi, A., Flaskerud, J. H., Leake, B., Dixon, E. L., & Lu, A. (2001). Evaluating the impact of peer, nurse case-managed, and standard HIV risk-reduction programs on psychosocial and health-promoting behavioral outcomes among homeless women. *Research in Nursing and Health, 24,* 410–422.

Poss, J. E. (2000). Factors associated with participation by Mexican migrant farmworkers in a tuberculosis screening program. *Nursing Research, 49*(1), 20–28.

## Resources

Lipman, T. H., Hayman, L. L., Favian, C. V., DiFazio, D. A., Hale, P. M., Goldsmith, B. M., et al. (2000). Risk factors for cardiovascular disease in children with type I diabetes. *Nursing Research, 49*(3), 160–166.

LoBiondo-Wood, G., & Haber, J. (1998). *Nursing research: Methods, critical appraisal, and utilization* (4th ed.). St. Louis: Mosby.

Polit, D. F., & Hungler, B. P. (1999). *Nursing research: Principles and methods* (6th ed.). Philadelphia: Lippincott.

CHAPTER

11

# The Research Process

## *How Is the Research Process Related to a Published Research Report?*

**KEY TERMS**

Aggregated data
Assumptions
Codebook

Dissemination
Pilot study

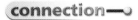

## CLINICAL CASE

In Chapter 8, an RN who worked in the pediatric intensive care unit (ICU) sought some research to help her to better understand and work with the parents of one of her patients. Shortly after reading the study about distress and growth outcomes in mothers of medically fragile infants (Miles, Holditch-Davis, Burchinal, & Nelson, 1999) the RN is invited to participate in a research group that is beginning. The goal of the group is to develop and implement a study of parent and staff relationships as a predictor of rehospitalization of children seen in the ICU. The RN is considering returning to school to earn her master's degree and decides that this group would provide her with a good opportunity to increase her knowledge about the research process. The research group is being led by a professor from the school of nursing affiliated with the RN's hospital and a pediatric clinical nurse specialist (CNS) who has a joint appointment with the RN's hospital and the school of nursing.

In the last eight chapters, we learned about the different sections of a research report and discussed the process of doing research, but we have not yet focused on the research process itself. Now that we are comfortable with much of the language of research and with some of the aspects of the research process that are reflected in a research report, it is time to look at the research process as a whole. This chapter describes the research process from beginning to end, links that process to the research report, and discusses the relationship between the research process and the nursing process.

## THE RESEARCH PROCESS

In Chapter 2, we briefly described the five steps of the research process:

1. Define and describe the knowledge gap or problem
2. Develop a detailed plan to gather information to address the problem or gap in knowledge
3. Implement the study
4. Analyze and interpret the results of the study
5. Disseminate the findings of the study

A process, whether it is the research process, the nursing process, or the critical-thinking process, is, by definition, fluid and flexible. All these processes refer to steps, because certain parts of the process are necessary before one can successfully move to the next part. However, the steps do not always follow one another in a step-by-step manner: at times, a step in the process leads to returning to the preceding step or two steps occur at the same time.

---

### CORE CONCEPT

*The steps of the research process are not always linear: they may overlap or be revisited during the research process.*

---

For example, a refined research purpose is necessary before one can begin to develop a detailed research plan, but it is possible that as a plan is developed, the research purpose may be revisited and refined further. Similarly, a research plan is needed before a study is implemented, but it is possible that as the study is implemented, the plan will be revised. In fact, in most qualitative methods, the methods are expected to change as the study progresses. Therefore, although this chapter discusses the steps of the research process in order, the process may be more fluid and flexible in action.

### Define and Describe the Knowledge Gap or Problem

The RN in our vignette finds that when she attends the first meeting of the research group, it is beginning the first step in the research process. The CNS who is helping to lead the group begins by describing a question that she has developed based on her work on the pediatric ICU. She has noticed that in some patient cases, the ICU staff and the parents of critically ill children develop warm and interactive relationships, whereas in other cases, the parent–staff relationship is poorly developed, with limited communication and contact. The CNS wonders why this difference occurs and how the differences in relationships may affect the patients. Another member of the research group states her belief that when the staff has better communication with parents, the children have shorter hospitalizations and are rehospitalized less frequently. Other members of the group begin talking about reasons why they believe that relationships between parents and staff differ: some focus on characteristics of parents, some on nursing staff, and some on medical staff. Then another member of the group suggests that length of hospitalization itself is an important factor in both what kind of relationship is established between staff and parents and rehospitalization. The RN in our vignette suggests that staff–patient ratio and whether a child is admitted on the weekend also affect nurse–parent relationships and hospital outcomes.

It is obvious to the RN that at this point in the group's process, there is no agreement about the knowledge gap that must be addressed. Creating a flowchart of all the ideas that have been discussed is suggested; Figure 11–1 illustrates the results that might have come from this effort. Once the group sees all its ideas in a flowchart, it begins to identify some of the areas that it must explore further. For example, the group identifies that it must find out what is known about staff–parent relationships. Relationships and communication are recognized as two separate but connected concepts. The group agrees that it will focus on the relationships between nursing staff and parents but will consider how physician–parent relationships may be a factor in the nurse–parent relationships. Beyond looking for information about nurse–parent relationships within ICUs, the group agrees that it needs to look for information about the effects of relationships on health care outcomes and information about factors that may affect relationships, such as staff–patient ratio and nurse and parent characteristics. The members of the group divide the list of various ideas they have discussed and agree to conduct a literature review focusing on a particular subset of ideas and return in 2 weeks to share what they have found. The process described in this hypothetical situation illustrates aspects of the first step in the research process.

**FIGURE 11-1**      **Possible flow chart developed during brainstorming about a research problem.**

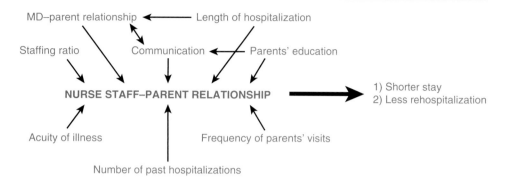

The information required for this first step in the research process will be acquired from existing theory and research to identify what is known about the problem and the relevant factors related to the problem. This step also requires thoughtful analysis, because rarely does theory or past research easily blend into an obvious research purpose. At this point in the research process, often what is needed is an explosion of ideas and information, all of which then must be thoughtfully analyzed and synthesized to develop a refined research purpose. The brainstorming session that the RN in our vignette experienced may be the first of several sessions in which many ideas are explored, validation and information about those ideas are sought and digested, and new ideas are generated. This step in the research process can be both exciting and frustrating: exciting because of the amount to be discovered about a problem of interest and frustrating because of the amount to digest and integrate to develop a refined research purpose.

For example, our hypothetical research group may find a great deal of research about nurse–patient communication, primarily with adult patients. However, perhaps little has been done examining nurse–parent communication in acute settings with patients who are children. Perhaps the focus primarily has been on communication rather than the broader concept of relationships. The group does find theory about the concept of relationship formation, in general, which certainly includes the concept of communication, as well as characteristics of the participants in a relationship. The group recognizes that several of the nurse theorists have focused on nurse–patient relationships and identified a range of concepts that are important to their development. They also found several studies that conclude by recognizing that the relationship between staff and parents of critically ill children is important.

---

## C ORE  C ONCEPT

*Whether a research problem or question has been identified from practice or from theory, the first step of developing a research study requires thoughtful and informed exploration of the problem to arrive at a refined purpose for a study.*

Yet, they find few research studies that link nurse–patient communication or relationships to longer-term outcomes, such as length of hospitalization or rehospitalization. Finally, nothing exists in either theory or literature about structural factors, such as overall staff–patient ratio or timing of admissions during weekends versus weekdays and nurse–parent relationships. Despite this lack of literature, the RN believes from her experience that when patients are admitted on the weekends, their parents often do not establish as good a relationship with the weekend staff as do parents who come in during the week with the regular weekday staff.

All these findings leave the group with even more information than they compiled when they brainstormed and with no immediately obvious connections between all the possible factors that it might consider. This is what was meant by an explosion of information: as ideas are analyzed in this step of the research process, they sometimes explode into multiple new ideas to explore.

Despite the potential explosion of information, notice that our hypothetical group has now acquired a foundation of knowledge about what is known, has been theoretically considered, or has been studied in the past. Developing that foundation of knowledge is the goal of the first step of the research process. That foundation of existing knowledge should include existing research, practice experience, and any appropriate and relevant theory. The challenge then becomes synthesizing the existing knowledge; critically examining practice experience, theory, and past research; and identifying a research purpose that includes specific factors or variables to be studied. Notice also that the foundation of knowledge found strongly supports the relevancy of the problem that this group has identified for nursing practice.

In addition to establishing a foundation of knowledge about the research problem, another part of this first step of the process entails identifying assumptions that are imbedded in the approach to the problem and the purposes being considered. **Assumptions** are ideas that are taken for granted or viewed as truth without conscious or explicit testing. Assumptions can be difficult to identify, because they are ideas that we "just know" or "all understand" and are usually unspoken. However, assumptions can sometimes color how a research problem is viewed, so that the approach to knowledge development is limited in some way. Several assumptions are often made in nursing research, and one researcher studied reports of research to describe some of these. Williams (1980) identified 13 assumptions that are commonly present in nursing studies. These included assumptions that stress is something to avoid, that health is a priority for most people, and that people operate on the basis of cognitive information. Identifying the assumptions imbedded in a study can be helpful, because we may realize that the assumptions must be researched and confirmed before we can move forward in knowledge development.

In the hypothetical study we are discussing, there is an assumption that relationships between parents and staff can be viewed as "good" or "bad." There is a second assumption that parents' experiences in the ICU will affect their child's health while the child is in the ICU and afterward. Because of these assumptions, the research group is not considering exploring whether the terms "good" and "bad" apply to relationships; it is beginning with looking at factors that make relationships good or bad. Perhaps this approach is too simplistic and there are only different types of relationships, some of which are more or less helpful in promoting positive health outcomes for the patients. If so, the study of factors that make relationships good or bad may miss some important types of relationships.

As the research problem is refined into a specific purpose, the types of questions that will be addressed and the approach likely to be taken to the study are often beginning to be identified. We previously discussed how research questions that address prediction or examine the effects of manipulation of a variable require a relatively large amount of background or foundation knowledge. It becomes increasingly clear to our hypothetical research group that not enough research or theory about factors affecting nurse–parent relationships or the effects of these relationships on outcomes exists to make predictions or to plan to manipulate any factor. Because the researchers cannot find studies and theory that convince them to predict that a certain variable will have a desired outcome, they realize that they must consider questions about relationships between variables in the nurse–parent relationship or questions that describe the nurse–parent relationship.

The group also begins to consider whether a qualitative, quantitative, or mixed method approach is most logical as it begins to refine the general problem of nurse–parent relationships. Some of the group argues that because so little has been studied about the parents' experiences in their interactions with nursing staff, the first study should be phenomenologic. Others suggest that a grounded theory approach might be taken, broadly based on Peplau's Theory of Interpersonal Relations (1952). A grounded theory approach based on Peplau's theory would aim to develop concepts and links that are grounded in nurses' and parents' experiences of developing and maintaining relationships. Others believe that nursing theory and existing theory about relationships in general, as well as past research about nurse–patient communication, provide a set of relevant factors that can be measured and tested to see how they affect nurse–parent relationships and think that a correlational study is what is needed. Everyone agrees about the need to discover whether staff–parent relationships can be linked to outcomes, such as a shorter total hospitalization or fewer rehospitalizations.

It is not uncommon that during the first step of the research process several potential research studies are identified that are relevant to the problem. Refining a problem clarifies the nature of the gaps in knowledge as well as the factors relevant to the problem. In many cases, the problems of interest to nursing are too complex to address in a single study. Let's assume, for now, that after several meetings and substantial discussion and review of theory and the literature, the hypothetical group in our vignette agrees upon a tentative purpose: to identify and examine factors that affect nurse–parent relationships in the pediatric ICU settings and the role these relationships have in patient outcomes. This purpose tells us that the variables in this study will be unspecific "factors," nurse–parent relationships, and patient outcomes. This purpose will probably need further refining, which will occur as the group moves into the second step of the research process. In this step, the group takes the purpose it has identified and develops a specific research plan that includes the research design and methods of measurement and sampling.

## Develop a Plan to Gather Information

As the purpose for a study is refined, ideas about gathering information about the problem being studied also begin to be generated. As researchers review past research studies regarding the problem, they consider not only the findings from that research but also the methods and samples used. This helps to clarify gaps in knowledge and identifies measures and approaches that previously have been successful in addressing the problem. For example, our hypothetical research group has found that most studies of nurse–patient communication have been conducted with adults who were the primary care recipients rather than with adults who were caregivers, such as parents. They also found that many of the communication studies have used videotaping as a method of data collection, with analysis of discrete episodes of communication as the focus of study. Because this group is interested in more than isolated episodes of communication, it knows that it needs a different research method.

The second step of the research process is complex and involves many considerations and decisions. This step includes deciding upon the general approach to be taken to the study, deciding on a specific research design, identifying and developing plans for the study sample or participants, and planning the measurement process, including specific techniques, measures, and timing. Finally, at the end of this step, an institutional review board (IRB) proposal must be written and submitted in preparation for actually implementing the study.

The group in our vignette intentionally left its preliminary statement of a research purpose broad, because it had not reached an agreement about whether this research needed to develop further knowledge about nurse–parent relationships or describe how factors that it has found in the literature and from practice affect that relationship. The group eventually decides that a mixed method approach makes the most sense, beginning with a grounded-theory study of the relationships between nursing staff and parents of the children in the ICU. It plans to follow this with a descriptive correlational study about how the factors they have identified from research and practice affect length of hospitalization and rehospitalization within the following 2 weeks. These factors include history of hospitalization, severity of illness, parent educational level, timing of initial admission and average staff–patient ratio during hospitalization, as well as any factors that are identified from the grounded-theory study that can reasonably be included. Following this overall decision about the study, the group is able to refine their purpose: to describe the perceptions of nurses and parents of their relationship during the hospitalization of an acutely ill child, including their perceptions of how that relationship does or does not impact health outcomes of the child, and to describe how nurse, patient, parent, and hospital unit factors impact length of hospitalization and need for rehospitalization within 2 weeks after discharge.

The refined purpose described reflects several decisions that have been made by the research group. It has decided that a grounded theory method is a better design for its purpose than a phenomenologic design, because it is examining interactions, has a general theory in Peplau's Psychodynamic Nursing Theory, and wants to develop knowledge about relationships. The group has ruled out doing a true longitudinal study, because it did not find strong research evidence about factors relevant to staff–parent relationships or the effect of factors on the outcomes of interest. A longitudinal study requires more time and resources than a cross-sectional correlational study, and the group members believe they do not have the knowledge base to justify that effort at this time. The group has also settled on two outcomes—length of hospitalization and occurrence of rehospitalization within 2 weeks of discharge—

partly for pragmatic reasons. They know that administration and insurance companies are interested in shortened hospitalization and avoiding unnecessary rehospitalization, so they expect they may be able to get support for this study from the hospital. Also, these two outcomes are easily measured. Other outcomes that the group discussed included parents' sense of control and efficacy, child's rate of recovery, and rate of complications. These are all still considered relevant by the group, but it agreed that potential difficulties with measurement precluded examining them in this study.

Thus, the second step of the research process requires critical thinking and decision making. Researchers must consider what is known, what has been shown to work, and what is feasible. The last consideration includes issues of time, cost, established measures or approaches, and other resources, such as space or access to samples. We will discuss these further when we discuss factors that affect research.

Decisions about the best possible methods for implementing the chosen study designs must also be made during this part of the research process. In the case of the grounded theory phase of the hypothetical study, for example, researchers must make decisions about methods of data collection, such as interviews, observations, or use of journaling, as well as the timing for the data collection. Similarly, to implement the descriptive correlational phase of the study, researchers will have to make decisions about measures, such as chart audits, and the use of a questionnaire or a structured interview. The issues of rigor, validity, and reliability that we discussed in Chapters 8 and 9 are central to making these decisions about methods and measurement.

Another important part of the second step of the research process is deciding on the sample for the study and approaches to the process of sampling, as discussed in Chapter 6. For example, the pediatric ICU sees a variety of patients in terms of both age and type of health problem. Although the group plans to measure severity of illness during the second phase of the study, it recognizes that the type of illness, type of insurance, and individual physician practices all also will affect length of hospitalization. The grounded theory phase of the study will benefit from researchers' talking to several parents, including those who have experience with the ICU and those who do not. However, parents whose children are on the unit for fewer than 24 hours will probably have limited time to participate. After some discussion of normal patient census and the most common types of patients seen, the research group decides to limit the study to children diagnosed with chronic diseases. This decision is based on the experience of our RN and several other group members who suggest that children and parents with one-time acute health crises have different needs and outcomes than those with recurrent health crises due to chronic disease. The decision also recognizes that parents of children with chronic diseases are likely to be more willing to assist in a research study of this type and, so, may more easily be recruited.

In addition to deciding who will participate in the study, the group in our vignette must consider how comfortable parents will be talking about their relationships with nursing staff and how nursing staff might change regarding their relationships with parents when they know there is a study in progress. This would be an example of the Hawthorne effect described in Chapter 9. Parents might be concerned about repercussions on the care their child will receive if they express any negative feelings, and staff might be concerned about negative effect on their performance evaluations. These issues could lead to a threat to internal validity from testing and to researcher effects threatening external validity. The research group decides to use individuals who are not associated with the ICU in any way as data collectors and to put extra effort into ensuring anonymity of participants and subjects to address this concern.

The hypothetical group in our vignette will make other specific decisions as it moves through the second step of the research process, and the details of these decisions could probably fill several chapters. Overall, this process is based on a further exploration of past research to identify research designs and methods that have been used, measures that are available, and sampling considerations. This research literature, along with the realities of the specific setting for the research, the knowledge and experience of the researchers, and resources such as time and money, all will be considered in developing a detailed plan to gather information about the research purpose. Box 11–1 summarizes these and other considerations affecting the development of the research plan.

Once a detailed plan is developed, the last part of this second step of the research process is to ensure the protection of human subjects and to acquire the resources needed for the study. We discussed informed consent and the role of IRBs in Chapter 7. The type of study we are discussing in this chapter would likely have to receive IRB approval from both a hospital board and from a university board. This will require two written proposals describing the study background, purpose, literature review, design, and measures and how the rights of subjects will be assured. Developing this type of IRB proposal often helps a researcher or research group to tighten the details of their plan of study but also takes time and must be considered when planning a timeline for a research study. In addition, many studies cannot be implemented without acquiring some outside resources to support the time and materials needed. Depending on the complexity of the proposed study and the resources inherent in the study site, researchers often must write and submit proposals for funding of a study before they can implement it. Again, the writing, review, and receipt of funding can take weeks to months. However, both the review of IRB proposals and the funding proposals provide outside input into the plans for a research study and often significantly improve those plans before the study is implemented.

## Implement the Study

The third step in the research process is to implement the study. This is when the advance planning and decisions can pay off and when unexpected issues can arise. One of the biggest responsibilities of the researcher during implementation is to maintain

---

**BOX 11-1 Considerations Affecting the Development of the Detailed Research Plan**

- Methods and samples used in previous research
- Potential setting(s) for the study
- Experience and knowledge of the researcher(s)
- Resources available, such as time and money
- Subject safety and rights
- Rigor, reliability, and validity

meticulous documentation of the sampling and data collection process. This documentation allows the researcher later to clearly identify any points in the study at which plans were changed and the rationale for decisions made during the implementation process. Areas that may need to be addressed and documented during this step of the process include: data about numbers and characteristics of those who were approached to be in the study but declined or later dropped out, any revisions in sampling criteria, any changes in the timing or the measurement process, and any anecdotal or incidental data that become relevant during the study implementation.

In Chapters 6 and 8, we discussed things that can "go wrong" with sampling and measurement and how important it is to consider those aspects when deciding on the usefulness of research for practice. The careful documentation kept by researchers during the study implementation is the basis for reporting information that will allow us to evaluate the sampling and measurement process. In addition, incidents or occurrences that are unexpected may have a big effect on the meaning of results of a study. For example, suppose that parents of children who had one particular physician all declined to be in our hypothetical study. Or suppose that as the study is implemented, parents start approaching the research staff and ask to participate before they have been recruited. Either of these observations suggests that there may be some underlying factor at work during the process of study implementation. In the first case, that factor may be a physician who has told parents not to participate because he is unhappy about the study, thus eliminating data about relationships with a provider who is controlling. In the second case, the underlying factor might be that parents have a strong need to talk about their experiences, which this study is meeting. This unmet need may be important to consider when gaining understanding about staff–parent relationships. One could speculate about the meaning of either observation, but what is important is to document the observation for future consideration as the results of the study are analyzed.

During the study implementation, the steps of the research process may be particularly fluid, moving back and forth between this step and the previous step of planning or to the next step of analysis and interpretation. As we discussed in Chapter 8, in the implementation step of the research process qualitative methods depend on a spiraling process of data collection followed by data analysis and interpretation that informs the next round of data collection. Sometimes during the study implementation, the plans for sampling prove to be unrealistic, perhaps because criteria are too strict or because the desired subjects for the study are not willing to participate. The researchers will then have to revise their sampling plan to implement the study. Or perhaps data collectors note that all subjects are confused and have difficulty answering some part of a questionnaire. The researchers will have to use this information to decide whether to change their measures in the middle of their study or continue with a measure that may have problems with reliability. These are just a few examples of the many kinds of problems that can be encountered during the study implementation. The process requires time, care, consistency, and ongoing monitoring.

## Analyze and Interpret the Results

The fourth step of the research process involves the analysis and interpretation of study results. As we indicated, this step may be interwoven with the step of implementation in a qualitative study. In contrast, most of the data analysis in a quantitative study is usually reserved until the entire data collection process is complete. This difference reflects the differences in philosophy behind the two types of approaches. A qualitative method uses data as it is generated to build additional data, with the goal of arriving at information that is dense and thick to inform our understanding of a phenomenon. Quantitative methods strive to control and isolate phenomena to understand each discrete element. Therefore, quantitative methods defer analysis of most of the data until the collection process is complete to avoid contaminating the data collection process with ideas generated from the analysis. The exception to this is in analysis of sample characteristics. A purposive sample or a matched sample, as discussed in Chapter 6, requires the analysis of subject characteristics during the study implementation to effectively implement the sampling plan.

Data analysis, whether carried out in a qualitative or quantitative study, requires the same level of meticulous care and documentation that is needed during the implementation step of the research process. In qualitative research, this is accomplished through the audit trail and notations within the software programs that are often used during data analysis. In quantitative research, decisions about data analysis are often documented in a codebook. A **codebook** in research is a record of the categorization, labeling, and manipulation of data about variables in a quantitative study. A codebook includes information about how each of the variables in the study was measured, how the data from the study were reviewed and transferred into computer files, and all decisions made regarding the management of problems, such as incomplete responses or confusing responses. Like an audit trail, a codebook provides a detailed description of how the data from a study were managed.

Qualitative data are often collected in an interview, so the first thing that must be done is to transcribe the data into a word-processing program. Once transcribed, the data can be either loaded into a qualitative analysis program or printed and analyzed on hard copy. In either case, data management often includes careful reading and listening to interviews that have been transcribed to ensure that the transcription is accurate and complete. Similarly, quantitative data have to be entered into computer software programs to be analyzed. This can be done in several ways, including direct entry of numbers from quantitative measurement into a data file or use of an optical scanner that reads and records numbers off a data collection measure into a data file. In either case, once it is in a data file, the data must be carefully examined for accuracy. Human error in keying numbers into a file or computer error in scanning answer sheets can significantly affect and even invalidate study results.

The researcher can proceed with the analysis and interpretation of the results once data have been put into a form that allows that process. As discussed in Chapters 4 and 5, data analysis is complex and challenging. It also is an exciting time in the research process, because the researchers begin to find out what their study says about the research problem that started this whole process. In addition to information about data management, codebooks in quantitative data analysis often include information about decisions regarding analysis approaches and the mathematic manipulation of the data. For example, a researcher can decide to use a mean score of items from a measure of a variable in the analysis or to use a score that is just the sum of all the items. Alternatively, a researcher may decide to study all subjects as one large group who have differences on a variable of interest or to divide subjects into two groups that clearly differ on that variable. All these types of decisions are usually documented in the codebook, so that, as the research progresses, the researcher can recall those decisions and the rationale behind them. Thus, both the audit trail and the codebook reflect documentation of data management and analysis, which are important aspects of the fourth step of the research process.

Interpretation is the last part of this step of the research process. Interpretation of the results of a study entails pulling the whole process together into a meaningful whole. The theory and research literature that served as a foundation for the study, the decisions made in the planning step of the process, and the decisions and observations that were made during the implementation step all must be considered and tied into the results of a study. At this point, the expertise of the researchers and their personal knowledge and experience are also used in interpreting results. For example, suppose that during the implementation of the hypothetical study of staff–parent relationships in the pediatric ICU subjects started hearing about the study and asking staff to be included. The research team will have to decide why this occurred and how it affected the data collected. The RN and research team in our vignette may decide that this interest in participating in the study reflected a strong need on the parents' part to feel included in the care of their children. Or they might conclude that parents needed an avenue for expressing their feelings about the nursing staff and the care of their children. These are different interpretations and would have different meanings for the results of the study.

## Disseminate the Findings

The last step of the research process brings us back to where we started in this book—to the research report. **Dissemination** of research findings refers to the spreading of knowledge and is an essential step in the research process, because knowledge development is wasted unless it becomes known so that it can be used. The dissemination of research findings may be accomplished in several ways. Findings may be disseminated through a report of the research to the agency or organization that funded or hosted the study. This type of dissemination is targeted at the specific groups that were closely involved in the study. Often, the results of a research study also are reported back to participants in that study. In addition, findings from a study may be verbally reported in the form of presentations to agencies or funding groups or at scholarly and professional meetings. Findings from research are reported in published journals in both print and online formats. Finally, research findings are sometimes disseminated to the public at large through the lay press, television, or other medium. Each of these types of approaches to dissemination of findings targets different groups of potential users of the research, with the report to those closely involved in the study clearly reaching a much smaller group than a published article in a major professional journal.

Because research dissemination targets different groups, the depth and detail of the dissemination varies. However, in all cases, the goal of dissemination is to share accurately the knowledge gained from the research so that it is useful and meaningful to the targeted recipients of that knowledge. For example, a summary of a research study that is being sent out in a regional newsletter will probably focus on a brief description of the problem, the sample, and one or two key findings. A presentation of a paper reporting the findings of a study at a professional meeting will usually be limited to 15 or 20 minutes, allowing inclusion of more detail than a newsletter column but less than what would be included in a published report in a research journal. A published report in a practice-focused journal will probably include fewer specifics about the research process than a report appearing in a research journal. However, in all cases, the researcher must ensure that the findings of a study are clearly and accurately stated.

The other consideration that is important for all types of dissemination is ensuring the anonymity of subjects or participants in a study. This requires that data primarily are reported in the aggregate, and careful scrutiny of even aggregated data to ensure that subjects will not be identifiable based on the information provided. **Aggregated data** means that the results from the study are reported for the entire sample rather than for individual members in the group. Usually, when data are aggregated, no specific result from the study can be attributed to any participant in the study. However, with a small sample, it is possible that even with aggregated data and elimination of any traditional identifiers, the anonymity of individual subjects might be lost.

For example, suppose that the hypothetical study of staff–parent relationships acquired a sample of 50 subjects in the descriptive correlational phase. One characteristic of subjects that will be reported is race, and perhaps only three subjects in the study were Asian. Further suppose that one finding was that there was a difference in parents' perceptions of staff by race, with Asian parents reporting much more negative experiences with staff. The staff on the ICU could read those results and likely know immediately which parents reported negative experiences, because they have so few Asian patients, thus eliminating the anonymity of those parents. In this type of circumstance, it is possible that a result may have to be withheld from dissemination to protect the rights of the subjects in the study. Given that the reason the results may breech anonymity is that the numbers of Asian patients was so small and, therefore, that the results may have happened by chance alone and must be confirmed with a larger sample, the withholding of such a result does not jeopardize knowledge development.

It should be noted that even at this last step in the research process, a researcher might revisit an earlier step. Sometimes only when writing up the findings of a study does a researcher discover the need to consider and report a specific descriptive result or conduct a particular statistical test. Sometimes after sharing findings from a study with others, suggestions are made for additional analysis that may shed further light on the research problem. Therefore, even in the last step of the process, there may be some reciprocal movement between the steps in the process. Of course, the findings from a study often raise new questions or suggest new research problems, bringing us back to the first step of the research process.

---

**BOX 11-2** **Characteristics of the Research Process**

- Systematic
- Complex
- Exacting
- Challenging

It should be clear from this description of the research process that it is complex, exacting, and challenging. The dissemination product of that research often does not provide a full picture of all the thought and work that went into a research study. Throughout this book, we have discussed common errors that can occur in a research report. However, any report of research deserves to be read with respect because of the effort and risk taken by the researcher to implement the research process and then make public the results of his or her efforts. Few research studies are perfect, and research reports certainly vary in their completeness and usefulness to practice. However, reports of research reflect a substantial time and commitment of one or more individuals to address a gap in knowledge through the use of the complex and, at times, strenuous process of research. The next section looks more closely at how and why publications of research do not always fully reflect the research process.

# RESEARCH PROCESS CONTRASTED TO THE RESEARCH REPORT

In Chapter 2, we discussed the relationship between the research process and the sections of a research report, as illustrated in Figure 11–2. Now that we have discussed the research process in more detail, a fuller comparison of the process to the research report is possible.

The first step of the research process of describing and defining the knowledge gap or problem is summarized in the background and literature review sections of a research report. These sections give us the context for a research problem and tell us about relevant theory and research regarding aspects of the problem. The information included in the research report is a synopsis of the much more extensive information that was gathered and synthesized during the first step in the research process. The research purpose and specific questions or hypotheses that conclude the first sections of a research report reflect the final refinement of the research problem into specific variables and a specific type of research question.

The second step of the research process is reflected in the methods section of a research report. The methods section of a report tells us the study design, sampling plan, methods of measurement, and procedures. Again, all the previous research, practicalities, and experience that enter into the decisions about settings for a study, the sample, and the measurement are distilled into a few paragraphs describing the final decisions that were reached about the study plan.

The third step of the research process of implementing the study is usually reflected in the results section of a research report, because it is in the results section that we learn who actually participated in the study. We also may see part of the implementation of the study reflected in the methods section of a report if what occurred during the study implementation process changed the sampling or measurement approaches taken. In either case, the information included in a report rarely reflects all the details of a study's implementation.

The fourth step of analysis and interpretation of the results of a study are reflected in both the results and conclusions sections of a research report. Of all the steps of the research process, probably this one is most fully described in the research report. However, even with this step, a great deal more goes into the process than is reflected in the results and conclusion sections of most reports.

**FIGURE 11-2**    **The relationship between the research process and the sections of a research report.**

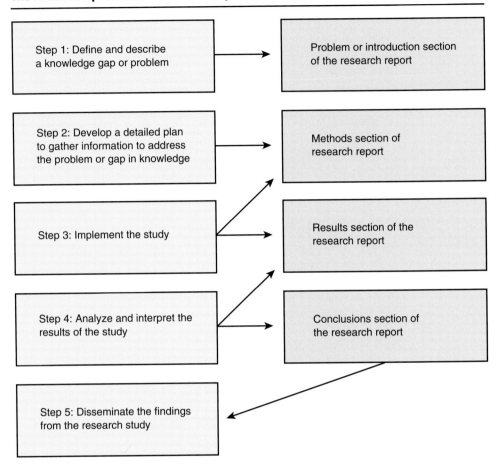

Finally, the fifth step in the research process is the research report itself. However, developing and publishing a research study report also requires more effort than may be obvious when looking at the final product. The publication of a research study depends on several factors. These include the fit between the purpose of the study and the emphasis of journals that publish research, the relevance and quality of the research study, and the ability of the researcher to express clearly and succinctly all the pertinent elements that are needed to fully understand and use the research. The first two factors primarily affect you as a user of research, because they affect what research is available to you through journals and online. Some research journals publish all types of research in each issue; others develop themes for different issues, limiting the types of studies they will publish at any particular time. Other journals reflect specialties, such as obstetric nursing, and are only interested in research that is relevant to that specialty. Some journals do not want to publish research that is highly theoretical, because they target readers who want practical and practice-focused information. To disseminate the study findings, a researcher first has to find journals that fit with the purpose of the completed study.

We mentioned in Chapter 10 that research reports from refereed or peer-reviewed journals are more respected, because they have been reviewed and critiqued by experts in the area of the research. Some research is not published because problems with the quality of the research are identified during the review process that decrease the meaningfulness or validity of the study's results. This does not mean that the research was bad but simply that some flaw or aspect of the study creates enough doubt about the findings or meaning of the results to preclude its warranting publication.

Another factor that affects publication of research studies is the ability of the researcher to express in writing adequate information to describe accurately the entire research process. As you will recall, many of the common errors in research reports that we discussed throughout this book were errors of omission or lack of complete information. We have now seen how much more thought and work goes into the research process than can go into a research report. The challenge for a researcher, then, and for the reviewers and editors who contribute to the final publication, is to describe clearly and completely all the aspects of the research process that were relevant to their particular study. The goal is to provide the readers with enough information to allow them to understand the study fully and to make intelligent decisions about the usefulness and meaning of the research for practice. One way this is accomplished is by using the language of research to limit the need to fully explain each study aspect. Yet, that very language of research may interfere with using research in practice, because the practitioner may not be familiar or understand that language.

## FACTORS THAT AFFECT THE RESEARCH PROCESS

In the previous section, we discussed factors that affect the publication of research studies. What about factors that affect whether a research study is implemented initially? Potential barriers to the implementation of research include lack of knowledge; lack of resources, such as money, time, or both; and lack of methods or measures.

Occasionally, research is not implemented because those who see a problem do not have the knowledge or skill to carry out the research process. An RN in practice, for example, may see an important problem but be unable to find others who have a similar interest with the skills to implement the research. Similarly, a community or a group of patients may see a problem that is not recognized as important by providers or by those who are prepared to implement research.

Research requires time and effort and is not without expense. Some research is not implemented because there are no resources to support the particular study. Expenses in research range from potentially small costs, such as copying, to potentially huge costs for sophisticated measures, such as ultrasounds or specialized laboratory testing. Costs are associated with the researcher's time and the time of others, such as data collectors or workers who enter data. Costs are associated with providing space and equipment needed for some research, and costs may be directly associated with subjects in the study, such as incentive payments or payments for travel or lodging.

Financial support for research can come from numerous sources, including individuals; local, regional, or national organizations; or the government. In almost every case, to receive financial support for a study, a researcher must prepare a proposal describing the study and identifying how the study will help to meet the goals of the funding source. Herein lies another limit or potential barrier to some research.

Sources of financial support for research usually have goals or initiatives that relate to the purpose of the group providing the support. Occasionally, these goals are specific, such as those of the National Alzheimer's Association, which are to support research into the mechanisms and treatment of Alzheimer's disease. Sometimes these goals are broad, such as the goal of the National Institute for Nursing Research (NINR) to support knowledge development in nursing. However, even the NINR, with its broad goal, has research priorities and target areas for research, such as studies with vulnerable populations, which may influence the success of a particular study in receiving funding. The Web site of a professional organization, such as Sigma Theta Tau or the NINR, usually publishes its research priorities. When developing a proposal for a research study, decisions about the study purpose, sample, or methods may be based, at least in part, on the goals and priorities of the potential funding source.

In addition to direct financial support for research, sources of indirect support also may affect the types of research implemented. In nursing, large health care organizations and nursing colleges in universities often employ individuals with the expectation that they will implement research as part of their role. These organizations pay for part of the time a researcher spends on research, because the results of research fit with the mission of the organization. A nurse researcher in a large metropolitan medical center, for example, may not need to find financial support for his or her time but may need to limit the types of research implemented to problems directly relevant to delivery of tertiary health care.

Another factor that affects the implementation of research is the availability of safe and tested methods and measures to study what we are interested in studying. For example, we may be interested in predictors of pancreatic cancer because it is so lethal, but have no effective way to identify the dependent variable of interest— pancreatic cancer—until an individual is so ill that it is no longer feasible to implement measurement of selected biologic or psychosocial parameters. Or, a researcher may be interested in a concept, such as empathy, but find that no instruments have been developed that can be used to measure empathy. Sometimes, it is unethical to implement a study using what might be the best design validity because of the need to protect the rights of human subjects, as discussed in Chapter 7.

One approach that researchers can take to address some of the limits related to measures and methods is to implement a pilot study. A **pilot study** is a small research study that is implemented to develop and demonstrate the effectiveness of selected measures and methods. Occasionally, a pilot study is used to demonstrate the potential importance of a selected factor to a research problem. At other times, a pilot study is used to demonstrate the reliability or validity of selected measures in a unique situation or sample. A pilot study also may be used to demonstrate the ability of the researcher(s) to implement a study. Because knowledge development regarding any particular gap in knowledge is a process that takes time and usually requires multiple studies, pilot studies can be an important first step in building a research program.

## GENERATING KNOWLEDGE CAN BE FUN!

We started this book by stating that the goal was not to make you a researcher but to give you the knowledge and tools needed to understand and use research intelligently. However, we do not want to end this chapter with an emphasis on how complex and arduous the research process can be or the many potential barriers there can be to both implementing and publishing research. The research process is a wonderful and exciting challenge. It is like a giant interactive puzzle, because as each piece is solved and fit into place, the rest of the pieces change and must be addressed in their new form, given what has already been completed. Fitting each piece into the puzzle can be extremely satisfying, and finishing small sections of the puzzle through completion of a research study can be rewarding.

Part of the reason the research process is fun is because it is a continuous learning experience for those involved. When one is trying to develop new knowledge, the challenges of planning and implementing a valid and meaningful study always require problem solving and creative solutions, so the opportunity to learn and create can be immense. More and more we are recognizing that most research is best approached using teams with members from different backgrounds and disciplines. This allows the knowledge brought to bear on a research problem to be wide ranging and to enhance the potential for a high-quality product.

It is the author's hope that as you read and use research, you will develop an interest in and excitement about the process of research, as well as for the problems that are addressed by research. Although the baccalaureate nurse is not expected to plan and implement research, there are several roles for nurses in the research process, such as participation in planning a study or in subject recruitment and data collection.

We started this chapter with the RN joining a newly formed group that hoped to address a research problem. We talked about the process employed by this group and how that process relates to the research report. As we discussed the research process, you may have noticed some similarities between it and the nursing process. For one thing, both are processes and both have been broken down into steps. In the broadest sense, the nursing process and the research process are similar because both are used to solve problems. Both a research problem and a patient care problem (whether the patient is an individual, family, or community) can be viewed as a complicated puzzle, where often only some of the pieces are available at any time point.

Both types of problems are initially addressed through gathering information. In the nursing process, this gathering of information is called assessment, and, in the research process, it is called describing and refining the knowledge gap or problem. However, in both cases, we are collecting information to guide us in understanding the problem and formulating a plan.

The second, third, and fourth steps of the research process and the nursing process also initially may appear similar, although they differ in some major ways. Although the second step of the nursing process is planning and the second step of the research process is developing a detailed plan, the two processes differ, because they have fundamentally different purposes. The purpose of the nursing process is to provide informed, scientifically based nursing care for human responses to potential or actual health problems. The purpose of the research process is to develop or validate knowledge. The goal of the nursing process is action to promote the established outcome of improved health. The goal of the research process is to acquire new knowledge, and the outcomes for that new knowledge cannot be known until the knowledge is established. Therefore, the second and third steps of the nursing process address planning and implementing care, whereas the second and third steps of the research process address planning and implementing acquisition of new information. As a result, the fourth steps of these two processes have different focuses, because evaluation in the nursing process is concerned with outcomes, whereas data analysis and interpretation are concerned with understanding. Table 11–1 summarizes the similarities and differences between the two processes. We discuss the roles of nursing in research more in the next chapter.

Although there are some similarities and differences in the processes of nursing and research, it is essential that there be a strong relationship between the two. The research process should provide knowledge that is the basis for the nursing process. This is why this entire book focuses on understanding and intelligently using research in practice. In addition, the nursing process will often be the source of problems that need to be addressed using the research process. As we plan, implement, and evaluate nursing care, we often find problems or face questions about the best ways to achieve our outcome of improved health. The nursing process and the research process differ in purpose, but they are closely linked and together ensure the growth and development of nursing as a profession.

## PUBLISHED REPORTS—WHAT DO YOU CONCLUDE NOW?

We have used 10 research study reports in this book as examples of how research can be used and related to clinical practice. In several cases, the studies examined a

**TABLE 11-1   Comparison of the Research Process and the Nursing Process**

|  | Research Process | Nursing Process |
|---|---|---|
| Similarities | A process with steps<br>A form of problem solving<br>Complex "puzzle" | A process with steps<br>A form of problem solving<br>Complex "puzzle" |
| Differences | Purpose is to develop knowledge<br>Plans and implements knowledge acquisition<br>Analysis and interpretation concerned with knowing | Purpose is to provide scientifically based care<br>Plans and implements delivery of care<br>Evaluation concerned with outcomes |

research problem from the two different approaches of qualitative and quantitative methods. None of the studies that we examined in this book could be called perfect, but each made a meaningful contribution to our knowledge about patients and patient care. No one study, however, gave us the full answer to our clinical questions. This is often a frustration for nurses in practice. With a better understanding of the research process, it should be clearer now why usually no one study fully answers a clinical question. Clinical questions are usually too complex, and too many variables and factors must be considered and examined for any one study to provide a complete answer. However, as research studies about a particular study accumulate, we should see answers to our questions begin to unfold. Evidence-based practice, which is discussed in Chapter 1 and Chapter 12, explicitly recognizes the need for an accumulation of knowledge regarding a problem to ensure the best and safest delivery of health care.

Therefore, what do you conclude now about what the RN in Chapter 1 needs to focus on in her discharge teaching with M.K.? What do you conclude about how the RN taking care of J.K. with his Parkinson's might decrease his risks of developing fecal incontinence? What should C.R. from Chapter 3 plan to teach to homeless women? How should the RN at the health department help his Latino families and improve tuberculosis screening? You can now ask and answer five questions as you read the research that may help you to answer these and other clinical questions intelligently.

- You can read and understand the background and literature review of a report to find out *why was the research question asked—what do we already know?*
- You can read the design and methods sections of a research report to find out *how were those people studied—why was the study done that way?*
- You can read the sampling section of the research report to find out *to what types of patients do these research conclusions apply?*
- You can read the results and conclusions sections of the report to find out *why the authors reached their conclusions—what did they actually find?*
- Finally, you can use the answers to these four questions to decide *what is the answer to the question—what did the study conclude?*

You also now know that finding the "answer" to your question will only be the beginning, and that it may give you new knowledge and insight into patient care, but may also leave you asking even more questions.

## OUT-OF-CLASS EXERCISE

### Critiquing the Whole

Before starting the last chapter of this book, exchange your abstract with another student. Read the abstract and critique it, giving at least two positive statements about it and at least two constructive suggestions for improvement. You may focus on the connections and links among the different parts of the abstract, how well each component was succinctly stated, the creativity of the abstract, or its usefulness for knowledge development. Return the abstracts to each other and see how well your effort to organize an abbreviated research report was understood. In Chapter 12, we discuss how nursing research has developed over time. We will examine the links between research, practice, and education, and we discuss evidence-based practice and quality assurance as two concrete areas where research is explicitly used in practice.

## References

Miles, M. S., Holditch-Davis, D., Burchinal, P., & Nelson, D. (1999). Distress and growth outcomes in mothers of medically fragile infants. *Nursing Research, 48*(3), 129–140.

Peplau, H. E. (1952). *Interpersonal relations in nursing: A conceptual frame of reference for psychodynamic nursing.* New York: G.P. Putnams' Sons. [Reprinted 1991, New York: Springer].

Williams, M. A. (1980). Editorial: Assumptions in research. *Research in Nursing & Health, 3*(2), 47–48.

## Resources

LoBiondo-Wood, G., & Haber, J. (1998). *Nursing research: Methods, critical appraisal, and utilization* (4th ed.). St. Louis: Mosby.

Locke, L. F., Silverman, S. J., & Spirduso, W. W. (1998). *Reading and understanding research.* Thousand Oaks, CA: Sage Publications.

Polit, D. F., & Hungler, B. P. (1999). *Nursing research: Principles and methods* (6th ed.). Philadelphia: Lippincott.

Tomey, A. M., & Alligood, M. R. (2002). *Nursing theorists and their work* (5th ed.). St. Louis: Mosby.

## CHAPTER 12

**LEARNING OUTCOME:**

*THE STUDENT WILL* relate nursing research to the development of the professional practice of nursing.

# The Role of Research in Nursing

**KEY TERMS**

Quality improvement
Research utilization

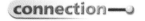

For additional activities go to
http://connection.lww.com/go/macnee.

S.J. is in the last semester of an RN-to-BSN program. One of her courses is nursing leadership. She has been assigned to present a review of a relevant research study on the nursing shortage in her next class. Of course, she also has several big papers due the same week!

S.J. notices the fictional article entitled "Demographic characteristics as predictors of

nursing students' choice of type of clinical practice" in her nursing association district newsletter. The article begins by addressing the nursing shortage. Because the article is research, S.J. decides it will fulfill her assignment for the nursing leadership class. She decides to read the article, using the five questions that organize this text.

**K**nowledge development through research is a core element in the development of the overall nursing profession. In this chapter, we step back to consider the history of nursing research and how nursing research relates to nursing practice, education, and theory. We move beyond the individual nurse's use of research in practice to consider the more structured process of evidence-based practice. Also, we examine how research is used and reflected in quality improvement studies. We finish by considering the future of nursing research and returning to how we started this book: considering the use of research in patient care.

## HISTORY OF NURSING RESEARCH

History helps us to understand the past and its continuing influence. Nursing research started slowly, but it has evolved at an ever-increasing and progressive rate. Figure 12–1 provides a timeline highlighting some major events within the history of nursing research.

It is widely accepted that the history of nursing research begins with Florence Nightingale and her studies of environmental factors that affected the health of soldiers in the Crimean War. During the last half of the 19th century, nurses, particularly in public health, continued to refine Nightingale's findings published in *Notes on Nursing* (1859). Little is known, however, of any nursing research during that time.

Between 1900 and 1940, nurses conducted research, but the larger focus was the preparation of nurses. During those years, the *American Journal of Nursing* began publication, baccalaureate nursing programs increased, and the first doctoral program in nursing opened at Teacher's College, Columbia University. Each of these developments helped to promote an increase in nursing research.

In the 1940s and 1950s, nursing research primarily focused on studying characteristics of nurses and nursing education. This probably occurred because nursing was relatively new to the university system and most doctorally prepared nurses had education degrees. Despite this focus, nursing research made significant progress during this time, as evidenced by the publication of the journal *Nursing Research*.

**FIGURE 12-1**  **Timeline showing important developments in the history of nursing research.**

| Historical Development | Research Focus of Development |
|---|---|
| • Florence Nightingale 1889 | Environmental factors that affect health |
| • 1900–1940 | |
|    Goldmark Report 1923 | Nursing preparation |
|    *American Journal of Nursing* published | |
|    First doctoral program in nursing | |
| • 1940s–1950s | Characteristics of nursing education and nursing students |
|    Publication of *Nursing Research* | |
| • 1960s | |
|    Development of theory in nursing | Research about clinical practice |
|    Began to teach research process | |
| • 1970s | |
|    Publication of three more research journals in nursing | Theory-based research |
|    Development of multiple doctoral programs in nursing | |
| • 1980s | |
|    National Center for Nursing Research started at NIH 1986 | Development of programs of research |
| • 1990s | |
|    National Institute of Nursing Research starts in 1993 | Priorities for research developed |
|    Five more research journals in nursing | Qualitative methods gain recognition |

During the 1960s, nursing began to recognize the need for theoretical foundations to its practice and research. Research also shifted away from the study of nurses toward the study of the clinical care provided by nurses. Within nursing education, nursing faculty began to teach the research process within baccalaureate nursing programs.

By the 1970s, nursing research examining clinical practice had increased significantly, as evidenced by the publication of three journals to disseminate research:

*Research in Nursing and Health, Advances in Nursing Science,* and *Western Journal of Nursing Research.* Doctoral nursing programs continued to emerge, leading to steady growth in nurses specifically prepared to be researchers. The emphasis in nursing research during this time was traditional quantitative methods, often testing theories borrowed from other fields. Despite this emphasis, nursing theory also was growing during this period, and qualitative methods were increasingly used.

The steady increase in both research itself and nurses prepared to do research reached a critical level in the 1980s, culminating in the establishment of the National Center of Nursing Research at the National Institutes of Health in 1986. The national recognition of nursing as a science, warranting funding for its own research agenda and center, was a major milestone. Nursing was now acknowledged as an important player among other "big" players, such as the National Institute for Medicine and the National Institute of Mental Health. In 1993, 7 years after its establishment, the National Center for Nursing Research became the National Institute of Nursing Research. This change placed nurses on equal footing with colleagues in medicine and other health-related fields. In addition, during the 1980s and 1990s, five more major nursing research journals were published and priorities for nursing research were developed. Nursing research had come of age.

At the beginning of the 21st century, nursing research continues to grow exponentially. Nurses prepared at the doctoral level, sources and opportunities for funding of nursing research, and diversity of topics examined in nursing research all have increased steadily. Since the 1990s, when qualitative approaches became recognized and respected as appropriate methods of scientific inquiry, nursing has begun to implement mixtures of quantitative and qualitative methods for study design and analysis that fit the unique research problems of the field.

Probably most important, as nursing research has grown, the body of nursing knowledge also has developed. As nurses, we have expanded our horizons to consider outcomes research, international research, and traditional laboratory research. We have replicated and expanded upon previous findings. Our researchers have completed multiple studies all related to the same problems, allowing us to truly build knowledge and to find real answers to complex questions. As a result, we now have Centers for Research housed in various universities, where groups of nurses with research expertise in specific areas (such as health-promoting behaviors) can work and build their research together to achieve a better-connected and deeper knowledge. Nurses also have recognized their limits as well as their strengths, moving increasingly toward the creation of and participation in interdisciplinary teams of researchers, capitalizing on the strengths inherent in the blending of many different disciplines.

## LINKING THEORY, EDUCATION, AND PRACTICE WITH RESEARCH

Although nursing research has made great strides, it still has a long way to go. The journey is linked with the past development of nursing education, practice, and theory, and these connections will continue in the future. In Chapter 10, we discussed the intertwining braid of research, practice, and theory. In fact, that "braid" contains four strands, the last of which is nursing education. Historically, nursing education occurred in an apprenticeship format, mostly within hospital schools of nursing. Only as nursing has moved into university education and begun to claim a unique body of knowledge have nurses started considering independent research. Nursing education has fostered nursing research, partly through the demand for faculty with credentials equivalent to those of other faculty in university settings and partly through the preparation of nurses who expect to use, participate in, and conduct nursing research. Doctoral preparation in nursing has given nurses the training and skills needed to become researchers. The existence of clinically based nursing has led to the education of nurses to use research in practice. Therefore, education has been, and remains, integral to the development and use of nursing research.

The four-stranded braid of nursing practice, education, theory, and research represents the future of the nursing profession (Figure 12–2). Nursing theory must be based on and applicable to nursing practice. Nursing research must test and refine nursing theory for practice. Nursing education must teach both theory and research as they relate to practice and develop in nurses a commitment to the understanding and use of research. Nursing practice must be based on an ever-developing body of knowledge derived from research and theory. Nurses must be educated to have an open, skeptical, and critical view of their practice to identify areas for using and problems to be addressed by nursing research.

The four-stranded braid is not without its symbolic "knots." As indicated within the discussion of the history of nursing research, early studies focused on nurses themselves and were not useful for direct practice. As practice-based research began, a real gap developed between nursing theory and nursing research. Nursing theory was highly conceptual and broad, focusing on the entire practice of nursing. Conversely, nursing research often was problem focused, addressing narrow and specific clinical situations. The two did not go hand-in-hand, and, as nursing research studies were completed, there often were no or few follow-up studies to build upon

**FIGURE 12-2**   **Four stranded braids of education, practice, research, and theory.**

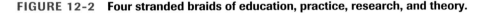

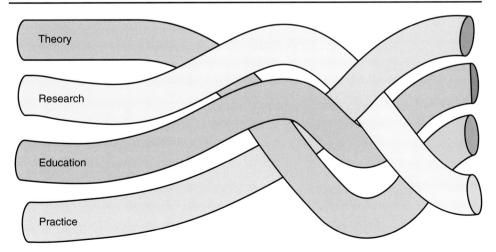

the initial knowledge developed. We have seen that it is unusual for a single study to fully answer a clinical question. Yet, at times, nursing has produced several single isolated clinical studies that failed to contribute to a coherent body of knowledge. One reason for this was the failure to use and to build theory relevant to the clinical problems of interest to nursing. Another problem has been limits in the dissemination of research. A third problem has been lack of funding for ongoing research programs. Finally, a gap has existed between researchers and practitioners of nursing. This gap occasionally has resulted from nurse researchers' limited connections with practice and occasionally from practicing nurses' discomfort with using research.

The gap between research and practice has been of particular concern to nursing. Since the 1970s, the profession has made a significant effort to facilitate research utilization. **Research utilization** means the use of research in practice. Several research studies have been completed to examine specifically whether research is assimilated into nursing practice. The results generally have been discouraging, although the extent to which research innovations are used has improved over time (Ketefian, 1975; Coyle & Sokop, 1990). Because studies continue to indicate that nursing often fails to use research in practice, nursing has looked closely at what may be causing this "knot" in the intertwining relationship between research and practice.

Many factors have been identified that affect research utilization, including limited applicability of some research to practice, resistance within health care organizations to make changes based on research, and difficulty understanding and using research among practicing nurses. The goal of this entire book is to address that last factor. Nursing has responded to the gap between findings from research and clinical practice by developing several different projects to increase the use of research findings in daily practice. Overall, the projects have demonstrated that research utilization can happen if the research relates directly to practice and is communicated broadly in ways that practicing nurses can understand and use (Horsley, Crane, Crabtree, & Wood, 1983).

One response in nursing to the problem with research utilization has been to develop models to describe and explain the process of using research. These models define phases or steps that may facilitate research utilization and include the Stetler model (1994), Rogers (1995) theory of research utilization, and the Iowa Model of Research Based Practice (Titler et al., 1994). Any of these models may help you to understand and to organize your use of research in practice. Rather than starting with an entirely new model for the use of research in practice, however, you may want to begin by using the five questions organizing this text.

To use research in practice, start by using your understanding about how to search for research as described in Chapter 1. Then use the five questions that organize the content of this text while reading the research you have found. This text has organized the presentation of content starting at the end of a research report and moving forward. Now that you have a better understanding of the language and process of research, it will be easier to read reports starting from the beginning and moving to the end. As you do so, ask yourself:

1. Why ask that question—what do we already know?
2. How were those people studied—why was the study done that way?

3.  To what types of patients do these research conclusions apply—who was in the study?
4.  Why did the author(s) reach that conclusion—what was actually found?
5.  What is the answer to the research question—what did the study conclude?

As you ask and answer these questions, always be openly questioning and critically regarding the study design, methods, sample, results, and conclusions. Doing so will help you to answer the overall question of how convincing the study is to use the results in practice. To help you read research, the end of this text includes a glossary, which provides definitions of terms and the page(s) in the book that describes them. The glossary also provides a lined column next to each term for you to use to make notes so that you will find it easier to understand the term the next time you encounter it. It is hoped that this glossary will be a real resource for you as you develop your skills at reading and understanding research. Using your understanding and knowledge about the language of research and the process of research, you will be able to make intelligent decisions about the use of research in practice.

In summary, we have examined the history of nursing research and how that has led to today's interacting relationships between education, practice, research, and theory. We have identified that although the relationships are essential to the ongoing development of nursing as a profession, there is still much to improve upon in the relationships. We have also seen that one of the biggest concerns in nursing has been and continues to be the dissemination of research results into practice. In the next section, we will explore evidence-based practice as currently used within nursing to strengthen the link between research and practice.

## EVIDENCE-BASED PRACTICE: PROS AND CONS

At the beginning of this book, we defined evidence-based practice broadly as nursing practice based on the conscious and intentful use of research and theory-based information to make decisions about care delivery to patients. The language "evidence-based practice" originated in the field of medicine. The concept often is considered to have been established by Dr. Archie Cochrane, a physician and epidemiologist. Cochrane was the developer of the "Cochrane Reviews," an electronic database similar to CINAHL, which consists of systematic reviews in various health care fields (French, 2002). If you search for topics in this database, you will find a short, focused systematic review, along with a list of relevant primary sources. Remember that a systematic review is the product of a process that includes asking a clinical question, conducting a structured and organized search for theory and research related to the question, reviewing and synthesizing the results, and reaching conclusions about the implications for practice.

Another important source for systematic reviews is the *Online Journal of Knowledge Synthesis in Nursing* (OJKSN) (Sigma Theta Tau International [STTI], 1993). The purpose of this recently developed online journal is to present "synthesized knowledge to guide nursing practice and research." The exercise in heart failure systematic review (Adams & Bennett, 2000) discussed in Chapter 9 came from the OJKSN. Both the Cochrane Reviews and the OJKSN serve an important function in improving the use of research in practice, because they pull together disparate studies into an easily accessible and organized form. This allows the nurse to find multiple studies on the same clinical question already synthesized into a single review that ends with recommendations for practice. Clearly then, systematic reviews address the issues of access to research and, to some extent, applicability of research to practice.

Use of systematic reviews for evidence-based practice has limits as well as strengths. As we saw in Chapter 9, just as a researcher implementing a traditional research study must make decisions about methods and sample, the author of a systematic review must make decisions about what research to include. This raises the question of what constitutes the "best" evidence. As demonstrated in the systematic review of exercise in heart failure, often the standard set for appropriate studies to include in a review is that they be clinical research using quasi-experimental or experimental designs. Although there is no question that studies using those designs are important and useful for answering some questions in nursing, many problems in nursing do not lend themselves to this level of quantitative study. Therefore, an overdependence on systematic reviews of clinical research may limit both the types of problems that practitioners consider appropriate for research utilization and the dissemination of important knowledge acquired using other research methods.

Systematic reviews as a type of research have an important place in using research in practice. Reading and understanding systematic reviews should be conducted using the same five questions mentioned throughout this book and keeping the same openly questioning and critical mind. The difference in reading and understanding systematic reviews is that you must answer the five questions at two different levels, rather than just at one level. For example, when considering the question "How were those people studied—why was the study done that way?" you must consider the methods for the different studies included in the review. However, you also must consider the rationale for use of a systematic review approach to this clinical question. Probably the toughest two-layered question will be "To what types of patients do these research conclusions apply—who was in the study?" To answer, you must consider the samples in the different studies in the review, as well as the sample of "studies" that comprise the review. The second layer becomes "Why did the reviewer include those studies and not others?" Table 12–1 provides an overview of how one might apply the five questions to a systematic review.

Systematic reviews are an important source of evidence for practice, but they are not the only evidence, and they are not even the only source of research evidence. Studies such as the one reported in the trajectory to certain death report (Steele, 2000) in Chapter 8 are not quasi-experimental nor experimental, yet they yield knowledge that can be useful to delivering thoughtful and understanding nursing care. As an intelligent reader and user of nursing research, you must find how the use of evidence in the form of systematic reviews can be most useful to you in your clinical practice.

## QUALITY IMPROVEMENT: FRAMED WITH THE RESEARCH PROCESS

Although systematic reviews are an important form of research that can be used in practice, quality improvement is a process that resembles, yet differs, from the research process. **Quality improvement** is a process of evaluation of health care serv-

| TABLE 12-1 | Five Research Questions Applied to Systematic Reviews and Quality Improvement Reports | |
|---|---|---|
| **Guiding Question** | **Application to Systematic Reviews** | **Application to Quality Improvement Reports** |
| Why ask that question—what do we already know? | What do we already know that suggests the need for a systematic review? | What is the basis for the standard or outcome to be examined? |
| How were those people studied—why was the study done that way? | Why was a systematic review used? Why were the studies that were included in the review done that way? | Why was the study done that way? What was the justification for the approach taken? |
| To what types of patients do these research conclusions apply—who was in the study? | What types of studies were included as evidence in the review? What types of samples were used in the studies reviewed? | What types of practices, settings, and patients are reflected by the information collected for the study? |
| Why did the author(s) reach that conclusion—what was found? | Why did the review reach its conclusions? What did the studies find? | Why did the report reach its conclusions? What was found about practice? |
| What is the answer to the research question—what did the study conclude? | What is the answer to the clinical question? | Were the standards or outcomes met—what does the report tell us about why or why not? |

ices to see if they meet specified standards or outcomes of care and to identify how they can be improved. As discussed in Chapters 1 and 2, quality improvement often is based on research, and the process and product resemble the research process. The question in quality improvement is whether a certain set of actions is occurring and how desirable outcomes can be facilitated. This is a form of a descriptive research question. The standard or outcome itself usually is based on earlier research that indicates the set of actions or outcome that can and should be achieved. Standards of care change as research findings suggest better approaches to and potential outcomes of care.

In addition to asking a descriptive question about the presence or frequency of a set of actions or outcomes, quality improvement studies also often examine relationships among factors that may affect the outcome or actions of interest. Just as we want to know what factors may influence a clinical problem of interest, we want to know what factors influence the consistency of achievement of standards or outcomes.

The usefulness of a quality improvement study can be understood using the same five questions discussed throughout this book. Table 12–1 outlines how they might be applied. We can consider why the standard or outcome was established—what is the evidence for that standard? We can ask about the manner by which the study was implemented, because various methods can be used to implement quality improvement, including chart review, observation, interviews, and questionnaires. Various approaches can be taken to the "sample" for a quality improvement study including convenience, random selection, and purposive sampling. Similarly, data from a quality improvement study can be handled and analyzed in several ways, making the fourth question about what was actually found appropriate to consider. The last question, what did the study conclude, is obviously also relevant to quality improvement studies. Just as an accurate and meaningful research study can inform clinical practice, an accurate and a meaningful quality assurance study can evaluate and strengthen practice. Findings from a quality improvement study that indicate standards are being met support continuation of existing practices. Findings that indicate that standards are not being met should guide revision of existing practices to improve care. As with traditional research, findings from a quality improvement study may lead to the need for another study to further clarify issues that may relate to meeting standards or outcomes.

In such ways, traditional research often serves as the basis for quality improvement standards. Moreover, many of the methods used in research directly apply to the process of evaluating quality. Finally, gaps in quality of care may indicate fresh areas requiring research, as well as needs for changes in practice.

## WHERE ARE WE GOING? ROLES OF NURSES IN RESEARCH

This text has focused on the baccalaureate-prepared nurse's role in understanding and using research in practice. It also has suggested some other ways that research may be part of the role of the baccalaureate nurse. For example, nurses may be asked to use research as the basis for decisions about the development of clinical programs. The vignette in Chapters 4 and 5 that used research as a basis for development of programs for Latino populations is an example. Nurses may be asked to participate in some step of the research process, particularly in acquiring informed consent and in collecting data, and we considered an example of that role in Chapter 7. Equally important, as the nursing profession recognizes the need for clinically relevant and informed research, baccalaureate nurses may be asked to participate in all phases of a research study, from development and refinement of the purpose to interpretation of the results. The vignette in Chapter 11 illustrated such a role for the baccalaureate-prepared nurse.

We began this book by saying that it was not the goal of this text to give you the tools to implement research independently. Doctoral-level nurses are expected to be the experts in the research process. Nurses prepared at the master's level are expected to be sophisticated consumers of research, able to critically evaluate and to actively participate in research. Nevertheless, baccalaureate-level nurses often are the foundation from which research is developed and are absolutely the focus for research utilization. Your understanding of the language and the process of research, coupled with your clinical experience, will allow you to be a contributor to a research team, should the opportunity arise. One hospital that perhaps best epitomizes the full extent of the potential role of the baccalaureate-prepared nurse in research is housed on the grounds of the National Institutes of Health. Every patient there participates in at least one research study, and the hospital employs only baccalaureate-prepared nurses. The nurses there not only participate in research but also can develop their own cooperative research projects, with support from researchers with advanced preparation.

Nursing not only has a role in research that directly addresses questions that the profession generates, but it also addresses larger questions in health care. We mentioned that nursing has moved increasingly to interdisciplinary teams to address research problems. Nurses also are being sought increasingly to participate in research teams led by researchers from other disciplines. Nursing's unique understanding of health as it affects the whole person, family, and community is a perspective that often contributes important ideas to research studies. Nurses are good at working with people. Thus, researchers from other disciplines often find that nurses can implement sampling plans effectively, with little subject loss.

Beyond generating and participating in research, nursing has an important role in formulating the national research agendas regarding health. The research supported and generated through the National Institute of Nursing Research at the National Institutes of Health has earned the respect of other, more established research disciplines. That development has contributed to ensuring that health concerns of particular concern to nursing have become part of national agendas for health-related research. Nursing research has made great progress since the days of Florence Nightingale, and we can be proud not only of our heritage of research but also of our current and future contributions to meaningful research that improves the care of our patients.

## FINDING ANSWERS THROUGH RESEARCH

What have we learned about reading and using research to answer questions about clinical practice? First, we have acknowledged that turning to research is not always the easiest way to get answers. We have identified that the language of research is unique. We have described how to find research and have examined each section of a research report in some detail. We have also considered the research process and how it is reflected in and relates to the nursing process, evidence-based practice, and quality improvement. Throughout the previous chapters, we have identified 31 core concepts, which are the foundation of ideas that can help nurses to understand and use research in practice. The concepts follow:

- Nursing research is the systematic gathering of information to gain, expand, or validate knowledge about health and responses to health problems. (Chapter 1)
- Abstracts from research reports can be helpful in narrowing or focusing on the appropriate research to acquire and to read. They cannot, and should not, be depended on to provide a level of understanding to support clinical decision making. (Chapter 1)

- The differences between results and conclusions is that results are a summary of the actual findings or information collected in the research study, whereas conclusions summarize the potential meaning, decisions, or determinations that can be made based on the information collected. (Chapter 2)

- Most research attempts to systematically gather information about a subset, or small group of patients or people, to gain knowledge about other similar patients or people. Many research methods are aimed at ensuring that what happens in the subset or sample studied is as similar as possible to what would happen in other larger groups of patients or people. (Chapter 2)

- Many terms used in research have a range of meanings rather than a single discrete locked-in meaning. (Chapter 2)

- The summary of findings in the discussion section of a research report contains only selected results from the study. It does not give the reader a complete picture of the results found in the study but does give information about some key or important results. (Chapter 3)

- The discussion section of a research report contains a debate about how the results of the study fit with existing knowledge and what those results may mean. (Chapter 3)

- Research results that only describe or explain cannot be used to predict outcomes or to identify directly the cause of the findings. (Chapter 4)

- Measures of central tendency and distribution are univariate statistics that summarize information about a variable. (Chapter 4)

- Inferential statistics are used to report whether the results found in the specific study are likely to have happened by chance alone. Statistical significance is *not* an absolute guarantee that the values are really different or related in the real world. Rather, statistical significance means that there is a less than 5% chance that the amount of relationship or difference happened by chance. (Chapter 5)

- Whether the report includes *p*-values or confidence intervals, the authors are telling you how likely it is that the results from the study happened due to chance and, therefore, how likely it is that these results can be used to infer similar results in future similar situations. (Chapter 5)

- Researchers use different types of statistics to test for the same kind of relationship depending on the form of the data collected. The research report may tell you why a particular type of statistical test was applied. (Chapter 5)

- A correlation between two variables tells us only that they are connected in some way and not the cause of that connection. (Chapter 5)

- The size of the sample, or number of cases in a study, affects the likelihood that the study will find statistical significance. (Chapter 5)

- Statistical significance does not directly equate with clinical meaningfulness. (Chapter 5)

- A researcher may define the population of interest for a study in one way but end up with a sample that differs from that defined population. (Chapter 6)

- Sampling strategies in qualitative and quantitative research differ in their goals and approaches, even when they are using a similar strategy. (Chapter 6)

- It is unethical and illegal to implement a research study using animal or human subjects without approval of the institutional review board. (Chapter 7)
- The goal of research with human subjects is always to minimize the risks and to maximize the benefits. (Chapter 7)
- The five human rights in research are first and foremost the responsibility of the researcher(s). (Chapter 7)
- The measures in a quantitative study should reflect the specific variables under study. (Chapter 8)
- Operationalizing variables is similar to translating a phrase from one language to another. The researcher translates an abstract and theoretical variable into a concrete measure or set of measures. (Chapter 8)
- Consistent measurement is reliable measurement. Accurate or correct measurement is valid measurement. (Chapter 8)
- The type of research question being asked affects the type of research design that will and can be used. (Chapter 9)
- Studies with problems in internal validity automatically will have problems with external validity. Having internal validity, however, does not guarantee that the study will have external validity. (Chapter 9)
- The labels for quantitative research designs usually are a combination of words or terms that define the design in terms of function, use of time, and use of approaches to provide control. (Chapter 9)
- Theory, theoretical frameworks, and conceptual frameworks all provide a description of the proposed relationships among abstract components that are aspects of the research problem of interest. (Chapter 10)
- The terms research purpose, research question, study or specific aim(s), or research objective(s) all refer to the statement of the variables to be studied that are related to the broad research problem. (Chapter 10)
- The literature review is guided by the variables that have been identified in the research purpose and aims to give the reader an overview of what is known about those variables, how those variables have been studied in the past, and with whom they have been studied. (Chapter 10)
- The steps of the research process are not always linear; they may overlap or be revisited during the research process. (Chapter 11)
- Whether a research problem or question has been identified from practice or from theory, the first step in developing a research study requires thoughtful and informed exploration of the problem to arrive at a refined purpose for the study. (Chapter 11)

Together, these core concepts form the backbone of your knowledge about the language and process of research.

One important idea that we have discussed throughout this text is the differences and relationships between qualitative and quantitative research approaches. Traditional science and medicine primarily have used and have supported the quantitative approach. As a result, nursing initially heavily emphasized quantitative approaches. Qualitative approaches, however, have been receiving steady recognition as being important to knowledge development in nursing. This text has attempted to present you with balanced information about both approaches so that you can read and understand research from both, as well as research that uses mixed methods.

Using research in practice has several advantages. The most obvious is that when research is used in practice, that practice is based on a clearly identifiable knowledge base. Using research in practice can open nurses to new ideas that are challenging and exciting to explore and to implement. It also can help nursing grow as a profession to achieve the broadest goal of promoting the health of patients. Using research in practice also has some disadvantages. First, time and effort are necessary to read and to understand research reports. Like any skill, the more one does it, the easier it becomes. Nonetheless, going to research to answer a question definitely necessitates more effort than does asking someone (assuming that he or she has the correct answer when you ask). Another potential disadvantage to using research in practice is that accessing research may not always be easy. Again, this problem is steadily becoming less important as more journals become available online. Nevertheless, for some nurses in rural settings, even online access to a system (such as a university library) may be difficult. The third disadvantage is the potential resistance to change that is inherent in the adoption of new or revised practices. Change, however, is both needed and inevitable in all aspects of life. Facing some resistance initially may simply be part of practicing as a professional nurse.

## FICTIONAL ARTICLE: WHAT WOULD YOU CONCLUDE?

The vignette at the beginning of the chapter provides an opportunity to take one final look at the fictional article discussed throughout this book. As S.J. reads that article, she starts by asking: Why ask that question–what do we already know? She finds that the background section of this report is brief. It does provide a broad context for the problem of varying extents of shortages in different fields of nursing. It also makes a somewhat limited case for targeting student recruitment efforts in a way that may increase the numbers of new graduates who will enter fields of nursing expected to have the greatest shortages.

S.J. finds that the purpose of the study is stated clearly and that the author gives three specific research questions that identify variables. S.J. can identify that this study asks a question about relationships. S.J. finds, however, several major gaps in the background section of the report. In particular, there is no literature review, so S.J. has no idea what other studies have been conducted to look at predictors of field of practice or what methods might have been used. In fact, although the purpose of the study is clear, the second and third research questions bring in two new variables that have not been mentioned: students' well-being and students' previous experiences. S.J. has a general answer to the question of why this study asked this question, but she also is somewhat confused about why this study included the particular variables. She does not have a clear picture of what is already known.

S.J. proceeds to read the methods section and finds that almost nothing in it tells her about the study design. Reading the abstract for the report, she learns that the study is identified as "descriptive," and she knows a descriptive study fits logically with the type of questions the study is to address. She skips the sample section and focuses on the measures section to see if she can clearly answer the second question:

How were those people studied–why was the study done that way? The measures section describes a questionnaire that asks specific closed questions. S.J. recognizes that this is a quantitative approach to description that again fits with the types of questions addressed in this study. The report gives S.J. a clear picture of the measure used, including some information about the reliability and validity of one scale included. This report includes no real theoretical or operational definitions, but most of the variables studied seem concrete. The exceptions are the two concepts, well-being and students' experiences, that also were not discussed in the literature review. Both are abstract; although the report is clear about their measurement, S.J. still is unclear about why they were included and why the author decided to add a more qualitative piece to the end of this questionnaire.

S.J. now returns to the sample section to try to answer: To what types of patients do these research conclusions apply? This section answers her question relatively clearly. S.J. finds that a convenience sample was used. She knows that such a sample opens the door to several potential threats to the validity of the study. She finds a clear description of the type of nursing program and students from which the sample was taken, giving her a good idea about both the strengths and the limits associated with those who participated. S.J. finds that the sample is small for a descriptive study. She notes that some effort was made to ensure the confidentiality of the students as subjects; however, there is no mention of informed consent. The sentence that indicates that subjects were told that the questionnaire was part of efforts to plan future programs suggests that students were, in fact, not fully informed of the purpose of the study, which truly concerns S.J. She believes that she has a clear answer to the question about who was in the study, but she also has some serious reservations about the ethics of this study.

The fourth question that S.J. wants to answer to understand this report is: Why did the author reach the conclusions—what was actually found? Reading the results section, she finds univariate statistics telling her the characteristics of the sample, which are also the variables included in the study. The variables in the analysis are the same as those discussed in the measures section, so a logical fit exists between these two sections. The report clearly tells S.J. the students' choices for fields of practice. The report then indicates that the nine fields identified in the table were categorized as either acute or nonacute; however, the report does not tell S.J. which fields were in each category. Although intensive care is obviously acute, S.J. wonders if the author counted obstetrics as acute or nonacute, given that women often deliver and go home the same day. S.J. understands from the results that, despite a small sample, which decreases the chance of statistically significant findings, there were differences in age and health rating that would have occurred fewer than 5% of the time by chance alone. Also, S.J. knows that regression means the author examined how a combination of more than two variables explained choice of acute and nonacute setting.

The results section starts with analysis that S.J. clearly recognizes as reflecting a quantitative approach to knowledge development. When the report starts to discuss "subjective findings," however, S.J. notes language that reflects a qualitative approach. The report discusses themes and gives some specific examples derived from students' answers to the open question about their experiences. S.J. realizes this study used a mixed methods approach, although this never was stated explicitly.

Finally, S.J. reads the discussion section considering the question: What is the answer to the research question–what did the study conclude? She finds that the summary of findings is clear. The report provides some interpretation or debate about the meaning of the results, suggesting age may relate to well-being and to type of experience, thus connecting findings that were separate before. Because no literature was at the beginning of the report, however, the author does not relate the findings to previous studies or to any existing theory. Therefore, although the ideas suggested in the discussion interest S.J., she realizes that they must be considered as informed speculation. She concludes that there is some limited evidence that older students particularly may be more likely to choose nonacute settings for practice after graduation than are younger students. She also concludes that health self-rating may be a relevant factor in setting choice. S.J. understands, however, that this report has several limits, and, as best as she can tell, the study itself had several limits. Therefore, she concludes that she would not make any recommendations based on the results except that further research should be done.

S.J. has been able to read and to understand this fictional example of a research report using the five questions that organized this text. As she answered these questions, she kept a critically open and questioning mind, looking for both strengths and weaknesses in the study that might be important in her decision about whether and how to use the study in the real world.

Reading and understanding research can be a positive and exciting challenge. The reality is that research, especially single research studies, almost never provides absolute and complete answers to real clinical questions, mainly because those types of questions have no simple and absolute answers. In practice, nurses must make decisions about what to do for each patient as problems arise. Nurses do not have time to examine the research literature at the moment that they are delivering care. Nevertheless, the research literature and the theory derived from and based on it comprise the foundation for daily clinical decisions. Reading and using research in practice is the hallmark of a professional nurse. The hope is that this text has given you a good start in your journey into the professional practice of nursing.

## References

Adams, C. D., & Bennett, S. (2000). Exercise in heart failure: A synthesis of current research. *The Online Journal of Knowledge Synthesis for Nursing, 7*(5).

Coyle, L. A., & Sokop, A. G. (1990). Innovation adoption behavior among nurses. *Nursing Research, 39,* 176–180.

French, P. (2002). What is the evidence on evidence-based nursing? An epistemological concern. *Journal of Advanced Nursing, 37*(3), 250–257.

Horsley, J., Crane, J., Crabtree, M., & Wood, D. (1983). *Using research to improve nursing practice: A guide.* New York: Grune & Statton.

Ketefian, S. (1975). Application of selected nursing research findings into nursing practice. *Nursing Research, 24,* 89–92.

Nightingale, F. (1893). *Notes on nursing.* London: Harrison & Sons.

Rogers, E. M. (1995). *Diffusion of innovations* (4th ed.). New York: Free Press.

Sigma Theta Tau International (STTI). (1993). Manuscript guidelines for *The Online Journal of Knowledge Synthesis for Nursing.* Available at: http://www.nursingsociety.org/library. Accessed August 10, 2002.

Steele, R. G. (2000). Trajectory of certain death at an unknown time: Children with neurodegenerative life-threatening illnesses. *Canadian Journal of Nursing Research, 32*(3), 49–67.

Stetler, C. B. (1994). Refinement of the Stetler/Marram model for application of research findings to practice. *Nursing Outlook, 42,* 15–25.

Titler, M. G., Kleiber, C., Steelman, V., Goode, C., Rakel, B., Barry-Walker, J., et al. (1994). Infusing research into practice to promote quality care. *Nursing Research, 43,* 307–313.

## Resources

LoBiondo-Wood, G., & Haber, J. (1998). *Nursing research: Methods, critical appraisal, and utilization* (4th ed.). St. Louis: Mosby.

Polit, D. F., & Hungler, B. P. (1999). *Nursing research: Principles and methods* (6th ed.). Philadelphia: Lippincott.

reduce**APPENDIX**

**A**

# Research Articles

The 10 articles contained in this appendix are referred to and discussed in various chapters throughout the text. While articles may be mentioned in several chapters, they normally correspond to topics specific to one or two chapters.

The following table will help link the articles to the chapters in which they are discussed:

| Article | Corresponding Chapter(s) |
|---------|--------------------------|
| A-1: Risk factors for cardiovascular disease in children with type I diabetes | 1—Using Nursing Research in Practice |
| A-2: Fecal incontinence in hospitalized patients who are acutely ill | 2—Components and Language of Research Reports |
| A-3: Homeless patients' experience of satisfaction with care | 3—Discussions and Conclusions |
| A-4: Evaluating the impact of peer, nurse case-managed, and standard HIV risk-reduction programs on psychosocial and health-promoting behavioral outcomes among homeless women | 3—Discussions and Conclusions |
| A-5: Mexican American family survival, continuity, and growth: The parental perspective | 4—Descriptive Results and 5—Inferential Results |

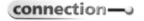

connection—⌐

reduceFor additional activities go to
http://connection.lww.com/go/macnee.

| Article | Corresponding Chapter(s) |
|---|---|
| A-6: Factors associated with participation by Mexican migrant farmworkers in a tuberculosis screening program | 4—Descriptive Results and 5—Inferential Results |
| A-7: Trajectory of certain death at an unknown time: Children with neurodegenerative life-threatening illnesses | 8—Data Collection Methods |
| A-8: Distress and growth outcomes in mothers of medically fragile infants | 8—Data Collection Methods |
| A-9: Exercise in heart failure: A synthesis of current research | 9—Research Designs: Planning the Study |
| A-10: Effect of positioning on $S\bar{v}O_2$ in the critically ill patient with a low ejection fraction | 9—Research Designs: Planning the Study |

# Risk Factors for Cardiovascular Disease in Children With Type I Diabetes

Terri H. Lipman, Laura L. Hayman, Carolyn V. Fabian, Diane A. DiFazio, Paula M. Hale, Barbara M. Goldsmith, Patricia C. Piascik

***Background***: *The major cause of morbidity and mortality in individuals with Type I insulin-dependent diabetes mellitus (IDDM) is premature and extensive atherosclerotic cardiovascular disease (CVD).*

***Objectives***: *To determine the prevalence and predictors of hypercholesterolemia and to examine the distribution and interrelationship of risk factors for CVD.*

***Methods***: *This observational (mixed-longitudinal) study, guided by an epidemiologic framework, assessed a sample of 140 children with IDDM. Total cholesterol (TC) and diabetes control were measured in the total sample. Standard CVD risk factors were measured in a subsample of 67 children.*

***Results***: *Observed frequency of TC greater than the 75th percentile and greater than the 95th percentile was significantly more than expected (p < 0.01 and p < 0.0001, respectively). In the total sample, TC-CVD risk factor associations were not observed. However, diabetes control and physical activity were correlated with TC in the risk sample of children at highest risk, as demonstrated by hypercholesterolemia.*

***Conclusions***: *Results demonstrate the importance of assessing the lipid profile in children with IDDM and monitoring CVD risk factors in hyperlipidemic children with IDDM. Future research should focus on prospective longitudinal studies in population-based multiethnic samples of children with IDDM.*

The major cause of morbidity and mortality in individuals with Type I insulin-dependent diabetes mellitus (IDDM) is premature and extensive atherosclerotic-cardiovascular disease (CVD) (Betteridge, 1989). The prevalence of CVD in this population points to the importance of early identification and treatment of known risk factors including dyslipidemias in children with IDDM.

Although recent recommendations for cardiovascular health promotion and risk reduction in children emphasize an integrated profile approach (Hayman & Ryan, 1994; Strong et al., 1992), minimal data exist regarding the distribution and interrelation of known risk factors for CVD in children with IDDM. Toward that goal, the purpose of this observational study of children with IDDM, designed within an epidemiologic-systems framework, was to determine the prevalence and predictors of hypercholesterolemia, and to examine the distribution and interrelation of risk factors for CVD: total cholesterol; systolic, diastolic, mean arterial blood pressures; body mass index; metabolic control (hemoglobin $A_1$ [$HbA_1$]); family history; Tanner stage of puberty; and patterns of physical activity and smoking behavior.

## CONCEPTUAL FRAMEWORK

The conceptual model guiding this study was the framework of epidemiology. The epidemiologic study of disease is extremely important for nursing because nursing and epidemiology share a common goal: the prevention of disease. Achievement of this goal, however, is a multiphasic process.

From a nursing perspective, the first phase of this process involves determining the distribution of disease in a population using epidemiologic methods. This approach allows for interpopulation comparisons, which facilitate the identification of risk factors. The ultimate goal in this line of research is to identify and define the environmental determinants of disease. Identifying and altering environmental factors may be effective in reducing the incidence of disease, or even preventing it.

Epidemiology uses an ecologic framework to study the relation of organisms to each other and to all other aspects of the environment (Mausner & Kramer, 1985). Therefore, epidemiologists propose that disease need not be attributed to any one factor, referring to such attribution as multiple causation or multifactorial etiology.

Epidemiology divides disease causation into three categories: agent, host, and environment. The *agent* is a factor that must be present for a disease to occur. Although the agent is a necessary factor, it is not sufficient to cause disease without the effect of the host and environmental factors. The *host* is the person with the disease, whereas the host factors (also called intrinsic factors) include one's genetic background, personality, and social class. *Environmental factors* (also called extrinsic factors) can be classified as biologic, social, and physical. The biologic environment involves the way individuals are integrated into the society, according to the society's economic and political organization. Physical environment normally includes heat, light, air, and water. The interrelation of the agent, host, and environmental factors, which cause disease, and each component must be analyzed and understood to ascertain the etiology of disease (Mausner & Kramer, 1985). The conceptual-theoretical-empirical structure for the research is depicted in Figure A1–1.

## RELATED LITERATURE

Knowledge of the established causal link between atherogenic lipids and CVD end points has prompted investigation of the lipid profile components in children with IDDM. Specifically, several observational studies have documented dyslipidemias, particularly elevated levels of total and low-density lipoprotein (LDL) cholesterol (LDL-C) as well as hypertriglyceridemia (Betteridge, 1989; Iwai et al., 1990; Ruderman & Hauderschild, 1984; Strobl et al., 1985). The association of diabetes duration and lipid levels (Couper et al., 1997; Rudberg & Persson, 1995) and the effect of glycemic and diabetes control (as measured by hemoglobin $A_1$ [$HbA_1$]) on dyslipidemias remain inconclusive. Whereas Lopes-Virella, Wohltmann, Mayfield, Loadholt, and Colwell (1983) demonstrated that intensive insulin therapy results in normalization of lipid and lipoprotein levels, results

**FIGURE A1-1**   **Conceptual-theoretical-empirical structure. Assessment of risk factors for cardiovascular disease in children with insulin-dependent diabetes mellitus. (Adapted with permission from Lipman, T. H., Hayman, L. L., Fabian, C. V., DiFazio, D. A., Hale, P. M., Goldsmith, B. M., et al. [2000, May/June]. Risk factors for cardiovascular disease in children with type I diabetes. *Nursing Research, 49*[3], 160–166.)**

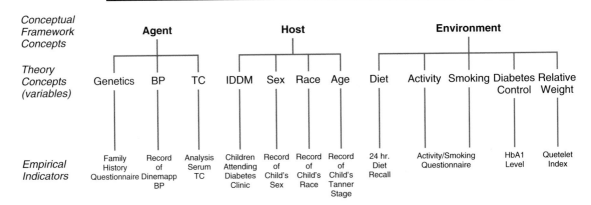

of more recent studies indicate no association between glycemic control and levels of lipids and lipoproteins in children with IDDM (Cruickshanks, Orchard, & Becker, 1985; Haffner, Tuttle, & Rainwater, 1991). Levitsky, Scanu, and Gould (1991) observed that enhancing diabetes control had no effect on total serum cholesterol in Black children and modest associations in White children. Methodologic differences notwithstanding, the results of these studies emphasize the need for additional data on the association between diabetes (metabolic) control and the lipid profile in children with IDDM.

Lipid levels increase with age because of interaction among both genetic and environmental factors. Quite low at birth, lipid levels approach young adult levels by the age of 2 years (Webber, Cresanta, Voors, & Berenson, 1983). At the time of puberty, partially because of hormonal changes, race- and sex-specific changes in the lipid profile become evident (Tell, 1985). Similar data from a cohort of children with Type I diabetes are not available.

Although levels of systolic, diastolic, and mean arterial blood pressure in children with IDDM have not been investigated extensively, data suggest an increased incidence of hypertension, which increases the risk and progression of nephropathy and atherosclerosis (Newkumet, Goble, Young, Kaplowitz, & Schieken, 1994). Relative to their nondiabetic counterparts, adolescents with IDDM have demonstrated higher resting and exercise-induced diastolic blood pressure levels (Newkumet et al., 1994; Nordgren, Freyschuss, & Persson, 1994).

In nondiabetic children, excess relative weight (used as a surrogate measure of adiposity) has been associated with adverse levels of lipids and lipoproteins (Aristimuno, Foster, Voors, Srinivasan, & Berenson, 1984) as well as systolic and diastolic blood pressure (Williams et al., 1992). Available data suggest similar associations in children with IDDM (Virdis et al., 1992). Although evidence indicates that physical activity has a positive influence on adiposity-lipid associations in nondiabetic children (DuRant et al., 1993), this has not been systematically investigated in children with IDDM.

Similarly, cigarette smoking, a major independent risk factor for CVD, has been extensively investigated and associated with both adverse lipid profiles and blood pressure in nondiabetic children and adolescents. Although less data are available on their diabetic counterparts, studies of adults with IDDM suggest similar atherogenic changes in smokers including lower levels of high-density lipoprotein cholesterol (HDL-C), the protective lipoprotein (Dullaart, Groener, Dikkeschei, Erkelens, & Doorenbos, 1991).

Because CVD aggregates in families, guidelines for targeted risk reduction in children and adolescents emphasize the importance of a reliable history of relevant diseases (National Cholesterol Education Program [NCEP], 1991). Although family history of CVD has not been investigated in relation to risk factor levels in children with IDDM, it has been examined in their nondiabetic counterparts (Dennison, Kikuchi, Srinivasan, Webber, & Berenson, 1989; Steiner, Neinstein, & Pennbridge, 1991). Data suggest that family history may fail to identify 40% to 60% of children with hypercholesterolemia, emphasizing the need for additional risk factor data to identify those at highest risk for CVD (Dennison et al., 1989).

Collectively, available data point to the importance of systematically investigating the total CVD risk profile in children with IDDM. Within the epidemiologic-systems framework, these data are requisite to timely, specific, preventive interventions. Therefore, this study was designed to examine the prevalence and predictors of hypercholesterolemia as well as the interrelation of CVD risk factors in children with IDDM.

## METHODS

### Sample

In the Section of Endocrinology at St. Christopher's Hospital for Children, 149 patients with IDDM were asked to participate in this study. Informed consent was obtained from 140 subjects. The criterion for inclusion was age between 1.5 and 20 years. This range of ages was chosen because it has been demonstrated that risk factors for CVD begin to track at 2 years of age (Lauer, Lee, & Clarke, 1989). Criteria for exclusion included ketosis, diabetes secondary to any other chronic condition (e.g., renal disease, cystic fibrosis), any known lipid abnormality, or the use of any medication known to influence lipids and lipoproteins.

In the first 73 children enrolled, data were obtained on demographics, total cholesterol, and $HbA_1$ levels. In a subset of 67 children, data were obtained on the total CVD risk factor profile, which included demographics, total cholesterol, $HbA_1$, pubertal stage, family history, activity, smoking, blood pressure, and body mass index. The second subset was a consecutive sample studied after the initial 73 children (Table A1–1).

### Procedure

After Institutional Review Board approval, the parents of all children with IDDM age 2 or older were asked to sign a consent form. Participants older than 12 years also gave assent. Parents who consented were asked to complete a questionnaire to assess family history and their children's activity and smoking behavior. At that visit, participants were weighed

---

**TABLE A1-1. Demographics of Children with IDDM**

| Group | n | Demographics | | | |
|-------|---|------|------|-----|---------------------|
| | | *Sex* | *Race* | *Age* | *Duration of Diabetes* |
| Subset 1[a] | 73 | 33F, 40M | 43W, 12B, 12H | $\bar{X}$ = 10.9 years | $\bar{X}$ = 4.1 years |
| Subset 2[b] | 67 | 30F, 37M | 53W, 8B, 9H | $\bar{X}$ = 10.2 years | $\bar{X}$ = 3.3 years |

Note: [a]The variables that were measured were demographics, total cholesterol, $HbA_1$.
[b]The variables that were measured were demographics, total cholesterol, $HbA^1$, pubertal stage, SBP, DBP, MAP, BMI, family history, activity, and smoking.
F = female.
M = male.
B = Black.
H = Hispanic.
W = White.

---

and measured for height. Blood pressure and Tanner staging also were determined. Blood was drawn to measure $HbA_1$ and nonfasting total cholesterol levels. Dietary history was not obtained in this study. The protocols were guided by the recommendations provided by the Report of the Expert Panel on Blood Cholesterol Levels in Children and Adolescents (NCEP, 1991).

### Measures

#### Lipids.
Venipuncture in the antecubital area was performed on all eligible subjects in the diabetes clinic. Participants were in a nonfasting state. Blood samples were centrifuged, and the serum was analyzed for total cholesterol using the Vitros-Ektachem (Model 700XR, Johnson & Johnson, Rochester, NY) coated on a clear polyester support. All total cholesterol (TC) values were converted from the serum values in the laboratory to plasma values (Lipid Research Clinic data). Because cholesterol levels measured in plasma are lower than in serum, the following conversion factor was used: serum value $\times$ 0.97 = plasma value (NCEP, 1991). Hypercholesterolemia was present if total cholesterol exceeded the 75th percentile for age, race, and gender.

#### Hemoglobin $A_1$ ($HbA_1$).
Glycosylated hemoglobin is measured routinely as an overall assessment of diabetes control in patients with diabetes mellitus. The concentration of a glycosylated hemoglobin in a cell reflects the average blood glucose levels in the cell during its 120-day life span. Normal nondiabetic individuals have $HbA_1$ levels of 5% to 8.5%. Patients

with diabetes in good control have levels below 10%. Using IMX (Model #9596, Abbott, La Jolla, CA), $HbA_1$ was assayed by separating it from other hemoglobin as the hemoglobin site passed through a prefilled column. The resin in the column was an affinity medium composed of boronate groups bound to agarose (Mullins & Austin, 1986).

#### Stage of pubertal development.
Stage of pubertal development was evaluated by an attending endocrinologist, advanced practice nurse, or endocrine fellow using the Tanner staging of pubic hair development (Tanner, 1975). Staging was from 1 (no development) to 5 (adult development).

#### Family history.
Family history was assessed and measured as in the coauthor's (L.L.H.) study of the CVD risk factor in twin families (Hayman, Meininger, Coates, & Gallagher, 1988). Health problems and how they were weighted for analysis included myocardial infarction (3), cardiovascular accident (2), diabetes (1), hyperlipidemia (1), and hypertension (1). Onset score was determined by age of onset (or death). Early onset (2) was defined separately for males ($\leq$50 years) and females ($\leq$60 years), with late onset was weighted 1 for both. The child's family history was based on a composite of the mother's and father's maternal and paternal histories. The range of scores was 0 to 32, with high scores indicating higher family history/risk.

#### Physical activity.
Items pertaining to physical activity on the questionnaire were based on a review of physical activity measures used in other epidemiologic studies (Paffenbarger, Wing, & Hyde, 1978; Taylor et

al., 1978). Items were developed into an index to measure level and type of physical activity. Responses to the single-item measure developed and used by Strazzulo et al. (1988) were summarized and used in data analysis. Parents were asked to indicate on a 1 (sedentary) to 4 (very active) Likert-type scale their perceptions of the child's leisure time physical activity. This measure of activity was pretested in the coauthor's study of CVD risk factors in twins. The items provide an overall interval-level index of physical activity.

Smoking. Questions relevant to the frequency of current cigarette smoking were included in the questionnaire. These data provide an ordinal scale index of cigarette smoking, which was used in the data analysis. This approach to quantifying tobacco consumption is similar to that used in the Bogalusa Heart Study (Hunter, Croft, & Parker, 1986).

Blood pressure. Three systolic blood pressure (SBP), three diastolic blood pressure (DBP), and three mean arterial blood pressure (MAP) measurements were recorded for each participant. The three SBPs, DBPs, and MAPs were measured with the Dinamap (Critikon, Tampa, FL: Model #1846). The participant was seated, and all measurements were taken from the right arm using the appropriate-size cuff (as determined by measurement of arm circumference) according to the criteria of the NHLBI Task Force on Blood Pressure Control in Children (1987). Although the participants did not rest before blood pressure measurements, three readings each of SBP, DBP, and MAP were recorded. The average value for each blood pressure variable was computed for each participant and used in the data analysis.

Relative weight. Height without shoes in children 3 years and older was obtained with a Harpenden Stadiometer (Holtain Ltd., Dyfed, Wales). In children younger than 3 years, height without shoes was obtained with a length board. Using a balance scale, weight was obtained with the children in light clothing wearing no shoes. An index of body mass (BMI) for the participants was computed using the Quetelet Index (weight in kg/height in $m^2$ [$kg/m^2$]) (LRC, 1980). For the purpose of data analysis, the BMIs were converted to percentiles for age, sex, and race based on Lipid Research Clinics population data (LRC, 1980). The average BMI for any age group was the 50th percentile.

### Statistical Analysis

Analyses were completed using StatView (SAS Institute Inc., Cary, NC). Means and standard deviations were computed for interval-level variables: age; total cholesterol; systolic, diastolic and mean arterial blood pressures; BMI; $HbA_1$; duration of diabetes; family history; physical activity; and Tanner stage. These computations were performed by total sample and by subsample (children with $TC \geq$ 75th age, race, and sex-specific percentile). According to $t$ tests (with Bonferroni-adjusted alpha level of 0.0045), there were no significant differences between the two groups on these variables.

In the total sample and subsample (children with $TC \geq$ 75th age, race, and sex-specific percentile), Pearson product-moment correlations were computed to examine the relation of the independent variables to the dependent variable (TC). In the subsample, regression analyses were conducted, with TC viewed as the dependent variable. An alpha level of 0.05 was used for the correlations and regression analyses.

### RESULTS

The sample included 70 males, 70 females, 96 Whites, 26 Blacks, and 18 Hispanics. The participants' mean age was 10.6 ± 4.6 years (range = 1.5–18.5 years). The mean duration of diabetes was 3.7 ± 3.3 years (range = 3 months to 14 years). Table A1–2 presents

---

**TABLE A1-2** Total Cholesterol Levels and Measurement of Risk Factors for CVD in Children with IDDM[a]

|  | TC mg/dL | $HbA_1$% | SBP mm/Hg | DBP mm/Hg | MAP mm/Hg |
|---|---|---|---|---|---|
| Mean ± *SD* | 164 ± 32.8 | 11 ± 3.2 | 106 ± 11.4 | 63 ± 8.7 | 78.9 ± 9.3 |
| Range | 86–272 | 6.2–21.7 | 85–131 | 45–86 | 61–101 |

Note: [a]$n$ = 140.
*SD* = standard deviation.

the mean, standard deviation, and range for TC, $HbA_1$, SBP, DBP, and MAP by total sample. The distribution of BMI of this population is skewed toward the higher percentiles (Figure A1–2). Most of the children had TC levels ranging from 120 to 200 mg/dl (Figure A1–3). The observed frequency of TC exceeding the 75th percentile ($n = 48; 34\%$) and 95th percentile ($n = 18; 13\%$) was significantly greater than expected ($p = 0.01$ and $p = 0.0001$, respectively). It is expected that 25% of the population would have TC levels exceeding the 75th percentile, and that 5% of the population would have TC levels exceeding the 95th percentile.

The results of the activity questionnaire showed that 33% of the children reported participating in sports or exercise three or more times per week (coded as 4), 21% two times per week (coded as 3), and 31% once a week (coded as 2), whereas 15% were described as sedentary (coded as 1) ($\mathbf{X} = 2.3 \pm 1.0$). The scores in the family history questionnaire ranged from 10 to 16 ($\mathbf{X} = 4 \pm 3.4$). Smoking history was noncontributory because the parents of all children except one reported that their children had never smoked.

For the total sample, no significant correlations were observed between TC and age, race, gender, duration of diabetes, $HbA_1$, Tanner stage, SBP, DBP, MAP, family history, BMI, or activity level. To determine if these associations were different in the subgroup of children with hypercholesterolemia, CVD risk factors were separately analyzed in children with TC that exceeded the 75th percentile. This subgroup did not differ significantly from the total sample in age, race, gender, duration of diabetes, $HbA_1$, blood pressure, Tanner stage, family history, BMI, or activity.

In linear regression analysis performed on children with TC exceeding the 75th percentile, $HbA_1$ was shown to be a significant predictor of TC ($R = 0.30; p = 0.03$), and activity level also was a significant predictor of TC ($R = 0.48; p = 0.02$). There was no interaction between $HbA_1$ and activity level in the regression analysis.

**FIGURE A1-2**  **Body mass index of children with insulin-dependent diabetes mellitus ($n = 67$). (Adapted with permission from Lipman, T. H., Hayman, L. L., Fabian, C. V., DiFazio, D. A., Hale, P. M., Goldsmith, B. M., et al. [2000, May/June]. Risk factors for cardiovascular disease in children with type I diabetes. *Nursing Research, 49*[3], 160–166.)**

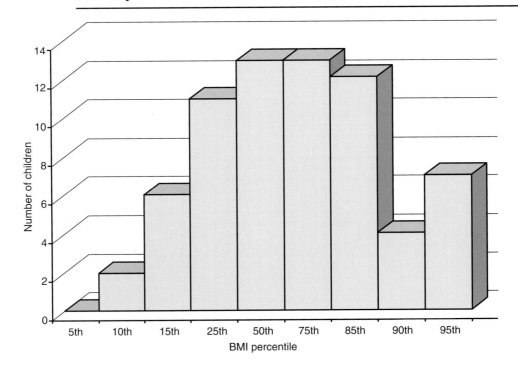

**FIGURE A1-3**    **Total cholesterol levels in children with insulin-dependent diabetes mellitus ($n = 140$). (Adapted with permission from Lipman, T. H., Hayman, L. L., Fabian, C. V., DiFazio, D. A., Hale, P. M., Goldsmith, B. M., et al. [2000, May/June]. Risk factors for cardiovascular disease in children with type I diabetes. *Nursing Research, 49*[3], 160–166.)**

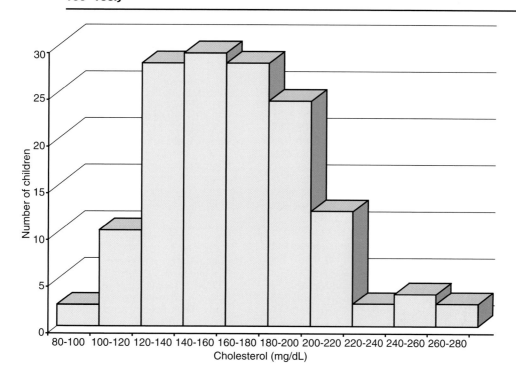

## DISCUSSION

The major purpose of this study was to examine the prevalence and predictors of hypercholesterolemia in children with Type I diabetes. The study was conceptualized within an epidemiologic-systems framework, with an emphasis on multifactorial determinants of disease causation. Consistent with this framework, the results of this study suggest an interaction of agent, host, and environment in the development and expression of Type I diabetes. Specifically, the results indicate that children with diabetes are at risk for hypercholesterolemia, an observation reported by others (Betteridge, 1989; Iwai et al., 1990; Strobl et al., 1985). Although no statistically significant TC-CVD risk factor associations were observed in the total sample, diabetes control (as measured by HbA$_1$) and levels of physical activity were correlated with TC in the subsample of children at highest risk.

The lack of association between HbA$_1$ and TC observed in the total sample of children with diabetes is consistent with results reported by Cruickshanks et al. (1985) and Haffner et al. (1991). Other studies have demonstrated that improved diabetes control results in normalization of lipid levels (Lopes-Virella et al., 1983). In practice, however, even diabetic children with 'very good' control do not have nondiabetic levels of HbA$_1$.

In the current study, an attempt was made to correlate TC with varying levels of abnormal HbA$_1$. As indicated in Table A1–2, the minimal variation observed in HbA$_1$ could account for the lack of association noted in this sample. Similarly, although blood pressure has been shown to correlate with TC in diabetic and nondiabetic children, minimal variation in levels of blood pressure was observed in the current study. It is noteworthy that only four children were hypertensive.

No association was found between family history of CVD and TC in the current sample. Therefore, if these children with diabetes had been screened solely on the basis of a positive family history, a number of children with elevated TC would have been missed.

There was no association between activity level and TC in the current sample, which also was demonstrated by Austin, Warty, Janosky, and Arslanian (1993). Campaigne et al. (1985) demonstrated that an exercise program significantly improved LDL levels in children with IDDM. The data are limited concerning the effects of activity on lipids in children with IDDM. Clearly, more studies are needed to elucidate the effect of exercise.

In the subgroup of children with TC exceeding the 75th percentile, TC was significantly predicted by $HbA_1$. However, the association was weak, and the underlying causal mechanism of the elevated cholesterol in this subgroup is unclear. Level of physical activity also significantly predicted TC in this subgroup. Previous studies have shown that exercise lowers lipid levels by decreasing body fat (DuRant et al., 1993), but in this study, the relation occurred independently of BMI. The mechanism is unknown, but it must be acknowledged that BMI is an indirect surrogate measurement of relative weight, and this relation should be reexamined with direct measures of adiposity.

Practice recommendations may advocate screening only children with a positive family history of CVD, but the lack of association between family history and TC in this study suggest that screening based on family history will not capture all children with elevated cholesterol. Additional research on population-based multiethnic samples of children with IDDM is needed. Although few statistically significant correlations and predictors among the measured variables were found, a total CVD profile approach in children with IDDM is advocated by the epidemiologic framework.

Methodologic limitations of this study (i.e., parental and self-report measures) could have influenced the range of scores and subsequently the lack of association between these risk factors and TC. A goal of epidemiologic research is to define risk factors most amenable to intervention. Improving diabetes control and encouraging exercise is a goal for all patients with diabetes, but the $HbA_1$/activity/TC association in the subgroup of hypercholesterolemic children with IDDM implies that exercise and metabolic control may be most beneficial for those at greatest CVD risk as defined by TC, and that these factors are amenable to intervention.

## References

Aristimuno, G. G., Foster, T. A., Voors, A. W., Srinivasan, S. R., & Berenson, G. S. (1984). Influence of persistent obesity in children on cardiovascular risk factors: The Bogalusa Heart Study. *Circulation, 69,* 895–904.

Austin, A., Warty, V., Janosky, J., & Arslanian, S. (1993). The relationship of physical fitness to lipid and lipoprotein (a) levels in adolescents with IDDM. *Diabetes Care, 16,* 421–425.

Betteridge, D. J. (1989). Diabetes, lipoprotein metabolism, and atherosclerosis. *British Medical Bulletin, 45,* 285–311.

Campaigne, B. N., Landt, M. J., Mellies, M. D., James, F. W., Glueck, C. J., & Sterling, M. A. (1985). The effects of physical training in blood lipid profiles in adolescents with IDDM. *Physician and Sports Medicine, 13,* 83–89.

Couper, J. J., Clarke, C. F., Byrne, G. C., Jones, T. W., Donaghue, K. C., Nairn, J., Boyce, D., Russell, M., Stephens, M., Raymond, J., Bates, D. J., & McCaul, K. (1997). Progression of borderline increases in albuminuria in adolescents with insulin-dependent diabetes mellitus. *Diabetic Medicine, 14,* 766–771.

Cruickshanks, K. J., Orchard, T. J., & Becker, D. J. (1985). The cardiovascular risk profile in adolescents with insulin-dependent diabetes mellitus. *Diabetes Care, 8,* 118–124.

Dennison, B. A., Kikuchi, D. A., Srinivasan, S. R., Webber, L. S., & Berenson, G. S. (1989). Parental history of cardiovascular disease as an indication for screening for lipoprotein abnormalities in children. *Journal of Pediatrics, 115,* 186–194.

Dullaart, R. P., Groener, J. E., Dikkeschei, B. D., Erkelens, D. W., & Doorenbos, H. (1991). Elevated cholesterol ester transfer protein activity in IDDM men who smoke: Possible factor for unfavorable lipoprotein profile. *Diabetes Care, 14,* 338–341.

DuRant, R. H., Baranowski, T., Rhodes, T., Gutin, B., Thompson, W. O., Carroll, R., Puhl, J., & Greaves, K. A. (1993). Association among serum lipid and lipoprotein concentrations and physical activity, physical fitness, and body composition in young children. *Journal of Pediatrics, 123,* 185–192.

Haffner, S. M., Tuttle, K. R., & Rainwater, D. L. (1991). Decrease of lipoprotein (a) with improved glycemic control in IDDM subjects. *Diabetes Care, 14,* 302–307.

Hayman, L. L., Meininger, J. C., Coates, P. M., & Gallagher P. R. (1988). *Biobehavioral cardiovascular risk factors: A twin family study.* Grant narrative (R01 NRO 1822, 1988–1993). National Institutes of Health, National Institute of Nursing Research, Bethesda, MD.

Hayman, L. L., & Ryan, E. A. (1994). The cardiovascular health profile: Implications for health promotion and disease prevention. *Pediatric Nursing, 20,* 509–515.

Hunter, S. M., Croft, J. B., & Parker, F. C. (1986). Biobehavioral studies in cardiovascular risk development. In Berenson, G. (Ed.), *Causation of cardiovascular risk factors in children: Perspectives on cardiovascular risk in early life.* (pp. 223–253). New York: Raven Press.

Iwai, M., Yoshino, G., Matsushita, M., Morita, M., Matsuba, K., Kazumi, T., & Baba, S. (1990). Abnormal lipoprotein composition in normolipidemic diabetic patients. *Diabetes Care, 13,* 792–796.

Lauer, R. M., Lee, J., & Clarke, W. R. (1989). Predicting adult cholesterol levels from measurements in childhood: The Muscatine Study. *Bulletin of the New York Academy of Medicine, 65,* 1127–1142.

Levitsky, L. L., Scanu, A. M., & Gould, S. H. (1991). Lipoprotein (a) levels in Black and White children and adolescents with IDDM. *Diabetes Care, 14,* 283–287.

Lipid Research Clinics. (1990). *Population Studies Data Book I: The Prevalence Study* (NIH Publication No.

80–1527). Washington, DC: U.S. Public Health Service. July, 1980.

Lopes-Virella, M. F., Wohltmann, H. J., Mayfield, R. K., Loadholt, C. B., & Colwell, J. A. (1983). Effect of metabolic control on lipid, lipoprotein, and apolipoprotein levels in 55 insulin-dependent diabetic patients: A longitudinal study. *Diabetes, 32,* 20–25.

Mausner, J. S., & Kramer, S. (1985). *Epidemiology: An introductory text.* Philadelphia: W.B. Saunders.

Mullins, R. E., & Austin, G. E. (1986). Sensitivity of isoelectric focusing, ion exchange, and affinity chromatography to labile glycated hemoglobin. *Clinical Chemistry, 32,* 1460–1463.

National Cholesterol Education Program. (1991). *Report of the Expert Panel on Blood Cholesterol Levels in Children and Adolescents* (NIH Publication No. 912732). Bethesda, MD: National Heart, Lung, and Blood Institute Information Center.

National Heart, Lung, and Blood Institute Task Force on Blood Pressure Control in Children. (1987). Report of the Second Task Force on Blood Pressure Control in Children—1987. *Pediatrics, 79,* 125.

Newkumet, K. M., Goble, M. M., Young, R. B., Kaplowitz, P. B., & Schieken, R. M. (1994). Altered blood pressure reactivity in adolescent diabetics. *Pediatrics, 93,* 616–621.

Nordgren, H., Freyschuss, U., & Persson, B. (1994). Blood pressure response to physical exercise in healthy adolescents and adolescents with insulin-dependent diabetes mellitus. *Clinical Science, 86,* 425–432.

Paffenbarger, R. S. Jr., Wing, A. L., & Hyde, R. T. (1978). Physical activity as an index of heart attack risk in college alumni. *American Journal of Epidemiology, 108,* 161–175.

Rudberg, S., & Persson, B. (1995). Association between lipoprotein (a) and insulin-like growth factor I during puberty and the relationship to micro albuminuria in children and adolescents with IDDM. *Diabetes Care, 18,* 933–939.

Ruderman, N. B., & Haudenschild, C. (1984). Diabetes as an atherogenic factor. *Progress in Cardiovascular Diseases, 26,* 373–412.

Steiner, N. J., Neinstein, L. S., & Pennbridge, J. (1991). Hypercholesterolemia in adolescents: Effectiveness of

screening strategies based on selected risk factors. *Pediatrics, 88,* 269–275.

Strazzullo, P., Cappuccio, F. P., Trevisan, M., DeLeo, A., Krogh, V., Giorgione, N., & Mancini, M. (1988). Leisure time physical activity and blood pressure in schoolchildren. *American Journal of Epidemiology, 127,* 726–733.

Strobl, W., Widhalm, K., Schober, E., Frisch, H., Pollak, A., & Westphal, G. (1985). Apolipoproteins and lipoproteins in children with type I diabetes: Relation to glycosylated serum protein and HbA$_1$. *Acta Paediatrica Scandinavica, 74,* 966–971.

Strong, W. B., Deckelbaum, R. J., Gidding, S. S., Kavey, R. E., Washington, R., Wilmore, J. H., & Perry, C. L. (1992). Integrated cardiovascular health promotion in childhood: A statement for health professionals from the Subcommittee on Atherosclerosis and Hypertension in Childhood of the Council on Cardiovascular Disease in the Young, American Heart Association. *Circulation, 85,* 1638–1650.

Tanner, J. M. (1975). Growth and endocrinology of the adolescent. In Gardner, L. J. (Ed.), *Endocrine and diseases of childhood* (2nd ed., pp. 14–64). Philadelphia: W.B. Saunders.

Taylor, H. L., Jacobs, D. R. Jr., Schucker, B., Knudsen, J., Leon, A. S., & Debacker, G. (1978). A questionnaire for the assessment of leisure time physical activities. *Journal of Chronic Diseases, 31,* 741–755.

Tell, G. S. (1985). Cardiovascular disease risk factors related to sexual maturation: The Oslo Youth Study. *Journal of Chronic Diseases, 38,* 633–642.

Virdis, R., Vandelli, M., Street, M., Zampolli, M., DeFanti, A., Cantoni, S., Bonacini, L., & Boselli, E. (1992). Blood pressure tracking in juvenile insulin-dependent diabetes mellitus: Preliminary data. *Acta Biomedica de Ateneo Parmense, 63,* 187–192.

Webber, L. S., Cresanta, J. L., Voors, A. W., & Berenson, G. S. (1983). Tracking of cardiovascular disease risk factor variables in school-age children. *Journal of Chronic Diseases, 36,* 647–660.

Williams, D. P., Going, S. B., Lohman, T. G., Harsha, D. W., Srinivasan, S. R., Webber, L. S., & Berenson, G. S. (1992). Body fatness and risk for elevated blood pressure, total cholesterol, and serum lipoprotein ratios in children and adolescents. *American Journal of Public Health, 82,* 358–363.

APPENDIX

A-2

# Fecal Incontinence in Hospitalized Patients Who Are Acutely Ill

Donna Zimmaro Bliss, Stuart Johnson, Kay Savik,
Connie R. Clabots, Dale N. Gerding

**Background:** Information about fecal incontinence experienced by patients in acute-care settings is lacking. The relationship of fecal incontinence to several well-known nosocomial or iatrogenic causes of diarrhea has not been determined.

**Objectives:** To determine the cumulative incidence of fecal incontinence in hospitalized patients who are acutely ill, and to ascertain the relationship between fecal incontinence and stool consistency, and between diarrhea and two well-known nosocomial or iatrogenic etiologies of diarrhea: Clostridium difficile and tube feeding. The relationship of fecal incontinence and risk factors for diarrhea associated with C. difficile and tube feeding in hospitalized patients was examined.

**Methods:** Fecal incontinence, stool frequency and consistency, administration of tube feeding and medications, severity of illness, and nutritional data were prospectively recorded in 152 patients on acute or critical care units of a university-affiliated Veterans' Affairs Medical Center. Rectal swabs and stool specimens from patients were obtained weekly for C. difficile culture. C. difficile culture and cytotoxin assay were performed on diarrheal stools. HindIII restriction endonuclease analysis (REA) was used for typing of C. difficile isolates.

**Results:** In this study, 33% (50/152) of the patients had fecal incontinence. The proportion of total surveillance days with fecal incontinence in these patients was $0.50 \pm 0.06$. A greater percentage of patients with diarrhea had fecal incontinence than patients without diarrhea (23/53 [43%] vs. 27/99 [27%]; $p = 0.04$). Incontinence was more frequent in patients with loose/liquid stool consistency than in patients with hard/soft stool consistency (48/50 [96%] vs. 71/100 [71%]; $p < 0.001$). The proportion of surveillance days with fecal incontinence was related to the proportion of surveillance days with diarrhea ($r = 0.69$; $p < 0.001$) and the proportion of surveillance days with loose/liquid stools ($r = 0.64$; $p < 0.001$). Multivariate risk factors for fecal incontinence were unformed/loose or liquid consistency of stool ($RR = 11.1$; 95% confidence interval [CI] = 2.2, 56.7), severity of illness ($RR = 5.7$; $CI = 2.6, 12.3$), and age ($RR = 1.1$; $CI = 1, 1.1$).

**Conclusions:** Fecal incontinence is common in hospitalized patients who are acutely ill, but the condition was not associated with any specific cause of diarrhea. Because loose or liquid stool consistency is a risk factor for fecal incontinence, use of treatments that result in a more formed stool may be beneficial in managing fecal incontinence. However, treatments that slow intestinal transit should be avoided in patients with C. difficile-associated diarrhea.

Fecal incontinence is a significant and costly problem. The condition ranks as the second leading cause for nursing home placement in the United States (Lahr, 1988), and its prevalence increases progressively with age (Campbell, Reinken, & McCosh, 1985; Johanson & Lafferty, 1996; Thomas, Ruff, Karran, Mellows, & Meade, 1987). Borrie and Davidson (1992) determined that an average of 52 minutes per day was spent by staff dealing with fecal, urinary, or double (i.e., fecal and urinary) incontinence in a long-term care institution, and that the associated annual cost was $9,771 per incontinent patient.

The prevalence of fecal incontinence associated risk factors have been described for persons in long-term care institutions and the community (Johanson & Lafferty, 1996; Nakanishi et al., 1997; Nelson, Norton, Cautley, & Furner, 1995; Thomas et al., 1987). Information about fecal incontinence experienced by patients in acute-care settings is lacking.

Previous studies of risk factors associated with fecal or double incontinence in institutionalized, long-term care patients focused on patients' mobility and cognitive status (Borrie & Davidson, 1992; Campbell et al., 1985; Issacs & Walkley, 1964). Diarrhea and liquid stools, reported to exacerbate fecal incontinence in community-dwelling adults (Read et al., 1979), may have a significant role in fecal incontinence among patients in both long-term and acute-care settings.

There are several well-known nosocomial or iatrogenic causes of diarrhea whose relationship to fecal incontinence has not been determined. *Clostridium difficile* is the most frequently identified organism responsible for nosocomial diarrhea (Bender et al., 1986; Cefai, Elliott, & Woodhouse, 1988; Siegel, Edelstein, & Nachamkin, 1990; Yannelli, Gurevich, Schoch, & Cunha, 1988). Diarrhea and liquid consistency of stools are common complications of tube feeding experienced by patients in acute- and chronic-care institutions (Bliss, Guenter, & Settle, 1992; Burns & Jairath, 1994; Guenter et al., 1991; Kelly, Patrick & Hillman, 1983).

Common risk factors implicated in diarrhea associated with *C. difficile* or tube feeding in patients who are acutely ill include medical therapies such as receipt of antibiotics or sorbitol-containing medications; patient characteristics such as older age, increased severity of illness, and malnutrition; and increased duration of hospitalization (Bliss et al., 1998; Edes, Walk, & Austin, 1990; Gerding et al., 1986; Gottschlich et al., 1988; McFarland, Surawicz, & Stamm, 1990). Whether these risks factors are associated with fecal incontinence in patients who are acutely ill is unknown.

The purpose of this study was to determine the extent and severity of fecal incontinence in hospitalized patients who are acutely ill, and to examine the relationship among fecal incontinence and stool consistency, diarrhea, *C. difficile*-associated diarrhea, tube feeding, and diarrhea during tube feeding. Risk factors for diarrhea associated with *C. difficile* or tube feeding also were examined for their relationship to fecal incontinence. These risk factors included exposure to antibiotics or sorbitol-containing liquid medications, age, severity of illness, nutritional status, duration of hospitalization before the study, and duration of surveillance. The relationship between the severity of fecal incontinence, as determined by the proportion of surveillance days with incontinence and the proportion of total stools that were incontinent, and the severity of diarrhea and loose or liquid stools was examined.

## METHODS

### Sampling

This study was a secondary analysis of data collected during a prospective cohort investigation of *C. difficile* infection in hospitalized tube-fed and non-tube-fed patients (Bliss et al., in press). Data about fecal incontinence were collected prospectively for this analysis in parallel to the original study. The original sample of patients included 184 adult patients in acute and critical care units at the Minneapolis Veterans Affairs Medical Center (MVAMC): 92 tube-fed patients who began nutritional support solely by tube feeding and a cohort of 92 non-tube-fed patients who were blocked or matched with the tube-fed patients on risk factors for *C. difficile* acquisition or associated diarrhea (Bliss et al., in press).

Sampling for the secondary data analysis included all patients from the original sample. However, 32 patients were excluded from the analysis: 7 patients with an enterostomy, for whom incontinence could not be determined, and 25 patients who were recruited into the epidemiologic study of *C. difficile* to pilot data collection procedures before prospective recording of fecal incontinence data. The blocking effect in the original sample thus was negated, and variables used for blocking then were assessed as covariates in this analysis.

### Surveillance Procedures

Fecal incontinence, stool consistency, and stool frequency or rectal bag volumes were recorded daily over at least 4 days for all patients on a stool record placed at the patient's bedside by the nursing staff or one of the investigators (D.Z.B.). Fecal incontinence was defined as the involuntary passage of stool from the rectum, resulting in soiling of clothing or bed linens or need for a rectal bag. Stool consistency was categorized as (a) hard and formed, (b) soft but formed, (c) unformed and loose, or (d) liquid. When these data were not reported on the stool record, the investigator checked the nurses' notes in the patient's chart or spoke with the nurses responsible for recording the patient's bowel movements.

Patients were monitored prospectively for *C. difficile* by obtaining a rectal swab (S/P Brand Culturette System, Baxter Diagnostics, Inc., Deerfield, IL) or stool specimen at baseline, at weekly intervals during tube feeding, and at the end of surveillance. For tube-fed patients, the baseline *C. difficile* culture was before the start of tube feeding, and the final culture was at cessation of tube feeding or at the time of their hospital discharge if tube feeding had been continued. Patients in the non-tube-fed cohort were monitored at least 80% of the time that the tube-fed patients were monitored.

Diarrhea was defined as three or more unformed or liquid stools per day or at least 250 ml liquid stool daily collected in a rectal bag (Bliss et al., 1992; Metcalf & Phillips, 1986). If a patient's stool met these criteria, a specimen for *C. difficile* culture, alcohol shock *C. difficile* culture, and cytotoxin assay was obtained every 48 hours until a positive culture or cytotoxin result was obtained or the diarrhea ceased. Episodes of diarrhea induced by medical therapy (e.g., laxatives, enemas, or preoperative bowel catharsis) were excluded from the analysis. A patient was considered to have *C. difficile*-associated diarrhea if a cytotoxin test result was positive or a toxigenic strain of *C. difficile* was recovered from a *C. difficile* culture, and if the diarrhea was concurrent with the positive *C. difficile* result or within the preceding week (range, 1 to 7 days). *C. difficile* colonization was defined as recovery of a toxigenic or nontoxigenic *C. difficile* strain from stool culture in a patient without diarrhea (asymptomatic colonization), or recovery of a nontoxigenic *C. difficile* strain from a patient with diarrhea (non-*C. difficile* diarrhea). Patients with *C. difficile*-associated diarrhea were excluded from analyses of the diarrhea during tube feeding and receipt of sorbitol-containing medications.

Clinical data about the patient's diagnosis, tube feeding, medications, and microbiologic test results were recorded daily from the patient's medical record. Exposure to antibiotics was recorded for 2 weeks before the study, then daily from the medical record. Nutritional data such as weight, percentage of ideal body weight, and serum albumin level were recorded from the patient's medical record. Severity of illness was determined using Horn's severity of illness index (Horn & Horn, 1986; Horn, Sharkey, & Bertram, 1983) and the MVAMC nursing care score.

The severity of illness index is a four-level index determined from the pattern of seven dimensions related to a patient's burden of illness: stage of principal diagnosis at admission, complications of the principal diagnosis, concurrent interactions affecting the hospital course, rate of response to therapy, dependency on care, non-operating room procedures, and remission of acute symptoms. The MVAMC nursing care score is a four-level, computer-determined score based on the types and number of nursing care needs of the patient related to activity, bathing, positioning, feeding, intravenous therapy, and frequency of patient observation. Higher values on both instruments indicate increasing severity of illness.

## Laboratory Procedures

Stool and rectal swab specimens were cultured anaerobically for *C. difficile* as described by Bliss, Johnson, Clabots, Savik, and Gerding (1997). *C. difficile* isolates were identified macroscopically and microscopically by characteristic colonial morphology and Gram-stain morphology (Holdeman, Moore, & Cato, 1977). Diarrheal stool samples were also tested for *C. difficile* by the alcohol shock culture method, as described by Clabots, Gerding, Olson, Peterson, and Gerding (1989). Diarrheal stools were tested for *C. difficile* cytotoxin by cell culture assay (Bliss et al., in press). *Hin*dIII restriction endonuclease analysis (REA) typing was performed on all isolates, using a rapid deoxyribonucleic acid (DNA) extraction method in conjunction with a comparison and grouping technique of known DNA types for profile analysis (Clabots et al., 1993).

## Statistical Analyses

The proportion of surveillance days with a specific symptom (fecal incontinence, diarrhea, unformed and loose or liquid stools) was calculated by dividing the number of days with the specific symptom by the number of days of surveillance. The proportion of incontinent and loose or liquid stools was calculated by dividing the number of each such stool by the total number of stools.

Bivariate comparisons were made using independent $t$ tests to compare differences in interval data between groups, and chi-square analyses to compare differences in categorical data between groups. A Mann-Whitney $U$ test was used to compare interval data when it was not normally distributed, or when there was inhomogeneity of variance between groups. The Mantel-Haenszel test was used to determine linear association among ordinal variables. A Pearson product-moment correlation coefficient was used to determine the existence and magnitude of a relationship between interval or ratio data. A $p$ value less than 0.05 was considered significant.

Multivariate analysis to determine a model for predicting fecal incontinence was accomplished using stepwise logistic regression analysis, appropriate for binary outcomes. The stepwise logistic regression analysis is useful because the important covariates are not yet known for the outcome of fecal incontinence in patients who are acutely ill, and associations with this outcome are not well understood.

The following variables were screened by chi-square analysis or *t* tests for inclusion in the logistic regression model: stool consistency, *C. difficile*-associated diarrhea, *C. difficile* colonization, tube feeding, diarrhea during tube feeding, age, type of unit, number of days of surveillance, number of days of hospitalization before the study, severity of illness index, treatment with sorbitol-containing liquid medications, and antibiotics or individual categories of antibiotics.

Antibiotics were categorized as follows: aminoglycosides, oral neomycin, antifungals, nystatin swish and swallow, antimycobacterials, aztreonam, bacitracin, first- and second-generation cephalosporins, third-generation cephalosporins, imipenem/cilastin, lincomycins, macrolides, intravenous metronidazole, penicillins, quinolones, trimethoprim/sulfamethoxazole, or intravenous vancomycin. Sorbitol-containing liquid medications were identified from the MVAMC formulary and available lists (Hauff 1993; Lutomski, Gora, Wright, & Martin, 1993; Miller & Oliver, 1993; Thomson & Rollins, 1997).

Variables with *p* values 0.1 or less were candidates for the multivariate analysis. Six variables were submitted originally to the stepwise regression analysis: age, presence of diarrhea, *C. difficile*-associated diarrhea, unformed and loose or liquid stool consistency, being in the intensive care unit (ICU), and severity of illness index. Coefficients of the regression variables were tested for significance using a Wald's chi-square statistic, and a *p* value less than 0.05 was considered significant. Data were analyzed using SAS for Microsoft Windows (v. 6.11, SAS Institute, Inc., Cary, NC) and SPSS for Windows programs (v. 7.0, SPSS Inc., Chicago, IL). Data are presented as means ± standard error of the mean (SEM).

## RESULTS

The study sample consisted of 152 patients (150 men and 2 women): 67 tube fed and 85 not tube fed. The primary diagnoses of the patients were categorized as follows: peripheral vascular disease ($n = 36$), head or neck cancer ($n = 34$), neurologic disorders ($n = 19$), pulmonary disorders ($n = 18$), gastrointestinal disorders ($n = 10$), cardiac disorders ($n = 10$), abdominal aortic aneurysms ($n = 9$), genitourinary or renal disorders ($n = 6$), and miscellaneous (e.g., leukemia, hip fracture) ($n = 10$). None of the patients had a primary or comorbid diagnosis of dementia at admission. A history of fecal incontinence was not documented in the medical record of any study patient on admission to the MVAMC. The patients were located on the following types of units: surgical ($n = 73$), medical ($n = 27$), mixed neurologic and neurosurgical ($n = 12$),

surgical intensive/transitional care ($n = 29$), medical intensive/transitional care ($n = 9$), and coronary care ($n = 2$).

Of the 67 tube-fed patients, 66 started tube feeding using continuous administration and 1 used intermittent administration. During the study, 29 patients changed the tube feeding method of administration. The following formulas were used when patients started tube feeding: Osmolite (Ross Laboratories, Columbus, OH) ($n = 52$), Osmolite HN (Ross Laboratories) ($n = 11$), and Impact (Sandoz Nutrition, Minneapolis, MN) ($n = 4$). The types of feeding tubes were nasogastric ($n = 30$), nasoduodenal ($n = 26$), nasojejunal or jejunostomy ($n = 6$), and percutaneous endoscopic gastrostomy ($n = 5$). At the time of the study, all nasoduodenal and nasojejunal feeding tubes were inserted using fluoroscopy. During the study, 14 patients changed types of feeding tubes.

### Fecal Incontinence and Its Severity

Fecal incontinence was present in 33% (50/152) of the patients. The proportion of days with fecal incontinence in these patients was 0.5 ± 0.06. The proportion of all stools found incontinent in these patients was 0.55 ± 0.04. Fecal incontinence was most common in patients with primary diagnosis categorized as a pulmonary (10/18 [56%]) or genitourinary/renal disorder (4/6 [68%]), and least frequent in patients with head or neck cancer (2/34 [6%]) or an abdominal aortic aneurysm (1/9 [11%]; $x^2$ (8) = 23.28, $p = 0.003$). Patients with fecal incontinence were older than patients without fecal incontinence (see Table A2–1). The length of hospitalization before surveillance was not significantly different between patients with fecal incontinence (13 ± 1 days) and those without fecal incontinence (11 ± 1 days) ($t[150] = -1.5$; $p = 0.13$). The duration of surveillance for patients with fecal incontinence (13 ± 1 days) was not significantly different than for patients without fecal incontinence (11 ± 0.5 days) ($t[71.4] = -1.97$; $p = 0.053$).

There was no significant difference in the nutritional assessment indices of patients with fecal incontinence and those without fecal incontinence (weight = 76 ± 3 kg vs. 78 ± 2 kg; $t[150] = 0.59$; $p = 0.55$; serum albumin = 3 ± 0.09 mg/dl vs. 3 ± 0.06 mg/dl; $t[104] = 1.2$; $p = 0.22$; percentage of ideal body weight = 103% ± 4% vs. 102% ± 2%; $t[47.7] = -.14$, respectively) for whom these values were available.

### Fecal Incontinence and Severity of Illness

The severity of illness index and nursing care score were greater in patients with fecal incontinence than in patients without fecal incontinence (see Table A2–1). A greater percentage of patients in the ICU had fecal incontinence than patients not in the ICU (23/40, [58%] vs. 27/112 [24%]; $x^2[1] = 14.9$; $p < 0.001$).

**TABLE A2-1** Patient and Stool Characteristics in Acutely-Ill Hospitalized Patients With and Without Fecal Incontinence

|  | Fecal Incontinence ($n = 50$) | No Fecal Incontinence ($n = 102$) |
|---|---|---|
| Age (years) | 70 ± 1[a] | 65 ± 1 |
| Severity of illness index | 2.6 ± .05[a] | 2.2 ± .03 |
| Nursing care score | 2.8 ± .04[b] | 2.5 ± .05 |
| Proportion of stools with unformed or liquid consistency | .60 ± .05[c] | .44 ± .04 |
| Proportion of surveillance days with diarrhea | .11 ± .02[d] | .06 ± .01 |

Values presented are means ± standard deviation.
[a]$p < .001$.
[b]$p = .02$.
[c]$p = .01$.
[d]$p = .04$.

## Fecal Incontinence, Diarrhea, and Stool Consistency

More patients with diarrhea had fecal incontinence than patients without diarrhea (23/53 [43%] vs. 27/99 [27%]; $x^2[1] = 4.1$; $p = 0.04$). The proportion of surveillance days with diarrhea was nearly twice as great in patients with fecal incontinence as in patients without fecal incontinence (see Table A2–1). There was a strong, positive association between the proportion of surveillance days with fecal incontinence and the proportion of surveillance days with diarrhea ($r = 0.69$; $p < 0.001$; see Figure A2–1).

Fecal incontinence was associated with stool consistency. More patients with unformed and loose or liquid stool had fecal incontinence than those with soft but formed or hard and formed stool (48/119 [40%] vs. 2/31 [6.5%]; $x^2[1] = 12.7$; $p < 0.001$). Two patients did not have a stool during the surveillance period. The proportion of loose or liquid stools in patients with fecal incontinence was greater than in patients without fecal incontinence (see Table A2–1). There was a significant association between the proportion of stools that were incontinent and the proportion of loose or liquid stools ($r = 0.29$; $p = 0.04$; see Figure A2–1). There was a significant relationship between the proportion of surveillance days with loose or liquid stools and the proportion of surveillance days with fecal incontinence ($r = 0.64$; $p < 0.001$; see Figure A2–1). The proportion of surveillance days with loose or liquid stools in patients with

fecal incontinence was $0.36 ± 0.04$ compared with $0.27 ± 0.03$ in patients without fecal incontinence ($t[150] = -1.87$; $p = 0.06$).

## Fecal Incontinence, *C. difficile* – Associated Diarrhea, and Diarrhea During Tube Feeding

*C. difficile* was isolated from rectal or stool specimens from 17% (26/152) of the patients. There was no difference in fecal incontinence between patients who had *C. difficile*-associated diarrhea and those who did not (4/8 [50%] vs. 46/144 [32%]; $x^2[1] = 1.1$, $p = 0.29$). A greater percentage of patients colonized with *C. difficile* had fecal incontinence than those who were not (11/18 [61%] vs. 35/126 [28%]; $x^2[1] = 8.05$; $p = 0.005$).

Fecal incontinence was not associated with tube feeding. The percentage of tube-fed patients with fecal incontinence did not differ significantly from that of non-tube-fed patients with fecal incontinence (26/67 [39%] vs. 24/85 [28%]; $x^2[1] = 1.9$; $p = 0.17$). After patients with *C. difficile*-associated diarrhea were excluded, there was no significant difference in the cumulative incidence of fecal incontinence between patients with diarrhea during tube feeding (12/29 [41%]) and those without diarrhea during tube feeding (34/115 [30%]) ($x^2[1] = 1.5$; $p = 0.2$).

## Fecal Incontinence and Medications

Fecal incontinence was not related to receipt of sorbitol-containing medications or antibiotics. There was no significant difference in fecal incontinence be-

**FIGURE A2-1**   **Relationship of fecal incontinence to diarrhea and stool consistency. There were strong correlations between the proportion of surveillance days with fecal incontinence and the proportion of surveillance days with diarrhea ($p < 0.001$), and between the proportion of surveillance days with fecal incontinence and the proportion of surveillance days with unformed and loose or liquid stools ($p < 0.001$). There was a significant relationship between the percentage of incontinent stools and the percentage of unformed and loose or liquid stools ($p = 0.04$). (Adapted with permission from Bliss, D. Z., Johnson, S., Savik, K., Clabots, C. R., & Gerding, D. N. [2002, March/April]. Fecal incontinence in hospitalized patients who are acutely ill. *Nursing Research, 49*[2], 101–108.)**

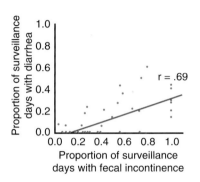 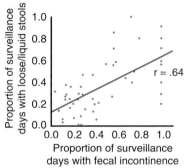 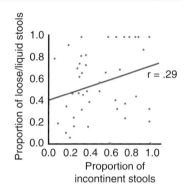

tween patients receiving liquid medications containing sorbitol (26/75 [35%]) and those not receiving such medications (20/69 [29%]) ($x^2[1] = 0.53$; $p = 0.47$). Antibiotics were received by 89% (135/152) of all the patients. There was no significant difference in fecal incontinence between patients receiving any antibiotics (46/135 [34%]) and those not receiving antibiotics (4/17 [24%]) ($x^2[1] = 0.76$; $p = 0.38$). A greater percentage of patients with fecal incontinence had received aminoglycosides or third-generation cephalosporins than patients without fecal incontinence (19/50 [41%] vs. 19/102 [21%]; $x^2[1] = 6.7$; $p = 0.01$; 15/50 [33%] vs. 12/102 [14%]; $x^2[1] = 7.6$; $p = 0.006$, respectively).

## Multivariate Analyses of Risk Factors for Fecal Incontinence

Variables associated with fecal incontinence in a multivariate stepwise regression analysis were unformed and loose or liquid stool, age, and severity of illness index (see Table A2-2). Patients with loose or liquid stool were 11 times more likely to have fecal incontinence than patients without such stool. For every increase of 1 on the severity of illness index, the likelihood of having fecal incontinence increased fivefold.

*Post hoc* analysis showed that *C. difficile* colonization and exposure to aminoglycosides or third-generation cephalosporins were significantly

associated with the severity of illness index. A greater percentage of patients colonized with *C. difficile* had a severity of illness index ≥ 3 than patients not colonized with this organism (10/18 [57%] vs. 36/126 [29%]; $x^2[1] = 5.2$; $p = 0.02$). A greater percentage of patients who received aminoglycosides (21/39 [54%]) or third-generation cephalosporins (19/27 [70%]) had a severity of illness index ≥ 3 than patients who did not receive them (28/113 [25%]; $x^2[1] = 11.2$; $p = 0.001$; 30/125 [24%]; $x^2[1] = 21.9$; $p < 0.001$, respectively).

### REA Typing

As shown in Figure A2–2, REA typing was performed on 118 *C. difficile* isolates from 26 patients, revealing 24 distinct REA types in 16 REA groups. Both toxigenic and nontoxigenic *C. difficile* strains were present in patients with fecal incontinence those without the condition.

## DISCUSSION

The results of this study indicate that fecal incontinence is a common problem in hospitalized patients who are acutely ill. One third of the patients in this study had fecal incontinence during an average surveillance time of 12 days. The severity of fecal incontinence can be estimated by the proportion of surveillance days with fecal incontinence and the proportion of total stools that are incontinent. Bliss et al.

**TABLE A2-2** Risk Factors for Fecal Incontinence in Acutely-Ill Hospitalized Patients Using Multivariate Stepwise Regression

| Variable (in order of entry) | β | SE | Wald$_2$ | p Value | RR | 95% CI |
|---|---|---|---|---|---|---|
| Severity of illness index | 1.738 | .395 | 19.324 | <.0001 | 5.686 | 2.62, 12.34 |
| Loose or liquid stool consistency | 2.404 | .834 | 8.319 | .004 | 11.069 | 2.16, 56.7 |
| Age | .079 | .029 | 7.701 | .006 | 1.082 | 1.02, 1.14 |

(1992) suggested that reported proportion of surveillance days with diarrhea was a more descriptive and discriminatory outcome measure and less influenced by duration of surveillance than reported incidence. This measure can be applied likewise to fecal incontinence. Patients were incontinent for approximately 50% of the surveillance time, and more than half of all stools of these patients were incontinent. The severity of fecal incontinence increased as the severity of diarrhea or loose or liquid stools increased.

The length of hospitalization or surveillance, which has been associated with other types of diarrhea, such as *C. difficile*-associated diarrhea and tube-feeding-associated diarrhea, was not significantly different between patients with or without fecal incontinence in this study (Bliss et al., 1992; Clabots,

**FIGURE A2-2** Frequency of *Clostridium difficile* restriction of endonuclease analysis (REA) groups recovered from continent and incontinent hospitalized patients who were acutely ill. The REA typing of isolates from 26 patients revealed 24 distinct REA types belonging to 16 REA groups. (Adapted with permission from Bliss, D. Z., Johnson, S., Savik, K., Clabots, C. R., & Gerding, D. N. [2002, March/April]. Fecal incontinence in hospitalized patients who are acutely ill. *Nursing Research, 49*[2], 101–108.)

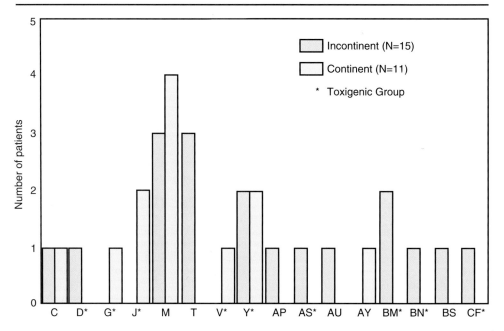

Johnson, Olson, Peterson, & Gerding, 1992). This may explain the lack of association between fecal incontinence and duration of hospitalization before the study or duration of patient surveillance.

In the multivariate analysis, fecal incontinence was associated with unformed and loose or liquid stool rather than any specific type of diarrhea such as diarrhea during tube feeding or *C. difficile*-associated diarrhea. The REA typing results illustrate a wide diversity of *C. difficile* strains, making the likelihood of a common-source outbreak of nosocomial *C. difficile* infection and associated diarrhea or fecal incontinence low. Fecal incontinence was not associated with exposure to antibiotics or sorbitol-containing medications.

The current results support those of Read et al. (1979), who reported that nonhospitalized patients with chronic diarrhea experienced fecal incontinence when stools were liquid, regardless of stool volume. When control was used for stool consistency, age and increased severity of illness were significant risk factors for fecal incontinence in the multivariate regression model. These results agree with those of Nelson et al. (1995), who reported that older age and poor general health were among the risk factors for fecal incontinence in community-living persons. The current results suggest that *C. difficile* colonization and exposure to third-generation cephalosporins and aminoglycosides are markers of a patient who is more severely ill. The association of increased illness severity with fecal incontinence implies alterations in both the cognitive and physiologic control processes of normal, voluntary defecation.

According to the results from this study, therapies that make stool consistency less loose or liquid may be useful in managing fecal incontinence. Studies of tube-fed formulas supplemented with dietary fiber provide evidence that dietary fiber can modify stool consistency. Zimmaro et al. (1989) reported that a pectin fiber supplement significantly reduced the percentage of loose or liquid stools in normal subjects ingesting a tube-fed formula. Heather, Howell, Montana, Howell, and Hill (1991) reported that tube-fed patients receiving a fiber supplement containing psyllium had firmer stools than tube-fed patients who did not receive the fiber supplement. Slavin, Nelson, McNamara, and Cashmere (1985) suggested that the amount of fiber ingested during tube feeding influences the consistency of stool. Healthy men who ingested a tube-fed formula with a moderate supplement of soy fiber (30 g/day) had stools more formed than when they ingested a larger amount of soy fiber (60 g/day). Controlled clinical trials comparing types and doses of dietary fibers and their effects on fecal incontinence and stool consistency in patients with fecal incontinence are needed. Medications that slow

intestinal transit, resulting in greater absorption of water and firmer stool consistency, may be beneficial for patients with fecal incontinence. However, in patients with inflammatory entericities such as *C. difficile*-associated diarrhea, agents that increase transit time are contraindicated.

Limitations of this study include the inability to determine more objectively than by history alone whether patients had fecal incontinence before admission because data collection began after admission of the patient. Nutritional status data were not available for some patients. Because risk factors for fecal incontinence in patients who are acutely ill were unknown before this study, it is possible that some risk factor was not included in this prospective surveillance.

In conclusion, the following risk factors for fecal incontinence are found among hospitalized patients who are acutely ill: loose or liquid stool consistency, an increased severity of illness, and older age. Treatments that result in a more formed stool may be beneficial in managing fecal incontinence and warrant further investigation.

## References

Bender, B. S., Bennett, R., Laughon, B. E., Greenough, W. B., III, Gaydos, C., Sears, S. D., Forman, M. S., & Bartlett, J. G. (1986). Is *Clostridium difficile* endemic in chronic-care facilities? *Lancet, 2*(8497), 11–13.

Bliss, D. Z., Guenter, P. A., & Settle, R. G. (1992). Defining and reporting diarrhea in tube-fed patients: What a mess! *American Journal of Clinical Nutrition, 55,* 753–759.

Bliss, D. Z., Johnson, S., Clabots, C. R., Savik, K., & Gerding, D. N. (1997). Comparison of cycloserine-cefoxitin-fructose agar (CCFA) and taurocholate-CCFA for recovery of *Clostridium difficile* during surveillance of hospitalized patients. *Diagnostic Microbiology and Infectious Disease, 28,* 1–4.

Bliss, D. Z., Johnson, S., Savik, K., Clabots, C. R., Willard, K., & Gerding, D. N. (1998). The acquisition of *Clostridium difficile* and associated diarrhea in hospitalized patients. *Annals of Internal Medicine, 129*(12), 1012–1019.

Borrie, M. J., & Davidson, H. A. (1992). Incontinence in institutions: Costs and contributing factors. *Canadian Medical Association Journal, 147,* 322–328.

Burns, P. E., & Jairath, N. (1994). Diarrhea and the patient receiving enteral feedings: A multifactorial problem. *Journal of Wound, Ostomy, and Continence Nursing, 21,* 257–263.

Campbell, A. J., Reinken, J., & McCosh, L. (1985). Incontinence in the elderly: Prevalence and prognosis. *Age and Ageing, 14*(2), 65–70.

Cefai, C., Elliott, T. S. J., & Woodhouse, K. W. (1988). Gastrointestinal carriage rate of *Clostridium difficile* in elderly, chronic care hospital patients. *Journal of Hospital Infection, 11,* 335–339.

Clabots, C. R., Gerding, S. J., Olson, M. M., Peterson, L. R., & Gerding, D. N. (1989). Detection of asymptomatic *Clostridium difficile* carriage by an alcohol shock procedure. *Journal of Clinical Microbiology, 27,* 2386–2387.

Clabots, C. R., Johnson, S., Bettin, K. M., Mathie, P. A., Mulligan, M. E., Schaberg, D. R., Peterson, L. R., & Gerding, D. N. (1993). Development of a rapid and efficient restriction endonuclease analysis typing system for *Clostridium difficile* and correlation with other typing systems. *Journal of Clinical Microbiology, 31,* 1870–1875.

Edes, T. E., Walk, B. E., & Austin, J. L. (1990). Diarrhea in tube-fed patients: Feeding formula not necessarily the cause. *American Journal of Medicine, 88,* 91–93.

Gerding, D. N., Olson, M. M., Peterson, L. R., Teasley, D. G., Gebhard, R. L., Schwartz, M. L. & Lee, J. T., Jr. (1986). *Clostridium difficile*-associated diarrhea and colitis in adults: A prospective case-controlled epidemiologic study. *Archives of Internal Medicine, 146,* 95–100.

Gottschlich, M. M., Warden, G. D., Michel, M., Havens, P., Kopcha, R., Jenkins, M., & Alexander, J. W. (1988). Diarrhea in tube-fed burn patients: Incidence, etiology, nutritional impact, and prevention. *JPEN Journal of Parenteral and Enteral Nutrition, 12,* 338–345.

Guenter, P. A., Settle, R. G., Perlmutter, S., Marino, P. L., DeSimone, G. A., & Rolandelli, R. H. (1991). Tube feeding-related diarrhea in acutely ill patients. *JPEN Journal of Parenteral and Enteral Nutrition, 15,* 277–280.

Hauff, K. (1997). *Sorbitol content of medications.* Unpublished report, Fairview University Medical Center, Minneapolis, MN.

Heather, D. J., Howell, L., Montana, M., Howell, M., & Hill, R. (1991). Effect of a bulk-forming cathartic on diarrhea in tube-fed patients. *Heart and Lung, 20,* 409–413.

Holdeman, L. V., Moore, W. E. C., & Cato, E. P. (Eds.). (1977). *Anaerobe laboratory manual* (4th ed.). Blackburg, VA: Virginia Polytechnic Institute and State University.

Horn, S. D., & Horn, R. A. (1986). Reliability and validity of the Severity of Illness Index. *Medical Care, 24,* 159–178.

Horn, S. D., Sharkey, P. D., & Bertram, D. A. (1983). Measuring severity of illness: Homogenous case mix groups. *Medical Care, 21,* 14–30.

Issacs, B., & Walkley, F. A. (1964). A survey of incontinence in elderly hospital patients. *Gerontology Clinics, 6,* 367–376.

Johanson, J. F., & Lafferty, J. (1996). Epidemiology of fecal incontinence: The silent affliction. *American Journal of Gastroenterology, 91,* 33–36.

Kelly, T. W. J., Patrick, M. R., & Hillman, K. M. (1983). Study of diarrhea in critically ill patients. *Critical Care Medicine, 11,* 7–9.

Lahr, C. J. (1988). Evaluation and treatment of incontinence. *Practical Gastroenterology, 12*(4), 27–35.

Lutomski, D. M., Gora, M. L., Wright, S. M., & Martin, J. E. (1993). Sorbitol content of selected oral liquids. *Annals of Pharmacotherapy, 27,* 269–274.

McFarland, L. V., Surawicz, C. M., & Stamm, W. E. (1990). Risk factors for *Clostridium difficile* carriage and *C. difficile*-associated diarrhea in a cohort of hospitalized patients. *Journal of Infectious Diseases, 162,* 678–684.

Metcalf, A. M., & Phillips, S. F. (1986). Ileostomy diarrhoea. *Clinics in Gastroenterology, 15,* 705–722.

Miller, S. J., & Oliver, A. D. (1993). Sorbitol content of selected sugar-free liquid medications. *Hospital Pharmacy, 28,* 741–744, 755.

Nakanishi, N., Tatara, K., Naramura, H., Fujiwara, H., Takashima, Y., & Fukuda, H. (1997). Urinary and fecal incontinence in a community-residing older population in Japan. *Journal of the American Geriatrics Society, 45,* 215–219.

Nelson, R., Norton, N., Cautley, E., & Furner, S. (1995). Community-based prevalence of anal incontinence. *JAMA, 274,* 559–561.

Read, N. W., Harford, W. V., Schmulen, A. C., Read, M. G., Santa Ana, C., & Fordtran, J. S. (1979). A clinical study of patients with fecal incontinence and diarrhea. *Gastroenterology, 76,* 747–756.

Siegel, D. L., Edelstein, P. H., & Nachamkin, I. (1990). Inappropriate testing for diarrheal diseases in the hospital. *JAMA, 263,* 979–982.

Slavin, J. L., Nelson, N. L., McNamara, E. A., & Cashmere, K. (1985). Bowel function of healthy men consuming liquid diets with and without dietary fiber. *JPEN Journal of Parenteral and Enteral Nutrition, 9,* 317–321.

Thomas, T. M., Ruff, C., Karran, O., Mellows, S., & Meade, T. W. (1987). Study of the prevalence and management of patients with fecal incontinence in old people's homes. *Community Medicine, 9,* 232–237.

Thomson, C. A., & Rollins, C. J. (1997). Nutrient–drug interactions. In J. L. Rombeau & R. H. Rolandelli (Eds.), *Clinical nutrition: Enteral and tube feedings* (pp. 523–533). Philadelphia: W. B. Saunders.

Yannelli, B., Gurevich, I., Schoch, P. E., & Cunha, B. A. (1988). Yield of stool cultures, ova and parasite tests, and *Clostridium difficile* determinations in nosocomial diarrheas. *American Journal of Infection Control, 16,* 246–249.

Zimmaro, D. M., Rolandelli, R. H., Koruda, M. J., Settle, R. G., Stein, T. P., & Rombeau, J. L. (1989). Isotonic tube feeding formula induces liquid stool in normal subjects: Reversal by pectin. *JPEN Journal of Parenteral and Enteral Nutrition, 13,* 117–123.

APPENDIX

A-3

# Homeless Patients' Experience of Satisfaction With Care

Susan McCabe, Carol L. Macnee, Mary Kay Anderson

*This article explores homeless individuals' experiences of satisfaction with health care, and explores the interrelationship among experiences of being homeless, health perceptions of participants, and experiences of satisfaction with health care. It presents the findings of a phenomenological study that was conducted using participants selected from five sites in one southeastern state. Participant interviews were conducted at a nurse-managed primary health care clinic for homeless, at a nighttime soup-kitchen, and at three private, not-for-profit, homeless shelters in two different towns. The study was part of a larger study designed to develop and validate a reliable measure of client satisfaction with primary health care among homeless individuals. Face-to-face in-depth interviews with 17 homeless individuals were conducted, with the semistructured interview constituting the primary data source. Common themes were identified and the interrelationship of theme clusters was explored. Analysis of the data yielded five distinct themes that represent the lived experiences of satisfaction with health care. These themes were mediated and directly informed by five themes of homelessness and three themes of health identified in the shared experiences of the participants. The themes identified suggest that satisfaction with health care for homeless persons differs from currently identified dimensions of satisfaction with care, and that some aspects of homelessness are seen by participants as positive and health promoting.*

Homelessness represents one of the most compelling social concerns and one of the largest health care dilemmas in America (Clarke, Williams, Percy & Kim, 1995). It has been estimated that between 350,000 and 2.5 million Americans are homeless, with evidence that this number is growing larger rather than smaller (Jackson & McSwane, 1992). Homeless individuals have difficulty in accessing health care, frequently lack preventive services, and often choose not to follow up on either return appointments or treatment recommendations. These health care issues have all been cited as explanations for homelessness constituting a significant risk factor for increased levels of illness and increased health care costs associated with this population (Aiken, 1987; Sheridan, Gowen & Halpin, 1993).

Patient satisfaction questionnaires have become a common form of outcome measurement in most areas of health care. There are a number of well-tested measures of patient satisfaction which have been shown to be reliable and valid with general populations of patients in a variety of outpatient settings (Marshall, Hays & Mazel, 1996; DiTommaso & Willard, 1991). While much emphasis has been placed on measurement of patient satisfaction, most of the commonly used measures have been tested in largely white, middle class populations, and have shown little variability when used in poorer or underserved populations (Avis, Bond & Authur, 1997).

*Archives of Psychiatric Nursing, Vol. XV, No. 2 (April), 2001: pp. 78–85*

This study was the first phase of a broader two-part study to develop a reliable and valid measure of homeless individuals' experiences of satisfaction with health care, and was designed to address the research question of what constitutes satisfaction with primary health care for homeless clients. The themes generated from this phase of the study were used to develop and validate a reliable measure of client satisfaction with primary health care among homeless individuals.

## REVIEW OF THE LITERATURE

Conceptually, patient satisfaction represents an individual's perceived experiences regarding the health care they receive and the extent to which these services meet the person's expectations and needs (Di-Tomasso & Willard, 1991). Patient satisfaction has been shown to be an important outcome measure of quality of health care services (Mahon, 1996; Ware, Snyder, Wright & Davies, 1983), and an important predictor of health and illness behavior (Marshall, Hays & Mazel, 1996). As a result, considerable effort has been made to develop reliable and valid measures of patient satisfaction, the most recognized of which is the PSQ, or Patient Satisfaction Questionnaire (Ware et al., 1983).

Despite demonstrations of both validity and reliability, a common finding in studies examining patient satisfaction is a lack of variability or a skew in ratings in disadvantaged and less educated populations (Avis, Bond & Arthur, 1997; Lindsey, Henly & Tyree, 1997; Rubin et al., 1993; Larrabee, Ferri & Hartig, 1997). In particular vulnerable populations (Lindsey, Henley & Tyree, 1997), disadvantaged populations (Ware et al., 1983), and less educated populations (DiTomasso & Willard, 1991) have shown less variability in responses or have been found to have less stability in their responses to patient satisfaction questionnaires. These findings have led several researchers to question the validity of current measures of patient satisfaction (Avis, Bond & Arthur, 1997; Williams, 1994), and to suggest the need for studies which directly explore the meaning of satisfaction from the client's standpoint (Bushy, 1995; Mahon, 1996).

Homeless individuals and families represent an extremely heterogeneous population with acknowledged special health needs (Drake, Osher & Wallach, 1991; Lehman, Myers & Corty, 1989). The literature supports that homelessness creates unique experiences, and it would seem reasonable that specific aspects of these experiences affect homeless persons' perceptions of satisfaction with health care. Studies examining the perceptions of homeless individuals have identified unique issues such as social isolation and uncertainty (Baumann, 1993; Dancy &

Barge, 1996; Reichenbach, McNamee & Seibel, 1998), a perceived sense of being different from the rest of society (Menke & Wagner, 1997), and strong privacy needs coupled with feelings of general mistrust (Baumann, 1993; Wagner & Perrine, 1994). Homeless persons have distinct and unique dimensions to their descriptions of what constitutes health (McCormack & Gooding, 1993), and in general homelessness is perceived by homeless persons as an unhealthy lifestyle (Jezewski, 1995; McCormack & Gooding, 1993). These studies support the need for measures of satisfaction with health care which reflect the distinct perspective and needs of homeless individuals.

Homelessness is unhealthy and homeless people are extremely vulnerable, with an increased incidence of acute and chronic health problems (Hodnicki, 1990; Vredevoe, Brecht, Shuler & Woo, 1992; Wright & Weber, 1987). Most of these chronic health problems require regular and ongoing health care, but despite this, homeless individuals remain one of the most underserved populations (Hodnicki, 1990; Gelburg, Gallagher, Andersen & Koegel, 1997). It has been recognized that homeless populations have multiple barriers to receipt of primary health care (Hunter, Getty, Kemsley & Skelly, 1991; Hodnicki, 1990; Mason, Jensen & Boland, 1992) with difficulty in both access and use of services. Because of the extensive health care needs in the homeless population, significant federal, state and local resources have been committed to provide primary health care services which are accessible and address the special needs of these patients. Evaluation issues in the homeless population are numerous (Hunter, Crosby, Ventura & Warkentin, 1997), and no studies were found in the literature specifically addressing patient satisfaction measurement among homeless clients.

## METHODOLOGY

This study was part of a larger triangulated study designed to develop and validate a reliable measure of client satisfaction with primary health care among homeless individuals. The researchers all work at East Tennessee State University, have faculty practice sites at a nurse-managed clinic which provides care exclusively for homeless and indigent clients which had nearly 10,000 patient visits in 1999. The authors' work with this population provided the impetus for the study, embedded the researchers within a homeless culture, and provided context for the study.

### Purpose

Because there are few studies explicating what constitutes satisfaction with care for homeless individuals, a Heideggerian phenomenological approach was chosen. The purpose of the study was to gain increased understanding of homeless participants lived experience of satisfaction with health care. A secondary purpose was to describe antecedental experiences that extended meaning and context of participant's experiences of satisfaction, including descriptions of health and of being homeless.

## Setting and Sample

The study was conducted at a nurse-managed primary health care clinic for homeless, at a nighttime soup-kitchen, and at three private, not-for-profit shelters for homeless in two different towns within a southeastern state. The clinic serves an average of 35 clients per day, whereas the soup-kitchen serves an average of 300 meals a day, and the shelters housed between 15 and 50 individuals, with one shelter exclusively housing men, and the other two housing families and individuals.

A total of 17 subjects were interviewed for this study, 3 women and 14 men, with an age range from 19 to 67 years. Their self-reported race or ethnicity included 10 White subjects, 3 Black subjects, 2 "White Indian" subjects, 2 Native American subjects, and 2 who did not identify a race. Length of time reported to be homeless ranged from 4 weeks to 41 years, with 12 subjects reporting being homeless for more than a year. Participant selection into the study continued until the data received became redundant and when data saturation was achieved with all data sets able to be classified into existent categorical coding structures.

## Data Collection Procedures

Phenomenological face-to-face, in-depth interviews with homeless individuals were conducted. The semi-structured interview constituted the primary data source. An interview protocol was established to serve as a guide to illuminate the meaning of four broad dimensional areas that assisted in structuring the interviews. The four areas discussed with participants were their (1) experiences of being homeless, (2) experiences of what health is, (3) experiences of satisfaction with health care, and (4) experiences of dissatisfaction with health care.

Participants were recruited from the four locations, with agency staff assisting with identification and introduction of individuals at the four locations who were thought to have experience with the phenomenon of interest. These individuals were approached, informed of the study and invited to participate. Informed consent was obtained, confidentiality issues explored, and all participants questions addressed before data collection. Interviews ranged from 40 minutes in length to 2 hours long, with most averaging 60 minutes. Data provided during the interviews were tape recorded, and later converted into typed textual data sets saved as an ASCII file. Verification of the accuracy of transcribed data

occurred, with each transcript being compared with the original tape sources by an independent reviewer. Extensive field notes were kept to establish an audit trail (Lincoln & Guba, 1985; Rogers & Cowles, 1993), and to provide contextual richness. To assist with later data analysis field notes described in detail the setting of each interview, the disruptions and intrusions to the interviews, other present in the environment, and participants' nonverbal behaviors.

## Data Analysis

Phenomenological interviewing produces rich amounts of data. The textual data transcribed from the interviews was examined using common phenomenological methods (Munhall & Boyd, 1993), focusing on analysis methods explicated by Miles and Huberman (1984, 1994). Analysis of the data occurred in three stages and was facilitated by use of QRS NUD.IST (Non Numerical Unstructured Data Indexing Searching and Theory building Multi-Functional) software program, using sentences as the text unit for analysis. Data reduction, a process of selecting, focusing, simplifying, abstracting and transforming data with the researcher finding meaning in the raw textual data (Miles & Huberman, 1994), was the first stage of the analysis process. Data reduction was done by careful listening and reading of the textual data describing the participant's lived experiences. The immersion into the data lead to initial coding of the data into inductively derived theme categories and tentative taxonomic labels which were applied to the emerging themes. As commonalities of data set units representing the lived experiences of homelessness, health, and satisfaction with health care became apparent, more abstractive interpretation and coding occurred, and clear operational definitions were established for the emerging data categories.

The operational definitions for coded categorical data sets provided the researchers with a guide for the second stage of analysis, data display, and allowed for further inclusion of textual data into or out of the emerging categories. These definitions were critically examined and continuously refined, establishing a process for internal consistency (Miles & Huberman, 1994) among the three researchers, and helping to identify the need for new theme development. Review and examination of both the data and the coding system was halted based on acceptable criteria of saturation and regularity (Denzin & Lincoln, 1994; Lincoln & Guba, 1985; Miles & Huberman, 1994; Munhall & Boyd, 1993) and when all incidents of data could be readily and repetitively categorized by all of the researchers. The third stage of analysis, conclusion drawing, occurred whereby identified themes were verified and confirmation of the data was done using accepted methods of rigor.

*Issues of Study Rigor.* Rigor was an issue of importance to this study. Credibility of themes was examined at two points during the study. The data and developing themes were taken to the source from which they were drawn for validation through the process of intermember checks (Denzin & Lincoln, 1994; Lincoln & Guba, 1985). Two homeless participants who had been interviewed early in the study were reinterviewed during member checks to assess their perception of emerging theme categories.

After final theme categorization was completed, a population group check process was used to assess the transferability of theme structure. Transferability as an issue of fit (Denzin & Lincoln, 1994) was checked with a group of homeless individuals who were residing in a private not-for-profit shelter in a neighboring city and who had not been involved in any aspect of the research. The group consisted of five men and three women, five White members and three Black members, with an age range from late 30s to middle 60s. The group was asked to comment on the themes as presented. The group was readily able to relate personal experiences that supported the identified themes, and assisted in enrichment of definitional attributes that gave expanded understanding of identified themes.

Consistency measures were used to ensure reliable findings and included use of QSR NUD.IST software to document, through memo functions, the process by which the researchers made decisions relevant to the development of the final theme structure. In a similar fashion, the qualitative software allowed for confirmability through documentation of an audit trail.

## Essential Theme Findings

Analysis of the data yielded distinct themes that represent the lived experiences of participants' satisfaction with health care. Understanding of this phenomenon was informed by the themes pertaining to homelessness and health. The full theme structure is identified in Table A3–1.

*Themes of Homelessness.* Five distinct themes were identified that describe what it meant to participants to be homeless. These five themes were uncertainty, resourcefulness, time splits, harmful, and distinctness.

Uncertainty was experienced as not being able to predict or anticipate the availability, course, and nature of routine life events. Uncertainty was experienced as constant changes and a lack of control over common events such as where they might sleep and eat. This theme was expressed by one participant in this way.

> You know you've got an apartment, whatever, you know what I'm saying. You pay your bills, you know for that month you're there, that's your place. You know if you pay your bills you

## TABLE A3-1 Themes

| Phenomenon of Interest | Themes |
|---|---|
| Homelessness | Uncertainty |
| | Resourcefulness |
| | Time splits |
| | Harmful |
| | Distinctness |
| Health | Ableness |
| | Self-knowing |
| | Well-being |
| Satisfaction with care | Committed care |
| | Respectful engagement |
| | Trust |
| | Assumption-free care |
| | Inclusion care practices |

get your two weeks notice. And living on the streets there's no such thing as two week notice. Living in a shelter, no such thing as that notice, your notice is when you come in and they tell you well, you know, whatever the captain [at the shelter] said, you don't stay here anymore.

The second theme, resourcefulness, was expressed as experiences of ingenuity and self-pride at being able to negotiate and survive being homeless. Resourcefulness was related to homeless individuals' own behaviors and to assistance from others, especially other homeless persons. This theme included such attributes as being able to take care of yourself, figuring out how to get needs met, not asking for much from others, and that it takes a lot for homeless to ask for help with certain things. Resourcefulness also included a sense that other homeless individuals served as both resource and support for one another. As one participant expressed, "But if the people on the street, if it wasn't for them I wouldn't have made it," whereas another said of homeless "It's a profession to some people—just like going to work for other people. You need to figure out how to get food, if it's going to rain, how to find a place out of the rain. It's a job you need to be good at to survive."

Time split was the third theme within homelessness and was expressed as experiences of dichotomous relevance of time where perceived health needs require an immediate response but, once feeling responded to, time became relatively unimportant with the individual willing to wait for a sustained time interval to be seen for care. Participants repeatedly expressed that they needed to know immediately that health care would be offered to them, but would wait for long time periods for that care once they knew their need had been understood. One participant expressed this as "You wait long, but when you know they'll take care of you and when its your turn they take as long as it takes so it all comes out ok."

Harmful, the fourth theme, was expressed as experiences that homelessness as a lived event is unhealthy. There was a general agreement in many participants that homelessness was not good for the person, exposed the person to abuse and victimization, could make a person sick, scared, lonely, and negatively impacted self-esteem and self-regard. One participant eloquently expressed the meaning of this theme.

It's scary [homelessness]. Never know what's coming next, a person coming to hurt you, a police to harass you, a virus cold to kill you. It's hard not knowing. Yea it ain't easy being homeless. Nothing but scared and worried followed by scared and worried. Them two words

[homelessness and healthy] don't even go together. Being homeless means being sick, sick in the head, sick in the body, and sick in the heart.

The last theme of homelessness, distinctness, was expressed as experiences that homelessness as a lived event gave individuals unique, separate, and different life-experiences that were characteristically unlike experiences of non-homeless individuals. As several participants stated, very simply, "We're different."

*Themes of Health.* Three distinct themes were identified that inform what health meant to homeless participants. The three themes were ableness, self-knowing, and well-being.

Ableness was a theme expressing that health is the relative presence or absence of capacity to function in daily life, and not the relative presence or absence of disease. As one participant said, "Health is being able to, when your body is able to do daily, things that you do daily. You know, know you can function good."

Self-knowing was expressed by participants as experiences of knowing when and why they are, and are not, healthy that is independent of objective data, and that they can quickly determine who will and will not be helpful to them. This theme encompassed several attributes including homeless people's belief that they know when they are ill, know immediately who will or will not be of help, know what is wrong, and know what is needed to make it correct. One participant shared her experience of presenting at a clinic during an asthma attack.

I went in there [health clinic] and I couldn't breathe and I told her I needed the breathing treatment. She told me sit down there's a bunch of people ahead of you and you need to be checked out to see if you need one. And she said no, she said sit down, and she said wait a minute. She said I've got so many names here, she said you're going to have to wait 'til after lunch. I said lady, if I stand here and die in your face, I'm not going to be able to have the breathing treatment after lunch.

Well-being was described as the experiences of health that are greater than just physical wellness and include the relative degree of self-regard from reflected appraisals. This theme included attributes of the link between mind and body, health being greater than the body being OK, and a perceived need to feel respected by others to be fully healthy. It was expressed in the following manner by one participant describing her experiences with getting care for a chronic health problem.

If you're treated badly, it does something to you inside. It eats at you. And, well I know just,

I can get depressed and get you know, just somebody picking at me and it makes me sick. And I think it does a lot of people.

*Themes of Satisfaction with Health Care.* Five themes informing satisfactory care experiences included committed care, respectful engagement, trust, assumption-free, and inclusionary care practices.

Committed care was expressed as experiences that providers do not give up on them, do not reject them if noncompliant, and would appraise for a range of health problems, not just expressed need at the time of care. Attributes of this theme included thorough care, sticking with the person even if they have not followed up on recommended care, working with the person until a problem is resolved, and not being punitive if appointments are missed. It was expressed by one participant as "People caring and working real hard with me, not over me." Another participant described an experience with health care that left him satisfied and seems to express this theme well.

> They take their time, they work with people. [Name] is the best and always stays working with me even if I screwed up and did something I shouldn't of. Doesn't tell me to go away if I didn't do my part like other places have told me.

The theme of respectful engagement was described as experiences of interpersonal interactions in health care settings that were characterized by perceptions of support, caring, empathy, acceptance, and respect towards the participant by the provider. These experiences were felt to enhance the individual's self-regard. This theme included attributes such as not feeling rushed, feeling respected as a person, being addressed by name, and feeling good about themselves because they were respected. One participant related how one clinic made him fell respected "And it's not just medical stuff. They don't, they don't care if I'm a little dirty or smelling, act like I'm just in my best suit. Offer me coffee, socks and other stuff I need." Respectful engagement was seen as significant to satisfaction with care, as expressed in the words of one of the participants. "If I feel better that's a start, I'll take it. But full satisfied, now that's different. I feel good 'bout myself not just my sickness when I'll be satisfied."

Trust was a third theme in satisfactory care experiences and was experienced as being able to believe and have faith and confidence in health providers. This trust was sufficient to allow the person to share sensitive data and to take as credible any health information and/or recommendations given by a provider. Trust attributes included homeless persons' perceptions that providers would believe what they were told, that shared information would not be used

against the person, that providers understand and accept the enhanced privacy needs of the homeless, and that providers' opinions of what is wrong and what treatment is required can be counted on as accurate. As one participant said, "I need to be sure that things stay private." The presence of trust appear to be related to respectful engagement as the following example shows. "If you're nice to me I know you wouldn't lie about what I needed so you're all the bosses." Another participant expressed that:

> Everyone is so nice to me here. I mean, you just help me out, you know. I just feel like I could talk to people here. Where I feel like if I went to another place I would have to, I would really have to, they would have to get to know me, I would have to get to know them.

Assumption-free as a theme represented experiences of being treated in a manner that does not reflect prejudgment and shows that the providers have not made negative assumptions, stereotyped, or have predetermined judgments about them as a homeless person. Participants shared many experiences of having felt prejudged and stereotyped. They believed that care practices responded to those prejudgments and was therefore different from the care given to non-homeless persons. One participant shared his experiences of feeling prejudged in this way,

> It's like, 'Your homeless man. Who wants to give you the time of day. You're nothing and a waste of energy. I don't believe a word you tell me so don't tell me any words. You not gonna do what I tell you so so long baby.' That's how they feel usually.

The last theme, inclusionary care practices, was experienced as being able to access needed care, being included in care decisions, and feeling able to reject treatment recommendations without penalty to further care. Attributes of this theme included limiting hassles like paperwork, a feeling of participation in care practices, feeling like a partner, treatment that reflected providers' awareness of homeless lifestyle issues, and respect for homeless persons' ability to prioritize their health care choices. Participants' experiences with this theme were often expressed as the absence of this aspect of care, in such ways as "They just didn't care about me, told me what to do and never asked me a thing 'bout me." Or as "And uhh, they say if you don't want our medication, you don't need us."

## Discussion and Directions for Future Research

Seven dimensions of satisfaction have been examined in the major satisfaction studies to date (Marshall et al., 1996; Ware et al., 1983). These dimensions include: general satisfaction, interpersonal manner, communication, technical competence, time spent with doctor, financial aspects, and accessibility/convenience of care. The themes identified in this study, although potentially overlapping, are different and suggest that the items which make up the commonly used measures of satisfaction have limited application to life situations and health care concerns of homeless clients.

The themes identified in this study represent five dimensions of satisfaction that are directly applicable to the homeless population, and cannot be separated from the themes representing the lived experiences of homelessness and health. For example, self-knowing and resourcefulness, identified as aspects of health and homelessness, underscore and explain why the satisfaction dimensions of respectful engagement and committed care matter in this population. The theme of uncertainty, identified as an aspect of homelessness, helps in explaining trust as a critical dimension of satisfaction; whereas the distinctness of homeless experiences aids in understanding the importance of inclusionary care practices as a dimension of satisfaction.

A significant finding of the study is that several of the identified themes represent strengths or positive facets of the participants' lived experiences. Resourcefulness, self-knowing, and distinctness were seen by participants as positive aspects of their lived experiences. These themes may function to provide insight into care practices that build on homeless individuals strengths, and decrease the common perception that all experiences of homelessness are negative.

The five dimensions of satisfaction with care may be useful in outcome measurement of homeless individuals' satisfaction with care, and may have broader clinical implications. Homeless individuals are a distinct population, and have unique health care needs that must be addressed through distinct structural and process considerations. The themes identified in this study highlight the need to develop a practice model for care of homeless individuals. Such a model would require alteration from traditional service delivery models, allowing for more consumer input, open and flexible structure, process activities facilitating respectful engagement, and the presence of committed, inclusionary care practices.

## References

Aiken, L.H. (1987). Unmet needs of the chronically mentally ill: Will nursing respond? *IMAGE: Journal of Nursing Scholarship, 19*(3), 121–125.

Avis, M., Bond, M., & Arthur, A. (1997). Questioning patient satisfaction: An empirical investigation in two outpatient clinics. *Social Science Medicine, 44*(1), 85–92.

Baumann, S.L. (1993). The meaning of being homeless. *Scholarly Inquiry for Nursing Practice: An International Journal, 7*(1), 59–73.

Bushy, A. (1995). Ethnocultural sensitivity and measurement of consumer satisfaction. *Journal of Care Quality,* (2), 16–25.

Clarke, P.N., Williams, C.A., Percy, M.A., & Kim, Y.S. (1995). Health and life problems of homeless men and women in the southeast. *Journal of Community Health Nursing, 12*(2), 101–110.

Dancy, B.L., & Barge, F.C. (1996). Homeless women's perceptions of their situation. *Journal of the National Black Nurses Association, 8*(2), 13–22.

Denzin, N.K., & Lincoln, Y.S. (Eds.). (1994). *Handbook of qualitative research.* Thousand Oaks, CA: Sage.

DiTomasso, D.A., & Willard, M. (1991). The development of a patient satisfaction questionnaire in the ambulatory setting. *Family Medicine, 23*(2), 127–131.

Drake, R.E., Osher, F.C. & Wallach, M.A. (1991). Homelessness and dual diagnosis. *American Psychologist, 46*(11), 1149–1158.

Gelburg, L., Gallagher, T.C., Andersen, R.M., & Koegel, P. (1997). Competing priorities as a barrier to medical care among homeless adults in Los Angeles. *American Journal of Public Health, 87*(2), 217–220.

Hodnicki, D.R. (1990). Homelessness: Health-care implications. *Journal of Community Health Nursing, 7*(2), 59–67.

Hunter, J.K., Getty, C., Kemsley, M., & Skelly, A. (1991). Barriers to providing health care to homeless persons: A survey of providers' perceptions. *Health Values, 15*(5), 3–11.

Hunter, J.K., Crosby, F., Ventura, M.R., & Warkentin, L. (1997). Factors limiting evaluation of health care programs for the homeless. *Nursing Outlook, 45*(5), 224–228.

Jackson, M.P., & McSwane, D.Z. (1992). Homelessness as a determinant of health. *Public Health Nursing, 9,* 185–192.

Jezewski, M.A. (1995). Staying connected: The core of facilitating health care for homeless persons. *Public Health Nursing, 12*(3), 203–210.

Larrabee, J.H., Ferri, J.A., & Hartig, M.T. (1997). Patient satisfaction with nurse practitioner care in primary care. *Journal of Care Quality, 11*(5), 9–14.

Lehman, A.F., Meyers, P., & Corty, E. (1989). Assessment and classification of patients with psychiatric and substance abuse syndromes. *Hospital and Community Psychiatry, 40,* 1019–1025.

Lincoln, J.M., & Guba, E. (1985). *Naturalistic inquiry.* Newbury Park, CA: Sage.

Lindsey, D.L., Henly, S.J., & Tyree, E.A. (1997). Outcomes in an academic nursing center: Client satisfaction with student services. *Journal of Care Quality, 11*(5), 30–38.

Mahon, P.Y. (1996). An analysis of the concept 'patient satisfaction' as it relates to contemporary nursing care. *Journal of Advanced Nursing, 24,* 1241–1248.

Marshall, G.N., Hays, R.D., & Mazel, R. (1996). Health status and satisfaction with health care: Results from the medical outcomes study. *Journal of Consulting and Clinical Psychology, 64*(2), 380–390.

Mason, D.J., Jensen, M. & Boland, D.L. (1992). Health behaviors and health risks among homeless males in Utah. *Western Journal of Nursing Research, 14*(6), 787–790.

McCormack, D., & Gooding, B.A. (1993). Homeless persons communicate their meaning of health. *Canadian Journal of Nursing Research, 25*(1), 33–50.

Menke, E.M., & Wagner, J.D. (1997). The experience of homeless female-headed families. *Issues in Mental Health Nursing, 18,* 315–330.

Miles, M.B., & Huberman, A.M. (1994). *Qualitative data analysis: An expanded sourcebook* (2nd Ed., Rev.). Thousand Oaks, CA: Sage.

Miles, M.B. & Huberman, A.M. (1984). *Qualitative date analysis: A sourcebook of new methods.* Beverly Hills, CA: Sage.

Munhall, P.L., & Boyd, C.O. (1993). *Nursing research: A qualitative perspective.* New York: NLN Press.

Reichenbach, E.M., McNamee, M.J., & Seibel, L.V. (1998). The community health nursing implications of the self-reported health status of a local homeless population. *Public Health Nursing, 15*(6), 398–405.

Rodgers, B.L., & Cowles, K.V. (1993). The qualitative research audit trial: A complex collection of documentation. *Research in Nursing & Health, 16,* 219–226.

Rubin, H.R., Gandek, B., Rogers, W.H., Kosinski, M., McHomey, C.A., & Ware, J.E. (1993). Patients' rating of outpatient visits in different practice settings. *Journal of the American Medical Association, 270*(7), 835–840.

Sheridan, M.J., Gowen, N., & Halpin, S. (1993). Developing a practice model for the homeless mentally ill. *Families in Society: The Journal of Contemporary Human Services,* 410–421.

Vredevoe, D.L., Brecht, M.L., Shuler, P., & Woo, M. (1992). Risk factors for disease in a homeless population. *Public Health Nursing, 9*(4), 263–269.

Ware, J.E., Snyder, M.K., Wright, W.R., & Davies, A.R. (1983). Defining and measuring patient satisfaction with medical care. *Evaluation and Program Planning, 6,* 247–263.

Wagner, J.K., & Perrine, R.M. (1994). Women at risk for homelessness: Comparison between housed and homeless women. *Psychological Reports, 17,* 1671–1678.

Williams, B. (1994). Patient satisfaction: A valid concept? *Social Science Medicine 38*(4), 509–516.

Wright, J.D. & Weber, E. (1987). *Homelessness and health.* Washington, DC: McGraw-Hill.

# Evaluating the Impact of Peer, Nurse Case-Managed, and Standard HIV Risk-Reduction Programs on Psychosocial and Health-Promoting Behavioral Outcomes Among Homeless Women

**Adeline Nyamathi, Jacqueline H. Flaskerud, Barbara Leake, Elizabeth L. Dixon, Ake Lu**

*Presented at the School of Nursing, University of California, Los Angeles, Los Angeles, CA*

   *Abstract: Investigators examined the 6-month impact of three cognitive–behavioral HIV risk-reduction programs on behavioral factors (substance use and sexual risk behaviors) and cognitive and psychological resources of 325 women who resided in emergency or sober-living shelters and their 308 intimate sexual partners. Participants were randomized by shelter to a peer-mentored, a nurse case-managed, or a standard care HIV risk-reduction program. Significant improvements were observed in all groups in all behavioral factors and cognitive and psychological resources except for self-esteem. Participants in the peer-mentored and nurse case-managed groups did not differ significantly from the standard group in self-esteem, life satisfaction, psychological well-being, use of non-injection drugs, sex with multiple partners, and unpro-tected sex at 6 months (n = 633). It was concluded that a standard approach by health care professionals appears to effectively modify HIV risk behaviors for a majority of homeless participants and may have important economic and policy implications. Further, the impact of short-term programs that address psychological vulnerabilities of impoverished population needs to be studied further.*

   Currently, the overwhelming majority of new cases of exposure to the human immunodeficiency virus (HIV) and of acquired immune deficiency syndrome (AIDS) cases in the United States are African American and Hispanic (Centers for Disease Control and Prevention [CDC], 2000). Injection drug use and unprotected sexual behavior are associated with 70% of all AIDS cases. Among minority populations, who comprise 28% of the U.S. population (U.S. Census Bureau, 1997), heterosexual transmission of HIV has

*Research in Nursing & Health, 2001, 24, 410–422, © 2001 John Wiley & Sons, Inc.*

steadily increased, particularly for women (CDC, 2000).

Homeless women constitute a vulnerable group whose behaviors have been particularly difficult to change as they deal on a day-to-day basis with problems of basic survival and lack of power. Poverty and drug use may predispose them to practice high-risk behaviors associated with AIDS as a result of trading sex for money, shelter, food, and drugs. Scarce personal, health, and social resources (Brickner et al., 1993; Koegel & Burnam, 1991; Nyamathi, Flaskerud, Bennett, Leake, & Lewis, 1994) and limited decision making in sexual relationships (Ulin, 1992) also may increase their vulnerability to HIV. Moreover, the selection of a significant other who is engaged in high-risk behaviors also can have a negative impact on health-promoting behaviors (Latkin, Mandell, Vlahov, Oziemkowska, & Celentano, 1996).

Researchers experienced in providing successful interventions for dysfunctional women contend that one of the most empowering techniques is the use of peer mentors, individuals who are respected and recognized as natural helpers, educators, and role models (Dearing, Larson, Randall, & Pope, 1998). At present, however, little is known about the ability of peer mentors, trained and supported by nurses, to provide effective AIDS education and prevention programs to homeless persons. Moreover, no studies to date have been reported in the literature on whether programs can be delivered successfully to intimate homeless couples, and whether programs can be effective in promoting behavior change in both partners despite gender differences.

This article presents the 6-month impact of three cognitive–behavioral HIV risk-reduction programs on substance use, sexual risk behaviors, and cognitive and psychological resources of homeless women and their intimate sexual partners. The three programs evaluated were a PEER MENTOR program, a nurse case-managed (NCM) program, and a standard care program.

Although the seroprevalence of HIV among the homeless is largely unknown at this time, minorities are overrepresented among the homeless. The latest data on the racial composition of the homeless reveal that African Americans and Hispanics comprise more than 68% of this population (U.S. Conference of Mayors, 1992). Homeless persons also are vulnerable to HIV because of high rates of engagement in risky behaviors. For example, Nyamathi, Leake, Flaskerud, Lewis, and Bennett (1993) found that a history of injection drug use is reported by 10%–20% of homeless adults. Compared to never homeless women, about twice as many homeless women reported a lifetime diagnosis of drug use (Caton et al., 2000). In addition, more than a third reported a history of sexually transmitted diseases and sexual activity with multiple partners (Nyamathi, Flaskerud, & Leake, 1997).

Broadhead et al. (1998) argue that peers are most effective in recruiting and educating drug users because the latter are more likely to listen to people whom they consider to be like themselves, and as trusted individuals, peers may carry more weight than health care professionals. Moreover, natural helpers are thought to be effective in promoting behavioral change by improving coping skills in dealing with difficult situations where unsafe behaviors commonly are used (Nutbeam, Blakey, & Pates, 1991). On the other hand, the nurse case-managed approach has been successfully applied in intervention studies aimed at risk reduction (Nyamathi, Stein, & Brecht, 1995). Its success appears to lie in the comprehensive approach used. Yet no investigators have examined whether nurses can be more effective than either peer mentors or nurses and trained counselors who provide standard community AIDS testing and counseling in reducing HIV-related drug and sexual behaviors or in improving the cognitive and psychological resources of homeless persons.

Less than half of homeless women report having a current partner or significant other (Nyamathi, Leake, Keenan, & Gelberg, 2000). Researchers have long recognized that a supportive person can provide encouragement to practice health-promoting behaviors (Norman, Talbott, Kuller, Krampe, & Stolley, 1991). However, significant others also can have a negative impact on the practice of health-promoting behaviors. For example, significant others may encourage drug use and provide barriers to entering drug treatment programs (Latkin et al., 1996; Neaigus et al., 1994). As a result, there has been mounting interest in including the intimate partners of homeless women in AIDS education and prevention programs in order to increase the effectiveness of those programs. Such couples are most elusive, however, as few shelters encourage women and their partners to live together. This policy appears to result from a pervasive philosophy of shelter directors that the sexual partners of homeless women are responsible for the women's drug use (Nyamathi, Bayley, Anderson, Keenan, & Leake, 1999).

The Comprehensive Health Seeking and Coping Paradigm (CHSCP; Nyamathi, 1989) has served as a framework to guide the assessment and the implementation of strategies relating to coping and health outcomes. In this model, adapted from the Lazarus and Folkman (1984) Stress and Coping Paradigm and the Schlotfeldt (1981) Health Seeking and Coping Paradigm, nursing intervention (conceptualized here as culturally competent AIDS education) is seen as exerting a direct influence on a number of outcome variables. For the purposes of this article, the outcome variables of interest will be labeled *psychological and cognitive resources* and *behavioral risk measures*.

Psychological variables include psychological well-being, depression, anxiety, and hostility. Cognitive resources are represented by self-esteem, life satisfaction, and AIDS knowledge, whereas risky behaviors include having used injection and noninjection drugs within the last 6 months, having multiple sexual partners, and having unprotected sexual activity. In previous research using this model the selection of variables was guided by findings that documented decreases in drug and sexual risk behaviors with interventions that enhance psychological well-being and improve depression, anxiety, and self-esteem (Nyamathi et al., 1995). Moreover, improved psychological variables were found to predict greater life satisfaction (Heckman, Somlai, Sikkema, Kelly, & Franzoi, 1997).

Theoretically grounded and systematic research on risk reduction and psychological well-being in impoverished women is rare (Smith & Williamson, 1991). A continued investigation is essential, therefore, to providing a clearer understanding of the factors that enhance these health domains among impoverished women and among significant others who may be highly influential in their lives.

Thus, the research question of interest in this study was whether three cognitive–behavioral HIV risk-reduction programs would have a positive effect on substance use, sexual risk behaviors, and cognitive and psychological resources of homeless women and their intimate partners at 6 months and whether the effectiveness would vary by type of program.

## METHOD

### Setting and Participants

A convenience sample of homeless African American, Hispanic, and Anglo women and their intimate partners living in an inner-city area of Los Angeles was enrolled from 1995 to 1998 into a longitudinal study in which women were randomized by shelter into a peer-mentored, a nurse case-managed, or a standard care HIV risk-reduction program. Additional women were recruited through street outreach activities by the research staffs of the respective programs. To be eligible to participate, women had to meet the following criteria: (a) 18–50 years of age, (b) homeless, and (c) having an intimate partner willing to participate in the study. A homeless woman was defined as one who spent the previous night in a shelter, hotel, motel, or home of a relative or friend and was uncertain as to her residence in the next 60 days or who stated that she did not have a home or house of her own in which to reside (Gelberg & Linn, 1989).

The intimate partners of the participating women were aged 18 and over and were determined as eligible if they had been in an intimate relationship with the women for at least 1 month. Potential participants were excluded if they were incoherent as a result of mental illness or drug use, as determined by the research nurse. In total, 948 participants were enrolled at baseline; 258 of the enrollees were in the peer-mentored program, 360 were in the nurse case-managed (NCM) program, and 330 were in the standard care program. Six-month follow-up data were obtained on 633 participants: 325 women (69% of the total number of women) and 308 partners (65% of the total number of partners). Overall follow-up rates were highest (78%) in the peer-mentored program, followed by 67% in the NCM program, and 64% in the standard care program. The vast majority of the intimate partners were male (94%); however, 7% of the partners were female.

### Procedure

Homeless women residing in 35 emergency and sober-living shelters whose directors approved their site as a participating shelter were recruited through informational presentations by the research staff and by flyers. Homeless women obtained through street outreach were presented with information and flyers on a one-on-one basis by the research staff. All interested women were provided with appointments to discuss the study with the research staff, composed of African American, Hispanic, and Anglo female nurses and outreach workers. Nurses largely were involved in implementing the education programs in the NCM and standard care programs, whereas peer mentors did this in the peer-mentored program. Outreach workers primarily administered baseline and 6-month follow-up questionnaires and assisted nurses or peer mentors in the organization of the program delivery. Informed consent was obtained from all eligible participants willing to be a part of the study. Quality assurance procedures were in place for both nurses and peer mentors in the three programs. Approximately 20% of the women encountered were ineligible to participate as they did not have a sexual relationship with an intimate partner.

The baseline instrument was a 45-min interview, which occurred in a private room in the shelters, administered separately to the women and their intimate partners by a research staff member well trained in working with homeless and drug-addicted persons. All women and their partners were offered HIV pretest and posttest counseling, had blood drawn for HIV antibody testing, provided a urine sample for drug testing, and received a list of available community resources. Few (2%) women refused HIV antibody testing, while 9% refused to provide a urine sample. Similarly, few (4%) partners refused HIV antibody testing, and 12% refused to provide a urine sample for drug testing. All participants were assured confidentiality and were paid $10 at the completion of the baseline interview and again at the completion of a 6-month follow-up interview. Tracking of the participants was conducted by the outreach workers based on locator information provided by the participant that detailed names of family and friends who were aware of their mobility patterns and of places where the participants commonly were known to congregate. The nature of the study always was kept confidential.

### Nurse Case-Managed Program

Women and their intimate partners in the nurse case-managed program engaged in a 2-hr session weekly for 6 weeks. The sessions were conducted by a female nurse and an outreach worker of the same ethnicity as the participants. Over the six weekly sessions the couple received, in group format with one or two other couples, information on HIV/AIDS, risk behaviors, and risk-reducing and health-protecting behaviors. Attendance by homeless women for the six sessions averaged 93%, with a range in the sessions from 85% to 98%. For partners the average attendance was 90% with a range in the sessions from 80% to 94%. Entry into needed agencies, such as outpatient services, clinics, and social services, was facilitated. Culturally and linguistically appropriate materials were distributed. Condoms and skill enhancement in condom placement were provided, along with discussion and demonstration through role play of the most and least effective coping enhancement strategies, a validated educational strategy (Nyamathi & Shuler, 1989) that depicted different situations homeless women deal with, such as negotiating condom use, survival sex, and loss of children. Research staff also assessed the partners' expectations regarding condom use, or use of dental dams for lesbian couples, and the effect of those protective aids on sexual pleasure; explored wellness benefits with the participants; and provided ongoing assistance in obtaining needed health care services.

### Peer Intervention

Women and their intimate partners assigned to the peer-mentored program received the same intervention as those in the nurse case-managed program, except that the role of the nurse was assumed by a female peer mentor who matched the participants' ethnicity. These individuals had led lifestyles similar to their clients, experiencing such things as homelessness and/or drug and alcohol addiction. Now sober and living in stable home environments, peer mentors were trained extensively by the research team to administer the peer-mentored program and questionnaires, as well as to facilitate referrals to

health and social services. Attendance by homeless women for the six weekly sessions averaged 88%, with a range from 77% to 98%. Partner attendance averaged 88%, with a range from 78% to 98%.

### Standard Care

Each participating women and her intimate partner who had been randomly assigned to the standard care program was administered the instrument packet by the research staff and received a standard traditional 15-min HIV antibody pretest as well as posttest counseling by the research nurses or outreach workers. HIV pretest counseling included an assessment and discussion of drug and sexual behaviors that place one at risk for HIV/AIDS and an explanation of the meaning of negative and positive HIV antibody test results. HIV posttest counseling reinforced this information, provided the result of the HIV antibody test, and reinforced the meaning of either the negative or positive test result.

### Instruments

All instruments except that measuring life satisfaction were pilot-tested using a focus group format to determine their clarity and sensitivity to homeless and drug-addicted women (Nyamathi & Lewis, 1991; Nyamathi & Vasquez, 1989). All instruments were translated into the Spanish language by a bilingual researcher of Hispanic ethnicity. The semantic validity of the instruments was well established and was assessed by having the instruments translated from English to Spanish by one bilingual professional and then back-translated from Spanish to English by another bilingual professional.

### Cognitive Resources

*Self-esteem* was measured using a revised version of the Coopersmith (1967) Self-Esteem Inventory (SEI), a 23-item scale in which subjects indicate whether self-esteem statements are "like me" or "unlike me." The original Cronbach's alpha for this scale was .89 (Coopersmith). Revisions in the measure consisted of simplifying the scaling for the homeless to "true" and "false," reflecting whether each feeling was experienced by the individual. The internal consistency for the SEI in the current study was .83. Responses to the 23 items were summed to form a scale score, with a range of 0 to 23. Higher means indicated greater self-esteem.

*Life satisfaction* was measured by a series of faces with expressions ranging from very happy to very sad. Participants were asked to circle a number under the face that most closely resembled how they felt about their life in general. Response choices ranged from 1 (*delighted*) to 7 (*terrible*).

*AIDS knowledge* was assessed using a modified 21-item scale developed by the National Center for

Health Statistics (1987) that covered a wide range of topics, including sources of AIDS information, knowledge about AIDS and its transmission, and experience with HIV testing. Modifications by researchers included the addition of a common response format that ranged from 1 (*definitely true*) to 4 (*definitely false*). A *don't know* response also was included. The internal consistency of the scale was .89. The measures were found to have face validity and to have support for convergent validity (Leake, Nyamathi, & Gelberg, 1997).

## Psychological Resources

*Psychological well-being* was measured by the Mental Health Index (MHI-5; Stewart, Hays, & Ware, 1988), which contains five items to which the respondent indicates a response on a 6-point scale that ranges from *all of the time* to *none of the time*. The MHI-5 has well-established reliability and validity and has been shown to detect significant psychological disorders, including major depression, general affective disorders, and anxiety disorders (Berwick et al., 1991). The original alpha coefficients for these scales ranged from .74 to .89 (Berwick et al.). The Cronbach's alpha for the MHI-5 in this sample was .82. The mean item scale scores were computed and linearly transformed to a 0–100 range in order to evaluate them in terms of an established clinical cut point. For the MHI-5, higher scores indicate greater psychological well-being. Individuals may be at high risk for mental health problems if they score less than 66 out of 100 (Rubenstein et al., 1989).

*Depression, anxiety,* and *hostility* were measured by the Brief Symptom Inventory (BSI; Derogatis & Melisaratos, 1983). Three subscales of the BSI were used to assess depression (six items), anxiety (six items), and hostility (five items). Each item of the BSI is rated on a 5-point scale of distress ranging from *not at all* to *extremely*. Internal consistency coefficients for the three subscales in this study ranged from .86 to .91. The original alpha coefficients for these scales ranged from .74 to .85 (Derogatis & Melisaratos).

## Behavioral Risk

*Drug and alcohol use* was assessed by a minimally revised Drug History Form (Simpson, 1991). The modification inserted by the researchers was a single item on use of injection drugs in the last 6 months. The form elicited information on: inhalants, marijuana, hallucinogens, crack/freebase, other cocaine, heroin, street methadone, other opiates, amphetamines and methamphetamine, valium, barbiturates, and other sedatives and alcohol. Items included lifetime use and frequency of recent use. The 2-week test-retest reliability for the modified daily narcotic use section of the form and for abstinence was in an acceptable range of .63 to .71 (Anglin et al., 1996).

*Sexual activity* was measured by two items that inquired about risky activities engaged in during the past 6 months. These items quantified the number of sexual partners of an individual and whether that individual had had sex without using a condom.

*Sociodemographic characteristics,* including age, education, ethnicity, length of time homeless, number of times homeless, usual living place in the past 30 nights, employment status, whether receiving public benefits, and whether receiving financial assistance from family or friends, were measured as part of a structured instrument developed by the researcher.

## Data Analysis

The baseline and 6-month differences between participants in the three programs were analyzed with chi-square tests for categorical variables and with analysis of variance (ANOVA) and/or Kruskal-Wallis tests for continuous variables, depending on their underlying distributions. These tests were conducted for participants who had both baseline and 6-month follow-up data. In addition, separate stratified comparisons were performed for women and for their partners. Time differences between baseline and 6 months and program by time, partnership status by time, and program by partnership status by time interactions were assessed with repeated-measures analysis of variance for continuous variables that were not highly skewed. Similar analyses for dichotomous outcomes were conducted using repeated-measures log-linear analysis. When significant interactions with time were found, the analyses were repeated for each group separately to examine changes over time within the group.

Because of its highly skewed distribution in some groups at 6 months, the AIDS knowledge scale was collapsed into two categories according to whether or not 17 or more questions were answered correctly. The cut point of 17 was chosen because it represents the median score at baseline. The dichotomous knowledge measure was used in repeated-measures and multivariate analyses. The three BSI subscales had similar distributional problems and attempts to apply normalizing transformations were not successful. Consequently, for repeated measures and multivariate analyses, these subscales were dichotomized according to whether or not they were above the respective mean scores of a population of 719 normal controls (Derogatis & Melisaratos, 1983). Self-reports of noninjection drug use were corrected by urinalysis results. In particular, negative baseline and 6-month follow-up self-reports of alcohol or noninjection drug use in the past 6 months were changed to positive if urine tests were positive for alcohol, marijuana, cocaine, amphetamines, barbiturates, or benzodiazepines. Injection drug use was not analyzed, as too few cases were identified by self-report or urine testing.

Linear regression analyses were used for further examination of the independent effects of program and partnership status on the continuous outcome measures at 6 months. These analyses controlled for the values of the outcome measures at baseline and for the variables listed in Table A4–1. For dichotomous variables, logistic regression analysis was used to assess the effects of the program and partnership

**TABLE A4-1** Baseline Sociodemographic Characteristics of Women and Their Intimate Partners as a Function of Program

| Characteristic | Nurse Case-Managed | | | | Peer-Mentored | | | | Standard Care | | | |
|---|---|---|---|---|---|---|---|---|---|---|---|---|
| | Women (n = 114) | | Partners (n = 106) | | Women (n = 100) | | Partners (n = 101) | | Women (n = 111) | | Partners (n = 101) | |
| | *M* | *SD* | *M* | *SD* | *M* | *SD* | *M* | *SD* | *M* | *SD* | *M* | *SD* |
| Age[a,b,c] | 35.8 | 8.4 | 38.4 | 8.4 | 30.0 | 7.6 | 32.5 | 8.2 | 37.0 | 8.5 | 39.3 | 9.3 |
| Year of education[a,d] | 11.2 | 2.8 | 11.1 | 3.1 | 10.5 | 2.7 | 10.8 | 2.6 | 11.4 | 1.8 | 12.1 | 2.4 |
| Ethnicity[e,f,g] | (%) | | (%) | | (%) | | (%) | | (%) | | (%) | |
| African American | 65.8 | | 69.8 | | 41.4 | | 47.0 | | 80.2 | | 82.2 | |
| Hispanic/Latino | 21.9 | | 21.7 | | 46.5 | | 46.0 | | 10.8 | | 13.9 | |
| Anglo American | 11.4 | | 8.5 | | 10.1 | | 7.0 | | 7.2 | | 3.0 | |
| Other | 0.9 | | 0 | | 2.0 | | 0 | | 1.8 | | 1.0 | |
| Usual living place[e,f,g] | | | | | | | | | | | | |
| Emergency shelter | 73.7 | | 71.4 | | 40.2 | | 39.2 | | 21.6 | | 18.0 | |
| Sober-living/residential drug treatment | 13.2 | | 8.6 | | 32.0 | | 24.7 | | 30.6 | | 24.0 | |
| Conventional housing | 14.04 | | 16.2 | | 22.7 | | 34.0 | | 55.9 | | 62.0 | |
| Other | 0.9 | | 3.8 | | 5.2 | | 3.1 | | 1.8 | | 6.0 | |
| Newly homeless[e,h,i] | 50.0 | | 53.5 | | 60.5 | | 53.2 | | 37.3 | | 33.7 | |
| Employed[e,g] | 8.8 | | 30.1 | | 16.0 | | 49.5 | | 10.8 | | 26.7 | |
| Lifetime history of substance abuse[e,f,g] | 61.4 | | 67.0 | | 28.0 | | 43.6 | | 59.5 | | 68.3 | |
| Receiving public benefits[i,j] | 81.6 | | 75.5 | | 74.0 | | 53.5 | | 78.4 | | 59.4 | |
| Receiving money from family or friends | 8.9 | | 5.8 | | 15.6 | | 13.1 | | 18.4 | | 14.0 | |

[a]*p* < .001, ANOVA for group differences.
[b]*p* < .001, ANOVA for group differences among women.
[c]*p* < .001, ANOVA for group differences among partners.
[d]*p* < .01, ANOVA for group differences among partners.
[e]*p* < .001, chi-square test for group differences.
[f]*p* < .001, chi-square test for group differences among women.
[g]*p* < .001, chi-square test for group differences among partners.
[h]*p* < .01, chi-square test for group differences among women.
[i]*p* < .01, chi-square test for group differences among partners.
[j]*p* < .01, chi-square test for group differences.

status, again controlling for baseline values and the potential confounders in Table A4–1. The regression models also were rerun to include the interaction of program and partnership status to determine whether any particularly marked program differences occurred among the women or their partners. In order to partially compensate for the large number of tests, the significance level for all main effects was set at .01.

## RESULTS

### Sociodemographic Characteristics

Sociodemographic characteristics of the women and their partners are shown in Table A4–1. The women in the peer-mentored group were significantly younger ($M = 30$ years) compared with women in the nurse case-managed ($M = 36$ years) and standard care groups ($M = 37$). Similar age differences were found among the partners. Overall, participants in the peer-mentored group reported fewer years of education than their counterparts in the other groups. African American women were most likely to be in the standard care (80%) and NCM groups (66%), whereas for Hispanic women it was the peer-mentored group (47%). This ethnic profile applied to the partners as well. Usual living places also differed among the groups. More than 70% of the participants in the NCM group resided primarily in homeless shelters, as compared to about 40% in the peer-mentored group and about 20% in the standard care group. More than half of the standard care group members had resided primarily in conventional housing over the past month. Persons in the NCM group were less likely than others to have resided in either conventional housing or sober-living shelters. Participants in the peer-mentored group were least likely to report substance use in their lifetimes. Finally, partners in the peer-mentored group were more likely to be employed than their counterparts in the other two groups, and partners in the NCM group were more likely to be receiving public benefits.

### Outcome Measures

*Baseline and 6-month profiles.* Means and medians for cognitive and psychological variables and frequencies and percentiles for behavioral variables are presented in Table A4–2 as functions of program and partnership status. Medians are presented instead of standard deviations (SDs) because distributions of many variables were skewed. Both the homeless women and their partners in the peer-mentored group had less AIDS-related knowledge but greater psychological well-being than those in the NCM and standard care groups at baseline. Members of the peer-mentored group were also less likely than their counterparts to report use of noninjection drugs or

alcohol, self-reporting corrected by urine toxicology. Participants in the NCM group were particularly likely to report having sex without condoms.

The 6-month comparisons revealed similar score patterns for AIDS knowledge and psychological well-being, although partners in both the peer-mentored and standard care groups reported relatively high levels of psychological well-being. Self-esteem at 6 months was somewhat lower among peer-mentored participants than the others, although they continued to be less likely to report noninjection drug and alcohol use. Hostility scores at 6 months were higher among NCM group participants, especially the women. Sexual risk behaviors were similar across the three groups at 6 months.

Modest to marked improvements among the women and their partners can be seen for all three groups, as confirmed by the statistical findings in Table A4–3. As shown, significant changes over time were found for all outcomes except self-esteem. However, differential program effects were found for self-esteem, as well as for being highly knowledgeable about AIDS and for depression and hostility. Within-group subanalyses indicated that NCM participants improved significantly in self-esteem, whereas their counterparts in the other two groups did not. The NCM group also improved somewhat more in AIDS-related knowledge. However, depression did not change significantly in the NCM group, whereas it lessened in the peer-mentored ($p < .01$) and standard care ($p < .001$) groups. In addition, hostility decreased significantly in the peer-mentored group ($p < .001$), but not in the other groups.

Shown in Table A4–4 are the results of linear and logistic regression analyses that examined program effects on the 6-month outcomes while controlling for baseline values and other potential confounders, which were cognitive, psychological and behavioral in nature. Compared to participants in the standard care group, those in the peer-mentored group were more likely to have higher levels of depression and anxiety and a lower level of AIDS knowledge at 6 months. NCM group participants were more likely to have high levels of hostility at follow-up compared to those in the standard care group. The NCM and peer-mentored groups did not differ significantly ($p < .01$) from the standard care group in self-esteem, life satisfaction, psychological well-being, use of noninjection drugs, sex with multiple partners, or unprotected sex at 6 months. Although overall effects were not found, analyses involving interaction terms indicated that partners in the NCM and peer-mentored groups had relatively low psychological well-being scores at 6 months and that women in the peer-mentored group had relatively low self-esteem.

**TABLE A4-2** Baseline and 6-Month Results for Cognitive, Behavioral, and Psychological Factors as Functions of Program and Partnership Status

| Variables/Time | Nurse Case-Managed | | | | Peer-Mentored | | | | Standard Care | | | |
|---|---|---|---|---|---|---|---|---|---|---|---|---|
| | Women (p = 114) | | Partners (n = 106) | | Women (n = 100) | | Partners (n = 101) | | Women (n = 111) | | Partners (n = 101) | |
| | M | Median | M | Median | M | Median | M | Median | M | Median | M | Median |
| Cognitive factors | | | | | | | | | | | | |
| Self-esteem | | | | | | | | | | | | |
| Baseline | 12.1 | (12) | 13.6 | (14) | 13.3 | (14) | 13.8 | (14) | 13.0 | (13) | 14.2 | (14) |
| 6 months[a] | 13.4 | (14) | 14.4 | (15) | 12.7 | (13) | 13.4 | (13) | 14.3 | (15) | 14.6 | (15) |
| Knowledge | | | | | | | | | | | | |
| Baseline[b,c,d] | 16.0 | (17) | 16.1 | (17) | 13.6 | (14) | 14.5 | (15) | 17.2 | (18) | 17.0 | (19) |
| 6 months[b,c,d] | 20.0 | (21) | 20.0 | (21) | 17.0 | (18) | 17.3 | (18) | 19.7 | (21) | 19.2 | (21) |
| Life satisfaction | | | | | | | | | | | | |
| Baseline | 3.19 | (3) | 3.23 | (3) | 2.94 | (3) | 2.86 | (3) | 3.06 | (3) | 3.02 | (3) |
| 6 months | 2.85 | (3) | 2.87 | (3) | 2.72 | (2.5) | 2.72 | (2) | 2.59 | (2) | 2.60 | (3) |
| Psychological factors | | | | | | | | | | | | |
| Psychological well-being | | | | | | | | | | | | |
| Baseline[e] | 62.3 | (66) | 70.0 | (76) | 75.2 | (80) | 76.9 | (80) | 65.2 | (68) | 72.4 | (76) |
| 6 months[a] | 71.4 | (76) | 74.0 | (80) | 77.9 | (84) | 79.3 | (88) | 72.2 | (76) | 80.7 | (84) |
| Depression | | | | | | | | | | | | |
| Baseline | 0.65 | (0.33) | 0.54 | (0.25) | 0.75 | (0.50) | 0.47 | (0.33) | 0.77 | (0.33) | 0.52 | (0.17) |
| 6 months | 0.52 | (0.33) | 0.42 | (0.17) | 0.43 | (0.0) | 0.46 | (0.17) | 0.48 | (0.08) | 0.30 | (0.0) |
| Anxiety | | | | | | | | | | | | |
| Baseline | 0.55 | (0.33) | 0.46 | (0.17) | 0.68 | (0.33) | 0.48 | (0.33) | 0.73 | (0.33) | 0.40 | (0.08) |
| 6 months | 0.50 | (0.17) | 0.37 | (0.17) | 0.42 | (0.17) | 0.42 | (0.0) | 0.44 | (0.17) | 0.28 | (0.0) |
| Hostility | | | | | | | | | | | | |
| Baseline | 0.65 | (0.40) | 0.53 | (0.30) | 0.79 | (0.60) | 0.55 | (0.40) | 0.86 | (0.40) | 0.53 | (0.20) |
| 6 months[f] | 0.66 | (0.40) | 0.52 | (0.20) | 0.50 | (0.0) | 0.50 | (0.0) | 0.51 | (0.20) | 0.47 | (0.0) |
| | N | % | N | % | N | % | N | % | N | % | N | % |
| Behavioral factors | | | | | | | | | | | | |
| Non injection | | | | | | | | | | | | |
| Drug use* | | | | | | | | | | | | |
| Baseline[g] | 74 | 65.5 | 74 | 70.5 | 31 | 32.6 | 52 | 53.1 | 70 | 63.6 | 71 | 71.7 |
| 6 months[g] | 56 | 49.6 | 68 | 64.8 | 21 | 22.1 | 36 | 36.7 | 58 | 52.7 | 58 | 58.6 |
| Multiple partners | | | | | | | | | | | | |
| Baseline | 28 | 24.6 | 16 | 15.1 | 25 | 25.2 | 29 | 29.3 | 31 | 28.7 | 28 | 27.7 |
| 6 months | 15 | 13.2 | 17 | 16.0 | 23 | 23.2 | 27 | 27.3 | 16 | 14.8 | 22 | 21.8 |

**TABLE A4-2** Baseline and 6-Month Results for Cognitive, Behavioral, and Psychological Factors as Functions of Program and Partnership Status (Continued)

| | Nurse Case-Managed | | | | Peer-Mentored | | | | Standard Care | | | |
|---|---|---|---|---|---|---|---|---|---|---|---|---|
| | *Women* (p = 114) | | *Partners* (n = 106) | | *Women* (n = 100) | | *Partners* (n = 101) | | *Women* (n = 111) | | *Partners* (n = 101) | |
| Variables/Time | *M* | *Median* | *M* | *Median* | *M* | *Median* | *M* | *Median* | *M* | *Median* | *M* | *Median* |
| Sex without condoms past 6 months | | | | | | | | | | | | |
| Baseline | 89 | 78.0 | 85 | 81.0 | 63 | 63.0 | 66 | 66.0 | 64 | 58.2 | 68 | 67.3 |
| 6 months | 69 | 61.1 | 61 | 58.1 | 59 | 59.0 | 54 | 54.0 | 59 | 53.6 | 54 | 53.5 |

*Corrected for urine test results.
[a]$p < .01$, ANOVA for group differences.
[b]$p < .001$, Kruskal-Wallis test for group differences.
[c]$p < .001$, ANOVA for group differences among women.
[d]$p < .001$, ANOVA for group differences among partners.
[e]$p < .001$, ANOVA for group differences.
[f]$p < .01$, Kruskal-Wallis test for group differences.
[g]$p < .001$, chi-square test for group differences.

# DISCUSSION

Except for self-esteem, significant improvements in all cognitive, psychological, and behavioral factors were observed in all three HIV risk-reduction programs, supporting the theoretical framework that culturally competent AIDS education can exert a direct influence on a number of outcome variables. Women in the NCM group demonstrated improved psychological, cognitive, and behavioral changes. For example, significant improvement in self-esteem and AIDS-related knowledge was demonstrated by these women. That nurses had an impact on improving self-esteem specifically and, along with other programs, on reducing risky behaviors of the participants may be explained by the comprehensive approach nurses use in their intervention programs. The finding that NCM participants did not significantly improve scores in hostility is difficult to explain given the reduced hostility scores of the participants in the peer-mentored and standard care groups. One consideration is that the NCM participants may have been challenged by the nurses when discussing painful experiences and, in the process, may have been exposed to psychological vulnerabilities not easily resolved within a short period of time.

The finding that the standard care approach effectively modified HIV risk behaviors for a majority of the homeless participants suggests its effectiveness and supports continued resource allocation for this approach. It is important to recognize that HIV antibody testing with pre- and posttest counseling in and of itself may represent a powerful intervention for homeless adults, who have limited access to health care professionals. Although other investigators have not found pretest and posttest counseling to produce similar results with HIV-negative individuals (Weinhardt et al., 1999), the addition of caring health care professionals may be an important consideration. In particular, details on the counselors and specifics of counseling were not provided in a meta-analysis of 27 published studied (Weinhardt et al.); thus, comparisons to the present study were not possible. Further, when those experienced in working with homeless persons conduct the HIV testing and counseling, the intervention results may be even more powerful. The key component is the creation of opportunities for the homeless population to access the health care system and to interface with health care workers (either professionals or trained lay workers). Many structures already in place, such as community-based organizations and local health departments, can—and do—provide these opportunities. Policies that facilitate and even enhance collaborative relationships between service providers to the homeless and the

**TABLE A4-3** Time Effects and Interactions With Program Type and Partnership Status for Cognitive, Psychological, and Behavioral Factors for Persons With Baseline and 6-Months[a] Data

| Variable | Time | Program × Time | Partnership × Time | Program × Partnership Status × Time |
|---|---|---|---|---|
| Cognitive factors | | | | |
| Self-esteem | 5.09 | 6.72** | 1.24 | 0.67 |
| High degree of AIDS knowledge | 197.85*** | 29.53*** | 0.21 | 1.31 |
| Life satisfaction | 29.73*** | 1.39 | 0.04 | 0.03 |
| Psychological factors | | | | |
| Psychological well-being | 34.50*** | 2.69 | 0.44 | 0.85 |
| High level of depression | 16.77*** | 7.71* | 1.11 | 3.78 |
| High level of anxiety | 22.99*** | 1.34 | 1.60 | 0.63 |
| High level of hostility | 16.21*** | 11.40** | 0.55 | 1.28 |
| Behavioral factors | | | | |
| Non injection drug use | 35.97*** | 0.27 | 0.08 | 2.74 |
| Multiple sex partners | 8.45** | 2.70 | 3.06 | 1.55 |
| Sex without condoms | 26.27*** | 5.62 | 2.30 | 0.19 |

[a]F statistics from repeated-measures analysis of variance for continuous variables and $x^2$ statistics from repeated-measure long-linear analysis for dichotomous variables.
*$p < .05$, **$p < .01$, ***$p < 0.001$.

health care system are vital. For example, many homeless shelters require a Mantoux test and/or chest x-ray on admission to ensure no individual entering the shelter has active tuberculosis. Through agreements with the tuberculosis screening providers, it would also be possible to offer voluntary HIV testing at admission if supportive policies and associated funding were in place.

The demonstrated success of the standard care group in reducing HIV risk behaviors, similar to the groups receiving the interventions from nurses or peers, may be understood from a number of perspectives, and important implications for research, economics, and policy may be drawn from this success. Our findings suggest that researchers and health care providers need to evaluate the effectiveness of different delivery modalities for HIV risk-reduction interventions and the impact of referrals for health and social services. Such evaluations need to include not only changes in risk behaviors and the multiple domains of health, but also the related costs of program delivery. Economic analyses that consider behavioral

and health status changes and their impact on reducing associated costs to the health care system (i.e., hospital admissions, drug treatment, and/or psychiatric services) have the potential to provide additional guidance for decision making about delivery modalities and to inform policy formation. A standard care approach clearly appeared to modify HIV risk behaviors effectively for a majority of the homeless participants in this study. However, its long-term effectiveness also needs to be studied, particularly for individuals with more serious psychological distress and those with substance addiction.

Despite the participants in the peer-mentored group being younger and less educated than their counterparts in other programs and having lower self-esteem scores at 6 months than the other participants, they were successful in reducing their substance use. However, the finding that self-esteem scores, particularly among the women, decreased in the peer-mentored group is difficult to interpret. It may reflect an inability of peer mentors to assist the participants in improving their self-worth. An alter-

**TABLE A4-4** Linear and Logistic Regression Results Comparing Nurse Case-Managed and Peer-Mentored Programs to Standard Care Program (*n* = 536)

| Outcome | Nurse Case-Managed | | | Peer-Mentored | | |
|---|---|---|---|---|---|---|
| | *B*[a] | *SE* | *p value* | *B*[a] | *SE* | *p value* |
| Cognitive | | | | | | |
| Self-esteem | 0.32 | 0.5 | .472 | −1.08 | 0.5 | .020 |
| High degree of AIDS knowledge[b] | 0.48 | 0.4 | .226 | −1.65 | 0.3 | .001 |
| Life satisfaction | −0.24 | 0.1 | .096 | −0.27 | 0.2 | .072 |
| Psychological | | | | | | |
| Psychological well-being | −3.34 | 2.1 | .115 | −5.17 | 2.2 | .019 |
| High level of depression[c] | 0.56 | 0.3 | .024 | 0.68 | 0.3 | .010 |
| High level of anxiety[c] | 0.42 | 0.3 | .118 | 0.76 | 0.3 | .008 |
| High level of hostility[c] | 0.89 | 0.3 | .001 | 0.44 | 0.3 | .111 |
| Behaviors Past 6 months | | | | | | |
| Non injection drug use[d] | 0.30 | 0.3 | .305 | −0.30 | 0.3 | .335 |
| Multiple sexual partners | −0.24 | 0.3 | .467 | 0.35 | 0.3 | .274 |
| Sex without a condom | −0.10 | 0.3 | .698 | 0.04 | 0.3 | .881 |

[a]Controlling for baseline values of the outcomes and the variables listed in Table 1.
[b]Knowledge score greater than the median at baseline.
[c]Scores above the mean of a normative sample.
[d]Self-reported use, but negative reports changed to positive if urine screening results were positive.

native explanation is that peer mentors may have focused more on the dangers and negative choices made by participants. Clearly, although low self-esteem has been related to lesser use of condoms and greater emotional distress among the homeless (Nyamathi et al., 1995), findings in this study have demonstrated that despite the vulnerabilities of this population, participants exposed to peer mentors demonstrated many other positive changes. It is possible that these outcomes were positively modeled by offering the homeless participants any successful stories about changing behaviors. By vicariously experiencing the hardships and subsequent successes of peer mentors who had managed to abstain from substance use, these participants may have been able to decrease their substance use, knowing that others like them had made it through and survived.

Both men and women mostly showed similar improvement on scores. Thus, programs designed for delivery to the dyad may have a successful impact on both partners simultaneously. Limitations of this design precluded evaluation of the 6-month impact of having an intimate partner present in the education program, as there were no control groups that excluded intimate partner participation. Additional limitations of this study include having a sample whose baseline characteristics differed across groups. However, these differences were controlled in the statistical analyses. Further, the impact of referrals offered to the participants was not assessed. Although self-report of drug use was validated at both baseline and 6-month follow-up by urine assays of drugs, the relatively short time period (24–48 hr) in which drugs are found in the urine may have led to an underestimation of drug use. In addition, some participants declined the assays. Finally, the West Coast perspective of this sample may limit generalizability of findings to other samples.

Homeless persons face many obstacles each day in their quest for survival. In addition to suggesting ways of helping to prevent the spread of HIV, our results suggest that overall psychological well-being can be improved through concerted efforts directed toward this vulnerable population.

## References

Anglin, M.D., Longshore, D., Turner, S., McBride, D., Inciardi, J., & Prendergast, M. (1996). *Studies of the functioning and effectiveness of treatment alternatives to street crime (TASC) programs.* Los Angeles: UCLA Drug Abuse Research Center.

Berwick, D., Murphy, J., Goldman, P., Ware, J., Barsky, A., & Weinstein, M. (1991). Performance of a five-item mental health screening test. *Medical Care, 29,* 169–176.

Brickner, P.W., McAdam, J.M., Torres, R.A., Vicic, W.J., Conanan, B.A., Detrano, T., Piantieri, O., Scanlan, B., & Scharer, L.K. (1993). Providing health services for the homeless: A stitch in time. *Bulletin of the New York Academy of Medicine, 70,* 146–169.

Broadhead, R.S., Heckathorn, D.D., Weakliem, D.L., Anthony, D.L., Madray, H., Mills, R.J., & Hughes, J. (1998). Harnessing peer networks as an instrument for AIDS prevention: Results from a peer-driven intervention. *Public Health Reports, 113*(Suppl. 1), 42–57.

Caton, C.L.M., Hasin, D., Shrout, P.E., Opler, L.A., Hirshfield, S., Dominguez, B., & Felix, A. (2000). Risk factors for homelessness among indigent urban adults with no history of psychotic illness: A case-control study. *American Journal of Public Health, 90,* 258–263.

Centers for Disease Control and Prevention (CDC). (2000, June). HIV/AIDS Surveillance Report (mid-year ed., Vol. 10, No. 1). Atlanta, GA: Author.

Coopersmith, S. (1967). *The antecedents of self-esteem.* San Francisco: Freeman.

Dearing, J.W., Larson, R.S., Randall, L.M., & Pope, R.S. (1998). Local reinvention of the CDC HIV prevention community planning initiative. *Journal of Community Health, 23,* 113–126.

Derogatis, L.R., & Melisaratos, N. (1983). The Brief Symptom Inventory: An introductory report. *Psychological Medicine, 13,* 595–605.

Gelberg, L., & Linn, L.S. (1989). Psychological distress among homeless adults. *Journal of Nervous and Mental Disease, 177,* 291–295.

Heckman, T., Somlai, A., Sikkema, K., Kelly, J., & Franzoi, S. (1997). Psychosocial predictors of life satisfaction among persons living with HIV infection and AIDS. *Journal of the Association of Nurses in AIDS Care, 8,* 21–30.

Koegel, P., & Burnam, M.A. (1991, November). The course of homelessness study: Aims and designs. Presented at the 119th annual meeting of the American Public Health association, Atlanta, GA.

Latkin, C., Mandell, W., Vlahov, D., Oziemkowska, M., & Celentano, D. (1996). People and places: Behavioral settings and personal network characteristics as correlates of needle sharing. *Journal of AIDS & Human Retrovirology, 13,* 273–280.

Lazarus, R., & Folkman, S. (1984). *Stress, appraisal and coping.* New York: Springer.

Leake, B., Nyamathi, A., & Gelberg, L. (1997). Reliability, validity and composition of a subset of the CDC AIDS knowledge questionnaire in a sample of homeless and impoverished adults. *Medical Care, 35,* 747–755.

National Center for Health Statistics. (1987). *AIDS knowledge and attitudes of black Americans.* Hyattsville, MD: Public Health Service.

Neaigus, A., Friedman, S., Curtis, R., Des Jarlais, D., Furst, R., Jose, B., Mota, P., Stepherson, B., Sufian, M., & Eward, T. (1994). The relevance of drug injectors social and risk networks for understanding and preventing HIV infection. *Social Science & Medicine, 38,* 67–78.

Norman, S.A., Talbott, E.O., Kuller, L.H., Krampe, B.R. & Stolley, P.D. (1991). Demographic, psychosocial, and medical correlates of pap testing: A literature review. *American Journal of Preventive Medicine, 7,* 219–226.

Nutbeam, D., Blakey, V., & Pates, R. (1991). The prevention of HIV infection from injecting drug use—A review of health promotion approaches. *Social Science & Medicine, 33,* 977–983.

Nyamathi, A. (1989). Comprehensive health seeking and coping paradigm. *Journal of Advanced Nursing, 14,* 281–290.

Nyamathi, A., Bayley, L., Anderson, N., Keenan, C., & Leake, B. (1999). Perceived factors influencing the initiation of drug and alcohol use among homeless women and reported consequences of use. *Women and Health, 29,* 99–114.

Nyamathi, A., Flaskerud, J., & Leake, B. (1997). HIV-risk behaviors and mental health characteristics among homeless or drug-recovering women and their closest sources of social support. *Nursing Research, 47,* 133–137.

Nyamathi, A., Flaskerud, J., Bennett, C., Leake, B., & Lewis, C. (1994). Evaluation of two AIDS education programs for impoverished Latina women. *AIDS Education & Prevention, 6,* 296–309.

Nyamathi, A., Leake, B., Flaskerud, J., Lewis, C., & Bennett, C. (1993). Outcomes of specialized and traditional aids counseling programs for impoverished women of color. *Research in Nursing & Health, 16,* 11–21.

Nyamathi, A., Leake, B., Keenan, C., & Gelberg, L. (2000). Type of social support among homeless women: Its impact on psychosocial resources, health and health behaviors, and health service utilization. *Nursing Research, 49,* 318–326.

Nyamathi, A., & Lewis, C. (1991). Coping of African-American women at risk for AIDS. *Women's Health Issues, 1,* 53–61.

Nyamathi, A., & Shuler, P. (1989). Factors affecting prescribed medication compliance of the urban homeless adult. *Nurse Practitioner, 14,* 47–54.

Nyamathi, A., Stein, J., & Brecht, L. (1995). Psychosocial predictors of AIDS risk behavior and drug use behavior in homeless and drug-addicted women of color. *Health Psychology, 14,* 265–273.

Nyamathi, A., & Vasquez, R. (1989). The impact of sex, drugs, and poverty on Latina women at risk for HIV infection. *Hispanic Journal of Behavioral Sciences, 11,* 299–314.

Rubenstein, L.V., Calkins, D.R., Young, R.T., Cleary, P., Fink, A., Kosecoff, J., Jette, A., Davies, A., Delbanco, T., & Brook, R. (1989). Improving patient function: A randomized trial of functional disability screening. *Annals of Internal Medicine, 111,* 836–842.

Schlotfeldt, R. (1981). Nursing in the future. *Nursing Outlook, 29,* 295–301.

Simpson, D.D. (1992). *TCU Forms Manual.* Ft. Worth, TX: Institute of Behavioral Research, Texas Christian University.

Smyth, K., & Williamson, P. (1991). Patterns of coping in Black working women. *Behavioral Medicine, 17,* 40–46.

Stewart, A.L., Hays, R.D., & Ware, J.E., Jr. (1988). The MOS Short-Form General Health Survey. Reliability and validity in a patient population. *Medical Care, 26,* 724–735.

Ulin, P.R. (1992). African women and AIDS: Negotiating behavioral change. *Social Science & Medicine, 34,* 63–73.

U.S. Census Bureau. (1997). *Resident population of the United States by race, and Hispanic origin.* Washington, DC: U.S. Government Printing Office.

U.S. Conference of Mayors. (1992). *A status report on hunger and homelessness in America's cities.* Washington, DC: U.S. Conference of Mayors.

Weinhardt, L.S., Carey, M.P., Johnson, B.T., & Bickham, N.L. (1999). Effects of HIV counseling and testing on sexual risk behavior: A meta-analytic review of published research, 1985–1997. *American Journal of Public Health, 89,* 1397–1405.

# Mexican American Family Survival, Continuity, and Growth: The Parental Perspective

Kathleen J. Niska

*An ethnographic study using Roy's adaptation model was conducted among 23 Mexican American families in Hidalgo County, Texas, from 1994 to 1998. The purpose was to characterize the family goals of survival, continuity, and growth from the parental perspective during early family formation. Parents affirmed that being healthy, being a united couple, having supportive parents, having a steady job, and having civic harmony were essential characteristics of family survival. Family continuity was characterized by mothers doing tasks inside the house, fathers doing tasks outside the house, and both parents performing toddler and early childhood tasks. Family growth was characterized by having shared communication, growing in togetherness, planning ahead, exerting joint effort, and helping the child become part of the family.*

Accurate data are needed about Mexican American family system goals for appropriate evaluation of outcomes achieved through nursing intervention (Castillo, 1996). Roy (1983) advises nurses to intervene in families by enhancing family processes of nurturing, support, and socialization, thereby helping families to achieve general goals of survival, continuity, and growth. The purpose of this part of the ethnographic longitudinal study reported here was to identify how Mexican American families in early fam-

ily formation establish basic patterns for family survival, continuity, and growth. The research question was, What characterized family survival, continuity, and growth in Mexican American families in early family formation? *Family survival* is defined as sustained organization of the family system. *Family continuity* is consistency of patterns in the family system over time. *Family growth* is change in the structure of the system allowing the family system to become more internally complex in adapting to changing needs of family members and changing relationships within the family. The change in structure of the family becomes more externally complex in responding to changes in the family environment. *Early family formation* spans the time from birth through the 4th year of life of the first child.

## Roy's Model of the Family as an Adaptive System

According to Roy (1983), the family is an adaptive system that responds to changes in the family environment, to changes in relationships within the family, and to changing needs of family members. The family adapts to these changes through family processes of nurturing, support, and socialization, thus achieving family goals of survival, continuity, and growth. Continual input to the family system comes through feedback mechanisms of member control and transactional patterns.

Roy's (1983) model of the family as an adaptive system has been used since 1994 to guide the research about Mexican American family transitions. During the first 10-month period of the study in 1994 to 1995, 26 Mexican American couples living in Hidalgo County, Texas, were followed from the third trimester of pregnancy until the firstborn child was 6 months old. This initial family study focused on parental concerns (Niska, Lia-Hoagberg, & Snyder, 1997), the meaning of family health (Niska, Snyder, & Lia-Hoagberg, 1999), and health-related decisions (Niska, Snyder, & Lia-Hoagberg, 1998). In 1996, the investigator returned for 8 weeks and interviewed 23 of the original 26 families to examine the distinctive nature of adaptive processes of nurturing, support, and socialization of the Mexican American family in early family formation (Niska, 1999b). The third part of the study, occurring from January to February 1998 and involving 25 of the original 26 families, investigated the similarity and acceptability of nursing interventions that enhance processes of nurturing, support, and socialization (Niska, 1999a) and also investigated basic patterns of survival, continuity, and growth within the family.

## RELATED LITERATURE

Roy's (1983) model of the family as an adaptive system references general system theory pioneered by Ludwig von Bertalanffy. Bertalanffy (1968) stated, "A system may be defined as a set of elements standing in interrelation among themselves and with the environment" (p. 252). Families are organized wholes. Bertalanffy wrote, "Characteristics of organization, whether of a living organism or a society, are notions like those of wholeness, growth, differentiation, hierarchical order, dominance, control, competition, etc." (p. 47). Whereas Bertalanffy cited a unitary conception of the world based on isomorphy of laws in different fields, such as biology, psychology, and sociology, he did not depart from regarding the individual person as the ultimate precept. He framed human society in terms of the achievements of the individual rather than viewing the individual as being "controlled by the laws of the superordinate whole" (p. 56).

Cultural communities invest family organizations with defined functions in childbearing, socialization of the young, sexual satisfaction of adults, and intimacy of family members. Family structure is the unique pattern of the family enacted to meet members' needs and to fit cultural precedents set for the family unit (Montgomery & Fewer, 1988). Montgomery and Fewer (1988) describe family patterns as

sequences of interactions and sequences of transactions that become typical ways the system behaves.

Family health is a state of being and becoming an integrated and whole family (Roy, 1983). Roy states that the family is an adaptive system that responds to the changing needs of family members, to changes occurring within relationships within the family, and to changes in the family ecosystem. Adaptational processes of support, nurturing, and socialization operate within the family to facilitate family integration. General goals of the family system are survival, continuity, and growth. Feedback mechanisms of member control and transactional patterns provide ongoing input to the family system.

Roy (1983) indicated, "To make diagnoses related to family adaptation . . . family behavior can be observed as it relates to the general family goals of survival, continuity, and growth" (p. 275). Roy stated that family behavior being observed may parallel the individual adaptive modes in the following way: Family survival behavior may parallel the physiological mode of the individual, family continuity may be aligned with the role function mode, and family growth may be analogous to the self-concept mode of the individual. Transactional patterns of the family may parallel the interdependence mode, and member control processes of the family may be aligned with both physiological needs and role function modes of the individual.

Regarding the Roy adaptation model, Roy and Andrews (1999) state, "In this model, the major processes for coping are termed the regulator and cognator subsystems as they apply to individuals, and the stabilizer, and innovator subsystems as applied to groups" (p. 37). Regarding the family, Roy and Andrews indicate,

> The *stabilizer subsystem* involves the established structure, values, and daily activities whereby participants accomplish the primary purpose of the group and contribute to common purposes of society. For example, within the family unit, specified members fulfill wage-earning activities; others may be primarily responsible for nurturance and education of children. The family members possess values that influence the way in which they respond to their environment and fulfill their daily responsibilities to each other and society. (pp. 47–48)

In contrast to the stabilizer subsystem, the innovator subsystem is described as "the structures and processes for change and growth in human social systems" (p. 48).

Within the Roy adaptation model (Roy & Andrews, 1999), the four group modes are distinguished from the four individual modes. The physical mode for groups "pertains to the manner in which the collective human adaptive system manifests adaptation relative to basic operating resources, that is, participants, physical facilities, and fiscal resources" to achieve resource adequacy (p. 49). Roy and Andrews state, "Group identity is the relevant term to use for the second mode related to groups," allowing the group to achieve a basic need for identity integrity (p. 49). The group role function mode is directed toward achieving expected tasks with role clarity as a basic need of members of the group. Roy and Andrews state that for groups, the interdependence mode "pertains to the social context in which the group operates. This involves both private and public contacts both within the group and with those outside the group" (p. 50). Thus, the physical mode, group identity, role function, and interdependence of a group are assessed when studying a variety of human social systems, such as a family, a police department, a manufacturing plant, or a local community.

The Roy (1983) model of the family as an adaptive system is at a midrange level of conceptualization uniquely suited for describing the family system. Parallels exist between the midrange theory of the family as an adaptive system and the Roy adaptation model (Roy & Andrews, 1999). The parallels established by Roy integrating the family model and the individual model suggest that family survival may parallel group physical status, family continuity may be aligned with group role function, family growth may be analogous to group identity, and transactional processes may coincide with the interdependence of a group.

## METHOD

A 170-square-mile area of Hidalgo County, Texas, was the setting for this longitudinal study. This rural area has a population of 12,352 persons (U.S. Bureau of the Census, 1991). From 1994 to 1995, data were gathered across 26 families. One family was lost to follow-up, and two families were working outside of the region during subsequent data collection, yielding 23 families with continuous data spanning 1994 to 1996. During the 3rd year of data collection in 1997 to 1998, 25 of the 26 families participated, but for purposes of this article only the data for the 23 families who have offered complete data sets from 1994 to 1998 will be reported.

During each of the three periods of data collection, the investigator lived within the research area with Mexican American families who were not study participants. The investigator used Spradley's (1979, 1980) Developmental Research Sequence. Spradley advised using grand tour questions in interviewing and doing card-sorting tasks later in the process of data collection. In 1994, the investigator used grand tour questions asking participants to describe a typical day from dawn until dark. Based on participant responses, the investigator developed a set of 34 typical household tasks and 12 child care tasks. Each task was written on a 3 by 5 inch index card with English on one side and Spanish on the other side. In meeting with the mother and father, the investigator asked them to sort the cards, placing each card in one of four piles according to the family member who performed the given task (i.e., "Mother," "Father," "Both," or "Neither").

In the 2nd year of data collection, 11 age-related child care tasks were added, such as "Pick up the child's toys" or "Read a story." In the 3rd year, 5 age-related child care tasks were added, such as "Toilet train the child," "Dance with the child," or "Play soccer with the child."

In the second and third periods of data collection in 1996 and 1998, parents were also asked two grand tour questions: "What is essential for a family to survive nowadays?" and "What is essential for a family to grow?" Parental responses were audiotaped and transcribed verbatim in English or Spanish, giving participants fictitious names on all the transcripts. Names were changed to honor privacy. The investigator translated the Spanish conversations into English using the Tannen (1984) style of conversation analysis, working to retain cultural features in both the Spanish and English (Levinson, 1983; Sanchez, 1994; Schiffrin, 1987). A bilingual consultant verified the accuracy of English translations of the Spanish transcripts.

From the responses to these two questions, the investigator developed a frequency distribution of characteristics that families offered. The investigator cross-checked the commonality of each characteristic of family growth and of family survival by creating a card-sorting task including each characteristic written on a 5 by 8 inch index card with English on one side and Spanish on the other. A set of 9 index cards related to family survival and 10 index cards related to family growth were created that could be shuffled in random order. During a subsequent visit with the family, the investigator asked each family to read each card related to family survival and to sort the cards into two labeled stacks: (a) "Yes, it's essential for family survival," or (b) "No, it's not essential for family survival." The investigator then asked each family to read each care related to family growth and to sort the cards into two labeled stacks: (a) "Yes, it's essential for family growth" or (b) "No, it's not essential for family growth." These card-sorting tasks were recorded in a data display.

## ANALYSIS

Grand tour questions about family activities elicited data appropriate for doing card-sorting tasks about household and infant care activities during the infancy period. Inquiry and updating the infant care tasks permitted ongoing assessment of continuity in the gendered distribution of child care during the 2nd and 3rd years of the child's life. Data summarizing the gendered distribution of performance of child care tasks were analyzed in this study using frequency distributions and percentages. Parental conversations about family survival and family growth were analyzed by content analysis, locating repeating characteristics. Card-sorting tasks regarding characteristics of family survival and growth were summarized by frequencies and percentages.

## FINDINGS

### Demographic Data

In 1998, maternal age ranged from 20 to 31 years with a mean of 24.4 years ($SD = 0.6$), and paternal age ranged from 23 to 36 years with a mean of 28 years ($SD = 0.8$). Firstborn children ranged in age from 31 to 44 months with a mean of 37.4 months ($SD = 4.4$). Nine second-born children ranged in age from 5 to 27 months with a mean of 12.5 months ($SD = 6.8$). One family had a third child aged 9 months. Maternal schooling was a mean of 11 years ($SD = 3.4$), and paternal schooling was a mean of 11.2 years ($SD = 2.8$). Only 7 mothers worked full-time outside the home. Seventeen fathers had full-time employment, 3 had part-time employment, and 5 were unemployed after returning from migrant labor. During the 3 years of data collection, mean family income in U.S. dollars was reported to be 7.69 thousand ($SD = 1.2$) from 1994 to 1995, 13.2 thousand ($SD = 3.0$) in 1996, and 13.5 thousand ($SD = 7.6$) from 1997 to 1998.

### Family Survival

In response to the question, "What is essential for a family to survive nowadays?" families initially responded with the following: having secure employment ($n = 19$), receiving some government help ($n = 4$), being a united couple ($n = 3$), having a supportive family of origin ($n = 2$), being healthy ($n = 1$), having child care ($n = 1$), and having harmony in the civic community ($n = 1$). Parents describe their struggles for family survival in terms of their needing to work. Timoteo, a carpenter, described how his family survived, stating,

> Trabajar, ahorrar, ahorrar,
> pues trabajando, ahorrar poquito lo
> más que se pueda
> porque pues a veces se acaba el
> trabajo,
> poquito carpenteria,
> como pues las verdures, hay muchas
> verdures,
> está todo barato aqui,

> a veces nos ayudan las estampillas un
> poquito, asi se vive bien,
> poquito, pero se vive por comer y
> todo,
> pero no para comprar casa ni nada.

> [Working, saving, saving,
> well working, saving, what little bit
> you are able,
> well, because at times the work stops,
> there's just a little carpentry,
> well, the vegetables, there are a lot of
> vegetables,
> everything is cheap here,
> at times they help us a little bit with
> food stamps,
> at least this way one manages,
> getting by, but one has food and all,
> but not enough to buy a house or anything.]

Parents also described how family survival depended on their working together in harmony within the family. Oscar stated, "What does it take? Apart from the money, a lot of patience, a lot of understanding really." Miguel stated, "The struggle to survive for a family really is child care, you know; it's hard to find jobs; there's not much work here; the work that is here is not that . . . it's not that good . . . the work."

When doing the card-sorting task across all 23 families so that families could respond to what other families had suggested as essential for family survival (see Table A5–1), "Being healthy," "Being a united couple," and "Having supportive parents" were affirmed by all 23 families. Twenty-two families affirmed that "Having a steady job" and 21 families affirmed that "Having civic harmony" were essential for family survival. Fifteen families responded affirmatively to "Having safe child care" and 13 families to "Having affordable child care." Ranking lowest were "Both parents have to work" and "Receiving government help," with only 10 families selecting these two as essential for family survival.

In summary, more than 90% of the 23 families affirmed that being healthy, being a united couple, having supportive parents, having a steady job, and having civic harmony were essential for family survival.

### Family Continuity

To uncover what characterizes family continuity, the investigator identified household tasks with a continual pattern of performance over the three data collection periods, that is, tasks performed by the mother over the 3 years, tasks performed by the father over the 3 years, tasks consistently performed by both parents all 3 years, and tasks performed by neither parent all 3 years (see Table A5–2). Tasks that

**TABLE A5-1** Percentages of Families Affirming Certain Characteristics as Essential for Family Survival (*N* = 23)

| Characteristic | *n* | % |
|---|---|---|
| Being healthy | 23 | 100 |
| Being a united couple | 23 | 100 |
| Having supportive parents | 23 | 100 |
| Having a steady job | 22 | 96 |
| Having a civic harmony | 21 | 91 |
| Having safe child care | 15 | 65 |
| Having affordable child care | 13 | 56 |
| Both parents have to work | 10 | 43 |
| Receiving government help | 10 | 43 |

neither parent performed over a 3-year period, such as using a baby-sitter, are included in tabulating continuity in households because continual omission of an activity constitutes a pattern of continuity in some cases as well as continual performance. For example, with respect to use of a baby-sitter, the tabulation includes the 7 families in which parents would not leave their infant or young child with a baby-sitter or day-care provider. One additional family would use a baby-sitter, but only in the family home, thereby never taking the child to a location outside the family home. Similarly, families that never vacuumed were poor and they damp mopped plywood floors or cement floors; however, that activity was continual over 3 years. In tabulating across families, the percentages of families in which continual performance of household tasks occurred across all three data collection periods were as follows: sew/mend clothes, change the oil on the car/truck ($n = 22, 96\%$); get a baby-sitter, iron clothes ($n = 20, 87\%$); wash clothes, vacuum, feed the animals ($n = 19, 83\%$); clean the kitchen, scrub the floor, fix lunches ($n = 18, 78\%$); paint the outside of the house, wash the car/truck, cut the grass ($n = 17, 74\%$); wash dishes ($n = 16, 70\%$); trim trees/shrubs, clean inside the car/truck ($n = 15, 65\%$); sweep the floor, fold dry clothes, paint inside of the house ($n = 14, 61\%$); clean the rooms, make the beds, work in the garden ($n = 13, 57\%$); set the table, shop for groceries, buy gas for car/truck, wash windows, and water trees/shrubs ($n = 12, 52\%$). These 25 tasks of the 34 household tasks had a pattern of continuity in more than half of the families during the 3 years of data collection.

With respect to the division of household tasks by gender, the investigator tabulated across families and noted the percentages of families in which the mother performed the tasks all 3 years; sew/mend clothes ($n = 21, 91\%$); wash clothes ($n = 19, 83\%$); iron clothes, scrub the floor, clean the kitchen ($n = 18, 78\%$); fix lunches ($n = 17, 74\%$); wash dishes ($n = 16, 70\%$); and sweep the floor, fold dry clothes ($n = 14, 61\%$). The percentages of families in which the father performed the household tasks across all three data collection periods were as follows: change the oil in the car/truck ($n = 22, 96\%$); cut the grass, wash the car/truck ($n = 16, 70\%$); clean inside the car/truck, paint the outside of the house ($n = 14, 61\%$); and trim trees/shrubs ($n = 12, 52\%$). With respect to household tasks shared by both parents over all 3 years, no tasks were shared by at least 50% of families. A division of household tasks by gender was the characteristic pattern that parents described.

Given these 34 household tasks, the range of tasks having continuity within families with respect to stability in performance of the task over the three periods of data collection ranged between 15 to 29 tasks that remained stable over a 3-year period. The mean number of stable tasks per family was 22 tasks ($SD = 4.4$), and the median number was 21 tasks per family. Not only was a division of household tasks by gender prevalent across families, but also an average of 22 of the 34 household tasks showed continuity within families.

The investigator also identified which of the 12 basic child care tasks had a continual pattern of performance across families over the 3 years of data collection (see Table A5–3) and which of the 16 age-related child care tasks had a continual pattern over the years of data collection (see Table A5–4). The percentages of families with continual performance of basic child care tasks over 3 years were as follows: hold the child ($n = 21, 91\%$); make the child's bed, go

**TABLE A5-2** **Number of Families Reporting Continuity in Household Task Performance Over 3 Years (_N_ = 23)**

| Task | Mother | Father | Both | Neither |
|------|--------|--------|------|---------|
| Change oil in car/truck | 0 | 22 | 0 | 0 |
| Sew/mend clothes | 21 | 1 | 0 | 0 |
| Get a baby-sitter | 7 | 0 | 6 | 7 |
| Iron clothes | 18 | 0 | 1 | 1 |
| Wash clothes | 19 | 0 | 0 | 0 |
| Vacuum | 9 | 2 | 4 | 4 |
| Feed the animals | 1 | 9 | 5 | 4 |
| Scrub the floor | 18 | 0 | 0 | 0 |
| Clean the kitchen | 18 | 0 | 0 | 0 |
| Fix lunches | 17 | 0 | 0 | 0 |
| Paint the outside of the house | 0 | 14 | 3 | 0 |
| Wash the car/truck | 0 | 16 | 1 | 0 |
| Cut the grass | 0 | 16 | 1 | 0 |
| Wash dishes | 16 | 0 | 0 | 0 |
| Trim trees/shrubs | 0 | 12 | 0 | 3 |
| Clean the inside of the car/truck | 0 | 14 | 1 | 0 |
| Sweep the floor | 14 | 0 | 0 | 0 |
| Fold dry clothes | 14 | 0 | 0 | 0 |
| Paint the inside of the house | 0 | 7 | 4 | 3 |
| Clean the rooms | 11 | 0 | 2 | 0 |
| Make the beds | 11 | 0 | 2 | 0 |
| Work in the garden | 1 | 5 | 4 | 3 |
| Set the table | 10 | 0 | 2 | 0 |
| Shop for groceries | 1 | 0 | 11 | 0 |
| Buy gas for car/truck | 0 | 8 | 4 | 0 |
| Water trees/shrubs | 0 | 3 | 6 | 3 |
| Wash windows | 5 | 0 | 5 | 2 |
| Go for the mail | 3 | 3 | 5 | 0 |
| Fix the toilet | 3 | 8 | 0 | 0 |
| Cook meals | 10 | 0 | 0 | 0 |
| Throw out the trash | 1 | 4 | 5 | 0 |
| Pay the bills | 1 | 1 | 5 | 0 |
| Return borrowed items | 2 | 0 | 4 | 0 |
| Plan the menu | 4 | 0 | 1 | 0 |

to Women, Infant, Children's Clinic (WIC) ($n = 20$, 87%); choose which toys to buy ($n = 18, 78\%$); go for a stroll with the child ($n = 13, 57\%$); and take the child to the doctor, rock the child, change diapers ($n = 12, 52\%$). The percentages of families in which 16 age-related child care tasks had a continual pattern of performance over the years of data collection were as follows for each task: play with the child ($n = 22$, 95%); talk to the child, take child to a baby-sitter ($n = 20, 87\%$); dance with the child, play catch with the

**TABLE A5-3** Child Care Tasks Among Families Who Maintained Continuity of Task Performance Over 3 Years (*N* = 23)

| Basic Care Task | Mother | Father | Both | Neither |
|---|---|---|---|---|
| Hold the child | 0 | 0 | 21 | 0 |
| Make the child's bed | 18 | 0 | 2 | 0 |
| Go to Women, Infant, Children's Clinic | 17 | 0 | 3 | 0 |
| Choose which toys to buy | 2 | 0 | 16 | 0 |
| Go for a stroll with the child | 2 | 0 | 11 | 0 |
| Take the child to doctor | 4 | 0 | 8 | 0 |
| Rock the child | 2 | 0 | 10 | 0 |
| Change diapers | 7 | 0 | 5 | 0 |
| Go to public health clinic | 5 | 0 | 6 | 0 |
| Bathe the baby/child | 5 | 0 | 3 | 0 |
| Sing songs to baby/child | 5 | 0 | 3 | 0 |
| Get the bottle ready | 4 | 0 | 2 | 0 |

child (*n* = 19, 83%); toilet train, listen to the child (*n* = 18, 78%); take the child for a ride in the car or truck (*n* = 17, 74%); cut up the child's food (*n* = 16, 70%); read the child a story, comfort the crying child, play soccer with the child, put the child to bed (*n* = 15, 65%); tell the child a story (*n* = 13, 57%); and put the child down to nap (*n* = 12, 52%).

With respect to the division by gender of child care tasks, the investigator identified which tasks were performed only by the mother in more than half of the families. Only the tasks of making the child's bed (*n* = 13, 57%) and taking the child to the WIC Clinic (*n* = 12, 52%) were performed exclusively by mothers in more than half of the families. Child care tasks continually performed by both parents over the 3 years of data collection were the following: holding the child (*n* = 21, 91%) and choosing which toys to buy (*n* = 12, 52%). Age-related child care tasks performed by both parents over the years of data collection were the following: play with the child (*n* = 22, 96%); talk to the child (*n* = 20, 87%; listen to the child (*n* = 19, 83%); dance with the child (*n* = 16, 70%); comfort the crying child, take the child for a ride in the car or truck (*n* = 15, 65%); and put the child to bed (*n* = 13, 56%). In looking across families for continuity in the performance by gender of child care tasks, the prevailing pattern was the shared performance of child care.

Given the 28 child care tasks, the range of continuity within families ranged from 8 tasks per family to 23 tasks per family. The mean number of continu-ously performed tasks within a family was 17.3 (*SD* = 3.03). Parents described these structured patterns for the performance of child care tasks over time.

**Family Growth**

Parents described the following factors that contributed to family growth: exerting joint effort (*n* = 9), having shared communication (*n* = 5), using coping strategies (*n* = 3), relying on family values (*n* = 3), planning ahead (*n* = 2), gaining inspiration from children (*n* = 2), receiving professional guidance (*n* = 1, and having social contact with extended family (*n* = 1). Yasinia commented,

> La comunicación entre los dos,
> este, la union entre,
> ah huh, la comunicación entre él y yo
> y que la niña, también, pues forma parte
> también en la familia,
> y como dice, la niña le da ánimos a trabajar y salir adelante.
> [The communication between us both,
> well, the union among,
> ah huh, the communication between him and me,
> and that the child becomes part of the family,
> and like they say, the child inspires him
> to work hard and get ahead.]

**TABLE A5-4 Age-Related Care Tasks Among Families Who Maintained Continuity of Performance Over 3 Years (N = 23)**

| Age-Related Task | Mother | Father | Both | Neither |
|---|---|---|---|---|
| Play with the child | 0 | 0 | 22 | 0 |
| Talk to the child | 0 | 0 | 20 | 0 |
| Take the child to baby-sitter | 4 | 1 | 7 | 8 |
| Listen to the child | 0 | 0 | 18 | 0 |
| Take child on car/truck ride | 0 | 2 | 15 | 0 |
| Read the child a story | 6 | 0 | 9 | 0 |
| Comfort crying child | 1 | 0 | 14 | 0 |
| Put the child to bed | 2 | 0 | 13 | 0 |
| Tell the child a story | 3 | 1 | 10 | 0 |
| Put child down to nap | 6 | 0 | 6 | 0 |
| Pick up child's toys | 3 | 0 | 5 | 0 |
| Dance with the child | 3 | 0 | 16 | 0 |
| Play catch with the child | 1 | 7 | 10 | 1 |
| Cut up child's food | 6 | 0 | 10 | 0 |
| Play soccer with the child | 1 | 3 | 10 | 1 |
| Toilet train the child | 11 | 0 | 7 | 0 |

Oscar stated, "Learning, ah, what to do, ah, learning how to cope with what you have." Jaime stated, "I'd just say never give up, because for us right now, money is tight big time; we're hurting for money right now; but, like I tell my wife, we just, we'll get through, we've done it before." Marta found planning ahead to be important for family growth saying, "Yah, one has to plan ahead, so you know what you are going to do in the future." Soraida said family growth occurs through adhering to values, "With old family values, just following family values." Similarly, Yasinia comments, "Pues que crezcamos la familia junta y unida, uno de los deseos, verdad, que siempre haya respeto, apoyo, amor, verdad; es ese el deseo [Well that we are as a family grow in unit and togetherness; that is one of the desires, right; that there may always be respect, helping each other, and love, right; that is the desire]." Ana stated that family growth depended on instilling in children the desire to belong to the extended family. Ana used the metaphor of the plant explaining, "Como si yo privo a mi hija de tener contacto con la familia, con el, con todo la familia que hay, y que yo no la llevo. . .allí la familia es está haciendo para abajo marchitándose en no tener contacto, en no tener éste con la familia [Like if I deprive my daughter of having contact with the relatives, with all the family that there is and I don't bring her. . .there the family wilts in losing contact, in not having contact with them]."

When doing a card-sorting task with all 23 families to clarify which characteristics were essential for family growth, all 23 families affirmed the essentialness of "Having shared communication," "Growing in togetherness," "Planning ahead," and "Helping the children become part of the family" (see Table A5–5). Of the 23 families, 22 affirmed as essential for family growth "Gaining inspiration from the children," "Relying on family values," and "Using coping strategies." Other highly affirmed characteristics were "Having social contact with extended family" and "Parents exerting joint effort." Ranking lowest was "Family receiving professional guidance."

By using the data obtained from doing card-sorting tasks about the gendered performance of household and child care tasks, the investigator obtained quantitative data about family growth. The investigator looked for changes from baseline performance of a task. For instance, the mother initially performed the following tasks in the 1st year, but then in subsequent years the father took over doing the task or shared in doing the task with the mother. The percentages of families in which fathers demonstrated this pattern of growth occurred with respect to the following types of household tasks: make the

**TABLE A5-5** Percentages of Families Affirming Certain Characteristics as Essential for Family Growth (*N* = 23)

| Characteristic | *n* | % |
|---|---|---|
| Having shared communication | 23 | 100 |
| Growing in togetherness | 23 | 100 |
| Planning ahead | 23 | 100 |
| Helping the children become part of the family | 23 | 100 |
| Gaining inspiration from children | 22 | 96 |
| Relying on family values | 22 | 96 |
| Using coping strategies | 22 | 96 |
| Having social contact with extended family | 21 | 91 |
| Parents exerting joint effort | 20 | 91 |
| Family receiving professional guidance | 14 | 61 |

beds, pay the bills (*n* = 7, 30%); return borrowed items (*n* = 6, 26%); and clean the kitchen, plan the menu, cook meals, sweep the floor, wash the dishes (*n* = 5, 22%). Likewise, the percentages of families in which mothers demonstrated this pattern of growth in assuming or sharing tasks previously performed only by fathers occurred with respect to the following household tasks: throw out the trash (*n* = 9, 39%); go for the mail (*n* = 7, 30%); water trees and shrubs (*n* = 6, 26%); and work in the garden (*n* = 5, 22%).

The percentages of families showing growth by fathers with respect to the child care tasks occurred with the following tasks: picking up the child's toys (*n* = 12, 52%); getting the bottle ready (*n* = 10, 43%); giving the child a bath (*n* = 9, 39%); and putting the child down to nap, making the child's bed, going with the child to the public health clinic (*n* = 7, 30%). Whereas mothers had performed all these tasks initially, by subsequent data collection periods fathers shared in doing the tasks or took over the tasks, but only the task of picking up the child's toys was shared in at least 50% of the families.

## CONCLUSIONS

This longitudinal study of basic patterns of Mexican American family survival, continuity, and growth yields some interesting results and suggests direction for future research. First, these 23 Mexican American family systems in early family formation linked family survival to being healthy, being a united couple, having supportive parents, and having a steady job with minimal dependence on the government for additional resources. This parental perspective of what

is essential for family survival is consonant with indicators of positive adaptation in the physical mode offered by Roy and Andrews (1999), that is, adequate participant capability (being healthy, being a united couple), adequate monetary resources (having a steady job, both parents work, government help), availability of physical facilities (supportive parents), and operational resources (having safe child care, having affordable child care). Second, family continuity is pervasive with respect to the continual pattern of performance of 25 of the 34 household tasks grounding family life. Maternal continuity in the performance of household tasks focused on tasks done inside of the house, and paternal performance focused on tasks done outside of the house. Both parents performed basic and age-related child care tasks. The data obtained by doing card-sorting tasks shed light on one of the indicators of positive adaptation in the role function mode, role clarity; however, these categorical data do not provide understanding about other indicators, such as accountability in role performance and effective processes of role transition (Roy & Andrews, 1999). Third, essential characteristics for family growth were shared communication, growing in togetherness, planning ahead, and helping the child become part of the family. The parental perspective coincides with positive indicators of adaptation in the group identity mode (Roy & Andrews, 1999), that is, effective interpersonal relationships (having shared communication, helping children become part of the family, planning ahead, using coping strategies, exerting joint effort, and relying on family values), supportive culture (having social contact with the extended family), positive morale (gaining inspiration from the children and growing in togetherness), and group acceptance (family receiving professional guidance).

Roy's (1983) model of the family as an adaptive system is useful for understanding patterns of survival of the family unit. The continuity of the patterns of the family system, and the emergent structural growth that ensues as family members respond to needs of other family members and to changing relationships in the family. This study has characterized Mexican American family survival, continuity, and growth among families in early family formation. The longitudinal design provides depth of detail about gendered performance of specific tasks across time. In working with similar families in clinical situations using Roy's model of the family, nurses can be confident in using these characteristics of family survival, continuity, and family growth as a foundation to start their discussion with a family about existing family goals and expected outcomes of nursing interventions that enhance family nurturing, support, or socialization.

The next step in this longitudinal study of family transitions is to assess parental concerns about the firstborn children making the transition to the community school system. One way that parental concerns might be lessened is by having the nurse work with the family to enhance family socialization within the community school system. The effectiveness of the nurse's efforts to enhance family socialization could be evaluated by observing the effect on family outcomes of continuity and growth. The foundation provided by the current study characterizing family survival, continuity, and growth provides baseline parameters for that measurement.

## References

Bertalanffy, L. von (1968). *General system theory: Foundations, development, applications*. New York: Braziller.

Castillo, H. (1996). Cultural diversity: Implications for nursing. In S. Torres (Ed.), *Hispanic voices: Hispanic health educators speak out* (pp. 1–12). New York: National League for Nursing.

Levinson, S. (1983). *Pragmatics*. Cambridge, UK: Cambridge University Press.

Montgomery, J., & Fewer, W. (1988). *Family systems and beyond*. New York: Human Sciences Press.

Niska, K. (1999a). Family nursing interventions: Mexican American early family formation. *Nursing Science Quarterly, 12,* 138–142.

Niska, K. (1999b). Mexican American family processes: Nurturing, support, and socialization. *Nursing Science Quarterly, 12,* 335–340.

Niska, K., Lia-Hoagberg, B. & Snyder, M. (1997). Parental concerns of Mexican American first-time mothers and fathers. *Public Health Nursing, 14*(2), 111–117.

Niska, K., Snyder, M., & Lia-Hoagberg, B. (1998). Family ritual facilitates adaptation to parenthood. *Public Health Nursing, 15*(5), 329–337.

Niska, K., Snyder, M., & Lia-Hoagberg, B. (1999). The meaning of family health among Mexican American first-time mothers and fathers. *Journal of Family Nursing, 15*(2), 218–233.

Roy, Sr. C. (1983). Roy adaptation model. In R. Clements & F. Roberts (Eds.), *Family health: A theoretical approach to nursing care* (pp. 255–278). New York: John Wiley.

Roy, Sr. C., & Andrews, H. (1999). *The Roy adaptation model*. Stamford, CT: Appleton & Lange.

Sanchez, R. (1994). *Chicano discourse*. Houston, TX: Arte Púbilico Press.

Schiffrin, D. (1987). *Discourse markers*. Cambridge, UK: Cambridge University Press.

Spradley, J. (1979). *The ethnographic interview*. New York: Harcourt, Brace, and Jovanovich College Publishers.

Spradley, J. (1980). *Participant observation*. Chicago: Rinehart and Winston.

Tannen, D. (1984). *Conversational style*. Norwood, NJ: Ablex.

U.S. Bureau of the Census. (1991). *1990 census of population and housing: Summary of population and housing characteristics Texas* (1990 CPH-1-45). Washington, DC: Department of Commerce.

# Factors Associated With Participation by Mexican Migrant Farmworkers in a Tuberculosis Screening Program

**Jane E. Poss**

**Background:** *Tuberculosis is an important public health concern among migrant farmworkers in the United States; providing appropriate screening and treatment is difficult due to their highly mobile existence.*

   **Purpose:** *To analyze the relationship between variables (susceptibility, severity, barriers, benefits, cues to action, normative beliefs, subjective norm, attitude, and intention) from the Health Belief Model (HBM) and the Theory of Reasoned Action (TRA) and participation by Mexican migrant farmworkers in a tuberculosis screening program.*

   **Method:** *A convenience sample of 206 migrant farmworkers were recruited after a presentation of a tuberculosis education program and were tracked during the administration and reading of the tuberculosis skin test. Participants were interviewed in Spanish by the principal investigator using the Tuberculosis Interview Instrument (TII) developed for this study.*

   **Results:** *Most subjects were male, aged 18–27 years, and had less than a sixth-grade education. Of the 206 subjects, 152 (73.4%) received the skin test, 149 (98%) had the skin test read, and 44 (29.5%) had positive skin tests. Based on logistic regression analysis, the model that best predicted intention included cues to action, subjective norm, susceptibility, and attitude. Participation in screening was best predicted by a model containing only two variables: intention and susceptibility.*

   **Conclusions:** *In this study, logistic regression analysis revealed that a more parsimonious model than the full HBM and TRA model accurately predicted both intention and behavior. The findings may be helpful in developing tuberculosis education and screening programs for Mexican migrant farmworkers.*

Approximately 4 million migrant and seasonal farmworkers work in the United States. Among migrant farmworkers, tuberculosis (TB) is one of the chief public health concerns. Studies have documented rates of positive TB skin tests in migrant workers as high as 37% on the peninsula shared by Delaware, Maryland, and Virginia (Jacobson, Mercer, Miller, & Simpson, 1987), 41% in North Carolina (Ciesielski, Seed, Esposito, & Hunter, 1991), 44% in Florida (Centers for Disease Control [CDC], 1992) and 48% in Virginia (CDC, 1986).

Because migrant workers are at high risk for TB, it is important to ensure that they receive appropriate screening, diagnostic studies, and treatment; however, this is difficult due to their highly mobile existence. TB screening requires administration of a Purified Protein Derivative (PPD) skin test that must be read after 48–72 hours. Treatment for TB infection requires 6–9 months of uninterrupted, carefully monitored chemoprophylaxis.

A review of the literature revealed no studies that have examined participation of migrant farmworkers in TB screening and treatment programs. The purpose of this study was to analyze the relationship between psychosocial variables from a framework comprised of the Health Belief Model (HBM) and Theory of Reasoned Action (TRA) and participation of Mexican migrant farmworkers in a TB screening program.

The HBM was developed in the 1950s to explain preventive health behavior (Rosenstock, 1960, 1966, 1974). The model postulates that in order for individuals to participate in screening, they must believe that (a) they are personally susceptible to the illness (perceived susceptibility), (b) contracting the illness would have a negative impact on their life (perceived severity), (c) taking a particular action would be beneficial by reducing the threat of illness (perceived benefits), and (d) taking action would not involve overcoming barriers (perceived barriers). In addition, the presence of an internal or external stimulus (cues to action) is postulated to trigger health behavior.

The TRA was introduced in 1967 by Fishbein and further developed by Fishbein and Ajzen (1975). According to the TRA, behaviors that are under volitional control are the result of intention (Ajzen & Fishbein, 1980), which is determined by two factors: attitude toward the behavior and subjective norm. Attitude is a person's overall evaluation of performing a behavior while subjective norm is the perception of social pressures to act. A person's attitude toward a behavior is in turn determined by (a) the belief that a given outcome will occur if he or she performs the behavior, and (b) the evaluation of the outcome of performing the behavior. The subjective norm is determined by a person's beliefs about what particular salient individuals want him or her to do and the motivation to comply with these referents.

The HBM and TRA have common characteristics and are combined to form the theoretical framework for this study (see Figure A6–1). Both are based on a value-expectancy theory of behavior and posit that beliefs about behavioral consequences predict behavior. The HBM has been used extensively to study health-related behaviors, and there is a substantial body of literature to support its use. The HBM has

been criticized because it lacks a normative component, and may not be applicable in cross-cultural research. Conversely, the TRA incorporates peer group norms, a concept that adds a more culturally based perspective on behavior.

When the HBM and TRA are integrated to form a new model, several concepts can be combined to maintain parsimony. The concepts *perceived barriers* and *perceived benefits* from the HBM are equivalent to *behavioral beliefs* from the TRA. In this study the resulting concept, *behavioral beliefs,* was operationalized following the well-delineated TRA guidelines.

## RELEVANT LITERATURE

Two studies of participation in TB screening were found. Other investigations of preventive health behaviors based on the HBM and TRA are discussed in this section because they provide relevant background information.

### Health Belief Model

An early study of TB prevention behaviors by Hochbaum (1956) found that those who felt susceptible to TB were more likely than those who did not have a screening chest x-ray. However, Hochbaum's study was not a test of the full HBM. A second TB-related study, conducted by Wurtele, Roberts, and Leeper (1982), analyzed compliance of participants with a TB detection drive. The authors added behavioral intention, a TRA-like concept, as a predictor variable. Stepwise discriminant analysis revealed that intention alone accounted for about 71% of the variance in behavior.

The HBM has been applied to studies of participation in immunization programs (Aho, 1979; Cummings, Jette, Brock, & Haefner, 1979; Larson, Bergman, Heidrich, Alvin, & Schneeweiss, 1982; Larson, Olsen, Cole, & Shortell, 1979; Rundall & Wheeler, 1979), and screening for breast cancer (Aiken, West, Woodward, & Reno, 1994; Calnan, 1984; Champion, 1985; Fulton et al., 1991; Hallal, 1982), colon cancer (Macrae, Hill, St. John, Ambikapathy, & Garner, 1984), genetic disease (Becker, Kaback, Rosenstock, & Ruth, 1975), hypertension (King, 1982), and general health status (Norman, 1993, 1995). Most studies have demonstrated support for the model.

Cummings et al. (1979) studied influenza vaccination in adults and added to the HBM two TRA-like concepts: behavioral intention and social influences. Stepwise multiple regression analysis revealed that a model without the HBM variables was able to explain 40% of the variance in behavior; however, path analysis showed that most of the influence of the HBM variables on behavior was mediated through their effect on intention.

Rundall and Wheeler (1979) also applied the HBM to a study of influenza vaccination. Logit analy-

**FIGURE A6-1**    **Combined Health Belief Model and Theory of Reasoned Action. (Adapted with permission from Poss, J. E. [2000, Jan./Feb.]. Factors associated with participation by Mexican migrant farmworkers in a tuberculosis screening program. *Nursing Research, 49*[1], 20–28.)**

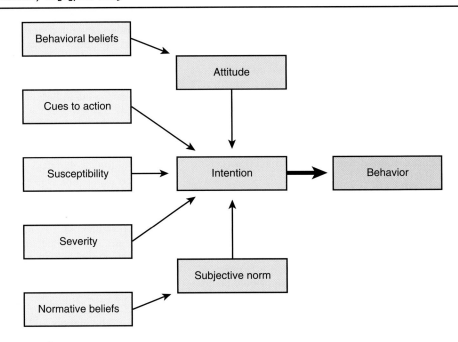

sis revealed that the model accounted for 34% of the variance in vaccination behavior. Bodenheimer, Fulton, and Kramer (1986) applied a modified version of the HBM (that included locus of control, knowledge, and intention) to healthcare workers' acceptance of hepatitis B vaccination. Stepwise multiple regression revealed that perceived benefits, susceptibility, and severity explained 20% of the variance in vaccine acceptance. Sixty-one percent of those who intended to receive the vaccination eventually did, while only 4% of those who did not intend to were ever vaccinated.

Champion (1985) used the HBM to study breast self-examination (BSE) frequency in women. Stepwise multiple regression revealed that 26% of the variance in BSE was accounted for by all the HBM variables tested together. In a study of compliance with mammography screening recommendations, Aiken et al. (1994) tested the original HBM concepts. Four of the HBM concepts plus an interaction term (susceptibility × barriers) accounted for 16% of the variance in compliance, and each of the individual concepts except severity added significantly to the predictive power of the regression equation.

Norman (1995) examined the predictors of attendance at screening examinations at general practi-

tioners' offices. Norman added two variables, intention to attend and general health value, to the HBM. Logistic regression analysis revealed that the HBM variables accounted for 56% of the variance in intention to attend, with benefits and barriers emerging as significant independent predictors.

**Theory of Reasoned Action**

The TRA has been used to study a variety of health-related behaviors including contraceptive choice (Adler, Kegeles, Irwin, & Wibbelsman, 1990; Davidson & Morrison, 1983), AIDS-preventive behaviors (Fisher, Fisher, & Rye, 1995), condom use (Boyd & Wandersman, 1991; Jemmott & Jemmott, 1991), vaccination behavior (Montano, 1986), and BSE (Lierman, Young, Kasprzyk, & Benoliel, 1990). An extensive literature review failed to uncover any TRA-based studies of TB screening behavior.

Jemmott and Jemmott (1991) applied the TRA to a study of condom use among Black female students. Multiple regression analysis revealed that 62% of the variance in intention was predicted by attitude and subjective norm. Boyd and Wandersman's (1991) study of condom use revealed that 38% of the variation in intention to use a condom was explained by the behavioral and normative beliefs concepts, while 34% was explained by the intervening variables of attitude and subjective norm. In this study, the best model for predicting behavior included all of the TRA variables plus two HRA-like concepts: susceptibility and fear of AIDS.

Morrison, Gillmore, and Baker (1995) applied the TRA and an augmented version of the TRA, the Theory of Planned Behavior, to a study of condom use. Separate multiple regressions were performed for respondents who had a steady partner and those who had casual partners, and revealed that attitude and subjective norm accounted for 44% and 25% of the variance in intention, respectively. Adler et al. (1990) used the TRA to study contraceptive use in adolescents and concluded that attitude and social norm contribute significantly to adolescent decision making about contraception. Intention, even when measured 1 year previously, was significantly related to future behavior.

Lierman et al. (1990) applied the TRA to a study of BSE practices among women. Multiple regression revealed that behavioral and normative beliefs accounted for 32% of the variance in intention and 39% of the variance in actual behavior. Montano (1986) used the TRA to study influenza vaccination and found that attitude and social norm accounted for 62% and 31% of the variance in intention and behavior, respectively.

## HBM and TRA

Several studies reviewed above incorporated components of one model into the other; for example, adding intention as a concept in HBM-based studies or including concepts such as perceived susceptibility in the TRA. Only one published study was found that synthesized the HBM and TRA to form a theoretical framework to study condom use among Thai men (VanLandingham, Suprasert, Grandjean, & Sittitrai, 1995). These researchers combined the HBM concepts severity, barriers, and benefits with the concept behavioral beliefs from the TRA. Logistic regression analysis classified 70% of the subjects into the correct condom-usage category.

The HBM, the TRA, and a model combining the two have been used successfully to study participation in screening programs as well as health behaviors and beliefs. The TRA includes a normative component and incorporates a methodology aimed at eliciting the basic concerns and beliefs of a group under investigation, making it useful for studying culturally diverse populations.

## Hypotheses

The study had two dependent variables (a) *intention* to participate in the TB screening program, and (b) *behavior* (participation in the program). When be-

havior was the dependent variable, intention was treated as one of the independent variables in the model. The following hypotheses were examined:

I.   There is a positive relationship between the following variables (susceptibility, severity, cues to action, attitude, and subjective norm) and intention to participate in a TB screening program.
II.  There is a positive relationship between behavioral beliefs and attitude.
III. There is a positive relationship between normative beliefs and subjective norm.
IV.  There is a positive relationship between intention to participate and behavior.
V.   There is a positive relationship between the following variables (susceptibility, severity, cues to action, attitude, and subjective norm) and behavior.

## Definition of Terms

The following definitions were applied in this study: *Mexican migrant farmworkers* were defined as individuals 18 years of age or older who establish a temporary abode to work in agriculture on a seasonal basis and who either were born in Mexico or who had one parent born in Mexico; *Susceptibility, Severity, Attitude, Subjective norm, Behavioral beliefs, Normative beliefs,* and *Intention* were scores obtained on the corresponding subscales of the TB Interview Instrument (TII); *Cues to Action* referred to attendance at the TB education program; and *Behavior* was participation in the TB screening program.

## METHOD

### Sample

A convenience sample of 206 Mexican migrant farmworkers was chosen from 20 migrant camps in Orleans and Monroe Counties. Subjects were excluded from the study if they had a history of a positive PPD skin test or active TB. Participation in the study was voluntary, and all explanations about the study, including the informed consent, were presented verbally in Spanish by the bilingual principal investigator. Subjects gave verbal consent to be interviewed, and the study was approved by the Human Subjects Review Committee of the State University of New York at Buffalo School of Nursing and the board of directors of the Oak Orchard Community Health Center (OOCHC). Participants were given a baseball cap at the conclusion of their interview.

### Procedure

The study was carried out in conjunction with an established TB education and screening program conducted by the OOCHC in northwestern New York state. All phases of the program took place in the migrant camps with the exception of chest radiographs which were performed at a local hospital. The optional education program was presented in Spanish on Monday evenings by bilingual, bicultural health promoters using popular education methods such as skits, demonstrations, and audience participation. Health promoters were Mexican migrant workers who have attended a series of classes and received on-the-job training about culturally appropriate, low-literacy educational techniques and health-related topics such as TB education, detection, and treatment.

Farmworkers were tested on Tuesday evenings with an intradermal injection of 0.1 ml of 5 tuberculin units (TU) of purified protein derivative (PPD) and the tests were read on Thursday evenings. Those with positive skin tests were transported to local hospitals for chest radiographs. The principal investigator, working with the OOCHC program, recruited subjects in the migrant camps and interviewed them in Spanish either on Monday, after the educational program, or on Tuesday. Subjects were then tracked to determine if they had a skin test on Tuesday and a skin test reading on Thursday. Participants who did not want to receive a skin test were interviewed only. The study was conducted between May and September, 1997.

### Interview Instrument

The 66-item Spanish-language TII was developed specifically for the present study. Development of the TII was guided by a qualitative study of migrant farmworkers' explanatory models about TB (Poss, 1998). Categories that emerged from the qualitative analysis were used to develop the closed-ended questions for the TII, according to the guidelines of Ajzen and Fishbein (1980).

The TII was developed in English and written at Flesch-Kincaid Grade Level of 4.6. It was translated into equivalent Spanish by a Mexican American bilingual outreach worker and then back-translated into English by a second bilingual Mexican American. The results were compared with the original English version, and necessary modifications were made. These procedures for establishing equivalency of instruments follow guidelines of Brislin, Lonner, and Thorndike (1973) and Marín and Marín (1991).

The TII consists of nine sections: demographic information and eight Likert-type subscales to measure the independent variables. The instrument was reviewed for content validity by Champion—an expert in instrumentation using the Health Belief Model. The TII was pilot tested on a sample of 20 migrant farmworkers, after which instrument subscales were tested for internal consistency reliability using Cronbach's alpha and revised. Final coefficient alphas for the subscales ranged from 0.71 to 0.96 based on responses of 206 subjects in the major study.

Items in the subscales were measured on a five-point Likert-type scale. The response format, formulated for populations with low literacy levels, was coded as follows: 'Definitely Yes' = +5, 'Probably Yes' = +4, 'No opinion' = +3, 'Probably No' = +2, and 'Definitely No' = +1. Negatively worded items were reverse scored. Items on the Behavioral Beliefs and Normative Beliefs Subscales were coded to allow calculation of a multiplicative score as proposed by Ajzen and Fishbein (1980, p. 66). For these subscales, items related to strength of belief were scored on the unipolar scale described above. Each belief question was followed by an evaluation question. The evaluation of each outcome was scored on a bipolar scale with anchors of +2 and −2. Each respondent's score on the strength of belief question was multiplied by the score on the evaluation question. The results for the entire subscale were then added to form a sum-of-products score (Lauver & Knapp, 1993).

### Data Analysis

The characteristics of the sample, including demographic and social data, were summarized using descriptive statistics. Pearson product moment correlation was used to study the relationships between the variables in the combined model. Logistic regression was applied to find the model that best predicted each dependent variable.

### RESULTS

The sample consisted of 206 migrant farmworkers—164 (79.6%) males—ranging in age from 18–67 years, with a mean age of 29 years ($SD$ = 10.7 years). Approximately 60% of the study participants were between the ages of 18 and 27 years. Fifty percent (103) of the participants were married, 39.3% (81) were single, 4.4% (9) reported living with a partner, and 6.3% (13) were divorced or separated. About one-third of the respondents had less than a 4th grade education and another third had attended school for 4–6 years. Fifty-two farmworkers (25.2%) had a 7th–9th grade education, and 28 (13.6%) had a 10th–12th grade education.

Study subjects had worked as migrant farmworkers 1–40 years ($M$ = 7 years, $SD$ = 7.73). The majority of subjects (80.1%) had worked between 1–10 years in agriculture. About one-third of workers (33.5%) reported that they lived in Mexico during the winter, while 56 (27.2%) resided in Texas, 45 (21.8%) lived in Florida, and 36 (17.5%) lived in New York state. PPD skin testing was performed on 152 (73.4%) subjects, 149 (98%) had their skin test read, and, of those, 44 (29.5%) had positive results.

### Testing of Hypotheses

Descriptive statistics for each of the TII subscales are shown in Table A6–1. Pearson correlation coefficients

## TABLE A6-1 Mean, Standard Deviation (SD), and Range for TII Subscales (*N* = 206)

| Subscale | Mean | SD | Range |
|---|---|---|---|
| Behavioral beliefs | 38.23 | 18.43 | −44–98 |
| Susceptibility | 16.72 | 6.01 | 5–25 |
| Severity | 33.15 | 6.42 | 12–40 |
| Normative beliefs | 17.01 | 12.14 | −14–30 |
| Subjective norm | 8.26 | 2.12 | 2–10 |
| General attitude | 17.55 | 2.75 | 5–20 |

between the model variables revealed significant correlations between intention to have the PPD skin test and all of the TII subscales (Table A6–2). There also were significant correlations between the predictor variables and intention to have the skin test read (Table A6–3). Hypothesis I was supported based on the significant correlations between the model variables and intention to participate in screening. Intention was most strongly related to subjective norm, but all variables had low to moderate correlations (Munro, Visintainer, & Page, 1986) with both intention to have the skin test and to have it read.

## TABLE A6-2 Correlations Among Predictor Variables, Intention to Have PPD, and PPD Given (*N* = 206)

| | Intention to Have PPD | PPD Given | Behavioral Beliefs | Education | Susceptibility | Severity | Normative Beliefs | General Attitude |
|---|---|---|---|---|---|---|---|---|
| Intention to have PPD | | | | | | | | |
| PPD given | .84** | | | | | | | |
| Behavioral beliefs | .36** | .38** | | | | | | |
| Education | .53** | .40** | .20* | | | | | |
| Susceptibility | .50** | .54** | .24** | .34** | | | | |
| Severity | .44** | .46** | .41** | .31** | .53** | | | |
| Normative beliefs | .55** | .48** | .42** | .30** | .36** | .41** | | |
| General attitude | .50** | .47** | .64** | .25** | .31** | .46** | .49** | |
| Subjective norm | .65** | .58** | .44** | .35** | .38** | .38** | .60** | .55** |

*p = 0.05 (2-tailed).
**p = 0.01 (2-tailed).

**TABLE A6-3** Correlations Among Predictor Variables, Intention to Have PPD Read, and Having PPD Read (*N* = 206)

| | Intention to Read PPD | PPD Read | Behavioral Beliefs | Education | Susceptibility | Severity | Normative Beliefs | General Attitude |
|---|---|---|---|---|---|---|---|---|
| Intention to read PPD | | | | | | | | |
| PPD read | .80** | | | | | | | |
| Behavioral beliefs | .36** | .36** | | | | | | |
| Education | .54** | .38** | .20* | | | | | |
| Susceptibility | .49** | .49** | .24** | .34** | | | | |
| Severity | .43** | .37** | .41** | .31** | .53** | | | |
| Normative beliefs | .55** | .51** | .42** | .30** | .36** | .41** | | |
| General attitude | .50** | .45** | .64** | .25** | .31** | .46** | .49** | |
| Subjective norm | .64** | .55** | .44** | .35** | .38** | .38** | .60** | .55** |

*$p$ = .05 (2-tailed).
**$p$ = .01 (2-tailed).

The developers of the TRA proposed that behavioral beliefs would be positively related to general attitude. In this study, a moderately strong, positive correlation was found between behavioral beliefs and general attitude ($r$ = 0.64, $p$ < 0.01), with the $r^2$ indicating that behavioral beliefs accounted for about 41% of the variance in general attitude, thus supporting Hypothesis II.

The correlation coefficient between normative beliefs and generalized subjective norm about screening showed a moderate, positive relationship ($r$ = 0.60, $p$ < 0.01) indicating that subjects who felt that specific others, including coworkers, friends, and family wanted them to have the skin test were more likely to believe that generalized others also believed they should be tested. Thus, about 36% of the variance in subjective norm was accounted for by specific normative beliefs. Therefore, Hypothesis III was supported.

Intention to participate in the screening showed a strong positive correlation with actual participation in the screening program. Specifically, intention to have the skin test was positively correlated with hav-

ing the test ($r$ = 0.84, $p$ < 0.01) and intention to have the test read was positively correlated with having it read ($r$ = 0.80, $p$ < 0.01), accounting for 70% and 64%, respectively, of the variance in actual behavior. These results provided support for Hypothesis IV.

There were positive, significant relationships between all the antecedent variables and actual participation in the screening program (see Tables A6–2 and A6–3). Therefore, the results of the Pearson correlations provided support for the association between the variables from the combined HBM and TRA model and participation in the screening program as posited in Hypothesis V.

### Testing the Model

The default setting in the SPSS Logistic Regression procedure was used to enter all the predictor variables simultaneously into the equation. The dependent variables in this study included (a) intention to have the skin test, (b) intention to have the skin test read, (c) having the skin test, and (d) having the skin test read. A separate logistic regression analysis was run for each variable, and the resulting models for each dependent variable were compared to determine which was best in terms of parsimony and interpretability.

First, intention to have the skin test was regressed on all of the predictor variables. The model chi-square (the difference between the $-2LL$ for the two models) was 135.44 ($df = 7, p < 0.00001$) indicating a statistically significant improvement in prediction using the model with all of the variables over using only the constant. Next, three variables (behavioral beliefs, severity, and normative beliefs) that showed nonsignificant Wald statistics were omitted from the logistic regression analysis and a new model was generated (see Table A6–4). The difference between the $-2LL$ for these two models was 4.37 ($df = 4$, not significant).

The goal of model testing in logistic regression analysis is to find a model that is *not* statistically different from the full model (Tabachnick & Fidell, 1996). Therefore, because there was no statistically significant difference between these two models, the reduced model was selected. Further reductions in this model did not improve its predictive ability.

The statistic labeled Exp (B) in Table A6–4 is the odds ratio. For education, the odds ratio was 9.93, indicating that subjects who attended the education program were about 10 times more likely to intend to be skin tested than those who did not attend. However, based on the model used in this study it is not possible to posit a causal relationship between attending the education program and participation. Overall, this four-variable model resulted in the classification of 89.8% of cases into the correct category. Of these cases, 94.9% of those who intended and 74.0% of those who did not intend to have the test were classified correctly.

Next, intention to have the skin test read was regressed on all of the predictor variables. The results

of this analysis were identical to the first regression analysis because the two variables (intention to have the test and intention to have it read) were highly intercorrelated ($r = 0.99, p < 0.01$).

Having the skin test was then regressed on all of the predictor variables. As was done previously, the variables that showed nonsignificant Wald statistics were omitted from the logistic regression and a new, two-variable model was generated (see Table A6–5). The difference between the model chi-square for these two models was 7.86 ($df = 6$), indicating no statistically significant difference between the full and reduced model.

The odds ratio for intention was 4.47, indicating that subjects who intended to have the skin test were four times more likely than nonintenders to actually be tested. Overall, this two-variable model resulted in the classification of 93.7% of cases into the correct category. Of these cases, 97.4% of those who had the skin test and 83.3% of those who did not were classified correctly.

Finally, actually having the skin test read was regressed on all of the predictor variables following the procedures outlined above (see Table A6–6). Overall, this two-variable model resulted in the classification of 92.7% of cases into the correct category. Of these cases, 97.3% of those who had the skin test and 80.7% of those who did not were classified correctly.

## DISCUSSION

The majority of migrant farmworkers in this study participated in screening. Seventy-five percent of the subjects received a skin test and 98% returned to have the test read. Of the participants whose skin test was read, 29.5% tested positive. These results are similar to the 1994–1995 OOCHC screening program in which 99% of workers had their skin test read, and 25% had a positive test (Poss & Rangel, 1997). This high rate of participation suggests that, given the

**TABLE A6–4** Logistic Regression Analysis: Four-Variable Model Dependent Variable = Intention to Have PPD ($N = 206$)

| Variable | B | SE | Wald | df | Sig | R | Exp(B) |
|---|---|---|---|---|---|---|---|
| Education | 2.295 | 0.550 | 17.446 | 1 | 0.0000 | 0.260 | 9.927 |
| Subjective norm | 0.532 | 0.136 | 15.194 | 1 | 0.0001 | 0.240 | 1.702 |
| Susceptibility | 0.148 | 0.050 | 8.720 | 1 | 0.0031 | 0.172 | 1.160 |
| General attitude | 0.274 | 0.109 | 6.308 | 1 | 0.0120 | 0.137 | 1.315 |
| Constant | −11.160 | 2.053 | 29.550 | 1 | 0.0000 | | |

TABLE **A6-5** Logistic Regression Analysis: Two-Variable Model Dependent Variable = Having PPD (*N* = 206)

| Variable | B | SE | Wald | df | Sig | R | Exp(B) |
|---|---|---|---|---|---|---|---|
| Susceptibility | 0.202 | 0.062 | 10.661 | 1 | 0.0011 | 0.191 | 1.224 |
| Intention | 1.500 | 0.213 | 49.310 | 1 | 0.0000 | 0.448 | 4.468 |
| Constant | −7.424 | 1.312 | 32.087 | 1 | 0.0000 | | |

opportunity to be tested in a culturally appropriate and geographically accessible program presented in Spanish by bilingual, bicultural health promoters, migrant farmworkers will participate in screening. Farmer (1997) has argued that structural barriers, inadequate access to care, racism, and environmental factors, not individual patient's beliefs, play a primary role in the TB epidemic that disproportionately affects the world's poor.

The results of this study cannot be generalized to settings where migrant farmworkers must travel to obtain healthcare services. In this study, all phases of the program were offered in the migrant camps, thus obviating the need to travel to distant sites or to use healthcare facilities staffed by providers with different cultural and linguistic backgrounds.

All of the research hypotheses were supported in this study. There were significant correlations in the predicted direction between the model variables and both intention and actual participation (Hypotheses I and V). In addition, relationships between the intermediate variables in the HBM and TRA model were in the predicted direction (Hypotheses II, III, and IV).

The correlation between behavioral beliefs and general attitude ($r = .64$) was somewhat stronger than that observed by other researchers. Morrison et al. (1995) found correlations between behavioral be-liefs and general attitude toward condom use of 0.37 ($p < 0.01$) and 0.48 ($p < 0.001$) for heterosexual adults with steady and casual partners, respectively. In Montano's (1986) study of vaccination behavior, the correlation between behavioral beliefs and attitude was 0.57 ($p < 0.01$).

The relationship between normative beliefs and subjective norm ($r = 0.60$) was slightly weaker than in other studies using the TRA. Morrison et al. (1995) found correlations between normative beliefs and subjective norm of 0.75 ($p < 0.001$) and 0.67 ($p < 0.001$) for adults with steady and casual partners, respectively. The correlation between these variables was 0.73 ($p$ value not reported) in the 1990 study by Marín, Perez-Stable, Otero-Sabogal, & Sabogal of Hispanic smokers and 0.8 ($p < 0.01$) in Lierman et al.'s (1990) study of BSE.

Based on the values of Hispanic culture, it was anticipated that subjective norm would contribute to the explanation of intention and behavior. One of the basic cultural values attributed to Hispanics is collectivism, evidenced by high levels of personal interdependence, conformity, and readiness to be influenced by others (Marín & Marín, 1991). In their research on smoking cessation, Marín et al. (1990) found that family-related reasons for quitting smoking were more important for Hispanic than for non-Hispanic White smokers.

TABLE **A6-6** Logistic Regression Analysis: Two-Variable Model Dependent Variable = Having PPD Read (*N* = 206)

| Variable | B | SE | Wald | df | Sig | R | Exp(B) |
|---|---|---|---|---|---|---|---|
| Susceptibility | 0.122 | 0.049 | 6.245 | 1 | 0.0125 | 0.132 | 1.130 |
| Intention | 1.337 | 0.188 | 50.501 | 1 | 0.0000 | 0.447 | 3.806 |
| Constant | −5.906 | 1.009 | 34.245 | 1 | 0.0000 | | |

Wurtele et al. (1982) found that intention to have a PPD skin test read accounted for about 71% of the variance in actual behavior. In their study, intention was measured only 48 hours before the behavior; this may account for the strong relationship. The timing was similar to the present study where intention was measured within 24 hours of having a skin test and 72 hours of having it read, and the correlations between intention and behavior were .84 and .80, respectively. Lierman et al. (1990) concluded that intention was strongly correlated with performing BSE ($r = 0.75$, $p < 0.01$), while Montano and Taplin (1991) found a moderate correlation between intention to have a mammogram and behavior ($r = 0.50$, $p < 0.01$) and Montano (1986) found a somewhat higher correlation between intention to be vaccinated and behavior ($r = 0.69$, $p < 0.01$).

In this study, logistic regression analysis revealed that a more parsimonious model than the full HBM and TRA model predicted both intention and behavior. Essentially, intention to take part in screening was best explained by four variables: subjective norm, general attitude, perceived susceptibility, and attending the education program. The model for actual participation included only two variables: intention and perceived susceptibility.

The findings of this study suggest several lines of future inquiry. The research instrument developed for this study, the TII, could be tested with migrant farmworkers in other settings or modified to study migrant workers' behaviors related to screening for diseases other than TB. The combined HBM and TRA model could be applied to study postscreening behaviors, including having a chest radiograph and, when indicated, initiating and following through with isoniazid (INH) prophylaxis. This application would test whether the model is able to explain behaviors that occur weeks to months after the initial interviews. This study should be considered an initial application of the combined model to a research problem. However, nurses who offer educational programs to migrant farmworkers may wish to incorporate some of the study results in designing such programs.

## References

Adler, N. E., Kegeles, S. M., Irwin, C. E., & Wibbelsman, C. (1990). Adolescent contraceptive behavior: An assessment of decision processes. *Journal of Pediatrics, 116,* 463–471.

Aho, W. R. (1979). Participation of senior citizens in the swine flu inoculation program: An analysis of Health Belief Model variables in preventive health behavior. *Journal of Gerontology, 34,* 201–208.

Aiken, L. S., West, S. G., Woodward, C. K., & Reno, R. R. (1994). Health beliefs and compliance with mammography-screening recommendations in asymptomatic women. *Health Psychology, 13,* 122–129.

Ajzen, I., & Fishbein, M. (1980). *Understanding attitudes and predicting social behavior.* Englewood Cliffs, NJ: Prentice-Hall.

Becker, M. H., Kaback, M. M., Rosenstock, I. M., & Ruth, M. V. (1975). Some influences on public participation in a genetic screening program. *Journal of Community Health, 1,* 3–14.

Bodenheimer, H. C., Fulton, J. P., & Kramer, P. D. (1986). Acceptance of hepatitis B vaccine among hospital workers. *American Journal of Public Health, 76,* 252–255.

Boyd, B., & Wandersman, A. (1991). Predicting undergraduate condom use with the Fishbein and Ajzen and the Triandis attitude-behavior models: Implications for public health interventions. *Journal of Applied Social Psychology, 21,* 1810–1830.

Brislin, R. W., Lonner, W. J., & Thorndike, R. M. (1973). *Cross-cultural research methods.* New York: Wiley.

Calnan, M. (1984). The Health Belief Model and participation in programmes for the early detection of breast cancer: A comparative analysis. *Social Science and Medicine, 19,* 823–830.

Centers for Disease Control. (1986). Tuberculosis among migrant farm workers—Virginia. *MMWR: Morbidity and Mortality Weekly Report, 35,* 467–469.

Centers for Disease Control. (1992). HIV infection, syphilis, and tuberculosis screening among migrant farm workers—Florida, 1992. *MMWR: Morbidity and Mortality Weekly Report, 41,* 723–725.

Champion, V. L. (1985). Use of the Health Belief Model in determining frequency of breast self-examination. *Research in Nursing & Health, 8,* 373–379.

Ciesielski, S. D., Seed, J. R., Esposito, D. H., & Hunter, N. (1991). The epidemiology of tuberculosis among North Carolina migrant farm workers. *JAMA, 265,* 1715–1719.

Cummings, K. M., Jette, A. M., Brock, B. M., & Haefner, D. P. (1979). Psychosocial determinants of immunization behavior in a swine influenza campaign. *Medical Care, 17,* 639–649.

Davidson, A. R., & Morrison, D. M. (1983). Predicting contraceptive behavior from attitudes: A comparison of within- versus across-subjects procedures. *Journal of Personality and Social Psychology, 45,* 997–1009.

Farmer, P. (1997). Social scientists and the new tuberculosis. *Social Science & Medicine, 44,* 347–358.

Fishbein, M. (1967). A behavior theory approach to the relation between beliefs about an object and the attitude toward the object. In M. Fishbein (Ed.), *Readings in attitude theory and measurement* (pp. 389–400). New York: Wiley.

Fishbein, M., & Ajzen, I. (1975). *Belief, attitude, intention and behavior: An introduction to theory and research.* Reading, MA: Addison-Wesley.

Fisher, W. A., Fisher, J. D., & Rye, B. J. (1995). Understanding and promoting AIDS-preventive behavior: Insights from the Theory of Reasoned Action. *Health Psychology, 14,* 255–264.

Fulton, J. P., Buechner, J. S., Scott, H. D., DeBuono, B. A., Feldman, J. P., Smith, R. A., & Kovenock, D. (1991). A study guided by the Health Belief Model of the predictors of breast cancer screening of women ages 40 and older. *Public Health Reports Washington, 106,* 410–420.

Hallal, J. C. (1982). The relationship of health beliefs, health locus of control, and self-concept to the practice of breast self-examination in adult women. *Nursing Research, 31,* 137–142.

Hochbaum, G. M. (1956). Why people seek diagnostic x-rays. *Public Health Reports, 71,* 377–380.

Jacobson, M. L., Mercer, M. A., Miller, L. K., & Simpson, T. W. (1987). Tuberculosis risk among migrant farm workers on the Delmarva Peninsula. *American Journal of Public Health, 77,* 29–32.

Jemmott, L. S., & Jemmott, J. B. III (1991). Applying the Theory of Reasoned Action to AIDS risk behavior: Condom use among Black women. *Nursing Research, 40,* 228–234.

King, J. B. (1982). The impact of patients' perception of high blood pressure on attendance at screening. *Social Science and Medicine, 16,* 1079–1091.

Larson, E. B., Bergman, J., Heidrich, F., Alvin, B. L., & Schneeweiss, R. (1982). Do postcard reminders improve influenza vaccination compliance? A prospective trial of different postcard 'cues.' *Medical Care, 20,* 639–648.

Larson, E. B., Olsen, E., Cole, W., & Shortell, S. (1979). The relationship of health beliefs and a postcard reminder to influenza vaccination. *Journal of Family Practice, 8,* 1207–1211.

Lauver, D., & Knapp, T. R. (1993). Sum-of-products variables: A methodological critique. *Research in Nursing & Health, 16,* 385–391.

Lierman, L. M., Young, H. M., Kasprzyk, D., & Benoliel, J. Q. (1990). Predicting breast self-examination using the Theory of Reasoned Action. *Nursing Research, 39,* 97–101.

Macrae, F. A., Hill, D. J., St. John, D. J., Ambikapathy, A., & Garner, J. F. (1984). Predicting colon cancer screening behavior from health beliefs. *Preventive Medicine, 13,* 115–126.

Marín, B. V., Marín, G., Perez-Stable, E. J., Otero-Sabogal, R., & Sabogal, F. (1990). Cultural differences in attitudes toward smoking: Developing messages using the Theory of Reasoned Action. *Journal of Applied Social Psychology, 20,* 478–493.

Marín, G., & Marín, B. V. (1991). *Research with Hispanic populations.* Newbury Park, CA: Sage.

Montano, D. E. (1986). Predicting and understanding influenza vaccination behavior: Alternatives to the Health Belief Model. *Medical Care, 24,* 438–453.

Montano, D. E., & Taplin, S. H. (1991). A test of an expanded Theory of Reasoned Action to predict mammography participation. *Social Science & Medicine, 32,* 733–741.

Morrison, D. M., Gillmore, M. R., & Baker, S. A. (1995). Determinants of condom use among high-risk heterosexual adults: A test of the Theory of Reasoned Action. *Journal of Applied Social Psychology, 25,* 651–676.

Munro, B. H., Visintainer, M. A., & Page, E. B. (1986). *Statistical methods for health care research.* Philadelphia: J. B. Lippincott Company.

Norman, P. (1993). Predicting the uptake of health checks in general practice: Invitation methods and patients' health beliefs. *Social Science and Medicine, 37,* 53–59.

Norman, P. (1995). Applying the Health Belief Model to the prediction of attendance at health checks in general practice. *British Journal of Clinical Psychology, 34,* 461–470.

Poss, J. E., & Rangel, R. (1997). A tuberculosis screening and treatment program for migrant farmworker families. *Journal of Health Care for the Poor and Underserved, 8,* 133–140.

Poss, J. E. (1998). The meanings of tuberculosis for Mexican migrant farmworkers in the United States. *Social Science & Medicine, 47,* 195–202.

Rosenstock, I. M. (1960). What research in motivation suggests for public health. *American Journal of Public Health, 50,* 295–301.

Rosenstock, I. M. (1966). Why people use health services. *Milbank Memorial Fund Quarterly, 44*(3, Supp.), 94–127.

Rosenstock, I. M. (1974). Historical origins of the Health Belief Model. *Health Education Monographs, 2,* 328–335.

Rundall, T. G., & Wheeler, J. R. (1979). Factors associated with utilization of the swine flu vaccination program among senior citizens in Tompkins County. *Medical Care, 17,* 191–200.

Tabachnick, B. G., & Fidell, L. S. (1996). *Using multivariate statistics* (3rd ed.). New York: HarperCollins College Publishers.

VanLandingham, M. J., Suprasert, S., Grandjean, N., & Sittitrai, W. (1995). Two views of risky sexual practices among northern Thai males: The Health Belief Model and the Theory of Reasoned Action. *Journal of Health and Social Behavior, 36,* 195–212.

Wurtele, S. K., Roberts, M. C., & Leeper, J. D. (1982). Health beliefs and intentions: Predictors of return compliance in a tuberculosis detection drive. *Journal of Applied Social Psychology, 12,* 128–136.

# Trajectory of Certain Death at an Unknown Time: Children With Neurodegenerative Life-Threatening Illnesses

Rose G. Steel

*Children with neurodegenerative life-threatening illnesses (NLTIs) account for a significant proportion of children requiring palliative care. Most of their care is provided at home by their families over many years, yet there is a paucity of research examining families' experiences when a child with an NLTI is dying at home. In this grounded theory study, data were collected from 8 families through observations and audiotaped interviews. Families moved through a process of navigating uncharted territory as they lived with their dying child. The illness trajectory of certain death at an unknown time was not a steady decline. Instead, families lived much of their lives on plateaus of relative stability where they often felt alone and isolated from health-care professionals. Inevitably, periods of instability originated in subsequent precipitating events in the process that led to families dropping off the plateau on the way to the child's inevitable death. Implications for research and practice are discussed.*

The numbers of children with a prolonged terminal illness are low when compared with adults. At any one time, there are over 200 children in the province of British Columbia living with progressive life-threatening illnesses (PLTIs) (Davies, 1992). One estimate from the United Kingdom is that 1:1000 children may be affected by PLTIs (Goldman, 1996). Although the numbers are relatively small, these children pose substantial management problems (Caring Institute of the Foundation for Hospice and Home Care, 1987). Additionally, the numbers are projected to increase as the incidence of life-threatening diseases rises and as advances in technology and medicine reduce mortality rates (Broome, 1998; Davies & Howell, 1998). Care for these children is typically provided at home by their families over an extended period of time, often years (Burne, Dominica, & Baum, 1984; Goldman, 1998; Stevens, 1998), yet there is little available research to guide professionals in assisting such families.

Children in pediatric palliative care suffer from a wide variety of diseases and syndromes. About 20% of these children have cancer. Many have progressive neuromuscular or neurodegenerative conditions (NLTIs) that will eventually cause their death (Ashby, Kosky, Laver, & Sims, 1991; Davies & Howell, 1998; Goldman, 1996). There is a lack of knowledge about the experiences of their families. Health professionals have barely begun to document the effects on families of caring for a child with an NLTI, and little is known about the most appropriate interventions.

## LITERATURE REVIEW

Some researchers (Davies, 1996; Martinson, 1993; Parker, 1996; Stein, Forrest, Woolley, & Baum, 1989; Stein & Woolley, 1990) have begun to investigate the impact on families of caring for a child with a PLTI at home. However, research in pediatric palliative care has been minimal. Only two studies were found that focused specifically on families and children with neurodegenerative disorders (Davies, 1996; Parker, 1996), and there is no published pediatric research documenting the illness trajectory of certain death at an unknown time—that is, a death that is inevitable but the timing of which cannot be predicted by anyone, including health-care professionals. The majority of available research has been published only within the past few years. It tentatively suggests, however, that a child's illness has a profound impact on every dimension of family life. The impact falls into five broad categories: emotional, physical, financial, and spiritual disruptions, and changes in family structure and patterns of interaction.

The emotional impact on families or caring for a child with a PLTI, including cancer, cystic fibrosis, HIV/AIDS, and NLTIs, is beginning to be documented (Bluebond-Langner, 1996; Clarke-Steffen, 1997; Davies, 1996; Gravelle, 1997; Parker, 1996; Stein et al., 1989; Stein & Woolley, 1990; Wiener, Theut, Steinberg, Riekert, & Pizzo, 1994). Most parents are anxious and worried (Parker, 1996; Stein et al.; Whyte, 1992). Many are depressed (Wiener et al., 1994) or experience varying levels of anxiety, insomnia, and social dysfunction as they struggle to balance the demands of their ill child with the management of everyday living (Stein & Woolley, 1990). Because some NLTIs are genetic, parents may feel responsible for causing the child's illness (Davies, 1996; Hunt & Burne, 1995; Parker, 1996).

A few authors have noted that parents of children with PLTIs are exhausted (Gravelle, 1997; Martinson, 1993; Stein & Woolley, 1990). In addition, exhaustion has been observed in mothers of chronically ill children (Stewart, Ritchie, McGrath, Thompson, & Bruce, 1994) and has been recognized as having a significant impact on their lives (Gravelle, 1997), although this effect has not been well described. Only one study provides some insight into the possible physical impacts of caring for a child with an NLTI (Leonard, Johnson, & Brust, 1993), reporting declining health in mothers of children with disabilities.

Families face many financial costs that are invisible to others yet drain family resources. High cumulative monetary costs are related to buying medications, special diets, and equipment, or frequent attendance at health-care facilities with the associated costs of travel, food, and telephone calls (Birenbaum & Clarke-Steffen, 1992; Stein et al., 1989; Stein & Woolley, 1990). There are also indirect costs, such as reductions in a mother's work hours resulting in decreased family income just as financial costs are increasing (Parker, 1996).

There is some evidence that parents seek spiritual guidance and support (Davies, 1996). Spirituality and faith provide both emotional and network support for many parents. Faith has been shown to be a key factor in a family's ability to keep an ill child at home (Davies, 1996).

A child's life-threatening illness may disrupt family patterns of interaction, require family reorganization, and impose shared adaptational changes. Management of the child's illness may necessitate changes in family roles (Clarke-Steffen, 1997; Gravelle, 1997; Stein, et al., 1989; Stein & Woolley, 1990). In addition, routines imposed by the child's needs may cause disruptions in the daily routines of family life (Parker, 1996; Stein & Woolley, 1990). Little is known about how family structure and interactions change over time. It is not unrealistic to expect that families will undergo many changes when a child has a terminal illness. However, little is known about when and how these changes occur, and the literature offers little guidance for professionals in providing care to such families.

## PURPOSE

This paper presents selected findings from a dissertation study (Steele, 1999). The purpose of the study was to enhance understanding among health-care professionals of the experiences of families with a child who has an NLTI. The specific aims were: (1) to describe families' perceptions and experiences of living with a child who has an NLTI, and how those experiences change over time; (2) to describe the impact on the family of living with a child who has an NLTI; and (3) to describe families' perceptions of the factors that influence their ability to care for their child with an NLTI. The purposes of the paper are to provide a brief overview of the grounded theory that emerged from the study and to describe the illness trajectory when families face a child's certain death at an unknown time.

## METHOD

### Procedure

Data were collected through a pediatric hospice-care program and a children's hospital after ethical approval had been obtained from each facility and from the researcher's university. Families were excluded if the child had been diagnosed within the previous month, because it was anticipated that they would lack the depth of experience required to act as key informants. Families were also excluded if the child was expected to die in less than 1 month, because of the potential stress of this period and because it was anticipated that they would have unique needs and experiences. This decision was made after careful deliberation with colleagues in pediatric palliative care and on the strong recommendation of four parents whose children had died. Further eligibility criteria were: that the ill child be no more than 17 years of age and be diagnosed with an NLTI; that at least one adult who lived with the child and provided care agree to participate; that participating adult family members understand English well enough to give informed consent and to be interviewed; that participating siblings be able to communicate in English; that in addition to parental consent, minor children aged 7 and older give their assent; and that the family be emotionally and physically capable of participating in the study. Families who were considered at risk were not approached.

Hospice and hospital staff made initial contact with families to explain that a study was in progress and that agreeing to talk with the researcher did not commit them to participating in the study. The researcher was clearly differentiated from the care provider, and verbal consent was obtained to allow the nurse to forward the family member's name and telephone number to the researcher. The researcher then contacted parents by telephone, described the study to them, invited them to participate, and followed up by obtaining written consent in the family's home.

## Participants

A total of eight families comprising 29 family members participated in the study. A total of 10 sick children (six boys, four girls) were observed, as two families had two children with an NLTI. The children's ages ranged from 3 to 13 years. At the time of the study, the children had been diagnosed for 2.5 to 6 years. While all of the children had an NLTI, the actual diagnoses will not be named to ensure anonymity. Most of these individual illnesses affect very few children throughout the world. Indeed, some of the study children represented the only known case of the particular illness in their geographic area. Identifying the diagnoses would effectively identify the children and their families. While the different illnesses are manifested in many ways, common attributes such as changes in verbal ability, changes in motor skills, and a proliferation of feeding disorders meant that these families experienced many of the same opportunities and challenges during the course of the illness.

There were siblings in only three of the families. Because the NLTIs are often genetic, most of the parents chose to have no more children once they learned of their child's diagnosis. Thus the small number of siblings was a result of a significant parental decision rather than serendipity. Out of four siblings, three—all female—had been born before the child was diagnosed. The other sibling was male. The siblings ranged in age from 2 to 9 years.

In the majority of families the parents were married and lived together, although there were difficulties in most of the marriages. The length of the marriages ranged from 8 to 15 years. The parents ranged in age from 28 to 48 years. Most had completed high school, although educational levels varied from Grade 6 to university degree. Occupations included both professional and non-professional. Some of the parents were currently unemployed, often because they were caring for the ill child.

Socio-economic diversity was apparent, with annual family incomes ranging from $11,000 to $112,000. Four families subsisted on incomes of less than $15,000 per year, while the others earned $50,000 or more. However, all families reported a substantial drop in actual or anticipated income due to the child's illness. All but one family identified with the dominant Caucasian Canadian culture; the other family came from an East Indian background.

## Data Collection and Analysis

The primary analytical method used was grounded theory (Glaser & Strauss, 1967; Strauss & Corbin, 1990), a qualitative research method in which theoretical explanations of participants' subjective experiences and situational meanings are generated. Because of its focus on social processes, grounded theory is particularly suited to family research. The main method of data collection was in-depth interviews with families supplemented by participant observations in the home. First each family member was interviewed individually; then the family was interviewed as a group. None of the ill children were interviewed because of their limited ability to communicate. Interviews were audiotaped and transcribed verbatim by the researcher. Data collection ceased when theoretical saturation was reached. Initial data collection occurred over a period of 1 year. During the following year, the evolving analysis was shared with the families. After the first interview and observations were completed with all eight families, each family was sent the preliminary analysis by mail. Second interviews took place by telephone, except for one in-home interview. Two families requested major iterations of the evolving theory so they could make comments; the data were sent by mail and these families were interviewed by telephone on a few occasions. The other families simply requested a copy of the completed research report.

Data analysis was carried out concurrently with data collection. Memos and diagrams were used to document the process and to capture relationships between categories and subcategories. Commonalities and differences both within and across data sources were checked through constant comparative analysis of each transcript and field note. The process involved in families' experiences was identified by linking action/interactional sequences. During "open coding," data were examined line by line to identify codes or words that captured the meaning of events. Similar phenomena were given the same conceptual name and these concepts were then grouped into preliminary categories. Connections between a category and its subcategories were made during "axial coding," when the researcher asked questions of the data and compared concepts. A coding paradigm was used to specify a category in terms of the conditions that gave rise to it: context, intervening conditions, action/interactional strategies, and resultant consequences. Finally, the core category was selected through a process of "selective coding." The researcher systematically related this central category to other categories, validated those relationships, and filled in the categories that needed further refinement and development. The core category was named with a high level of abstraction, and the chosen conceptual label fit the story it represented.

## FINDINGS

### Overview

The basic social process of navigating uncharted territory characterized the experience of the families. Strong emotions of fear, uncertainty, and grief gave the process momentum. While these emotions were always present, they changed in intensity over time. *Navigating uncharted territory* comprised four dimensions: *entering unfamiliar territory, shifting priorities, creating meaning,* and *holding the fort.* Each dimension, in turn, involved strategies that the families used to manage the experience. The context of the illness experience included *acute, curative healthcare system* and *sociocultural environment.* In addition, the families' experiences were moderated by four intervening conditions: *relationships with healthcare providers, availability of information, gender differences,* and *communication between parents* (see Figure A7–1).

Families sought ways of dealing with the unfamiliarity, uncertainty, and unpredictability in their lives. Parents tried to describe an experience they perceived as unique, filled with poignancy, and indescribable. Their grief encompassed many losses, such as their lost dreams for their child and their loss of re-

lationships with extended family and friends. Some parents underwent a transformation that resulted in personal growth. Those parents who made peace with their emotions, accepted the situation, and formed positive meanings from the experience felt more in control of their lives, were not overwhelmed by their emotions, and believed that they had gained from the experience.

The illness placed heavy demands on families, taxing them cognitively, emotionally, and physically and requiring them to undertake extensive work to manage the experience. Many parents suffered from exhaustion, injuries, migraine headaches, anemia, or hives. Parents also experienced extreme emotional distress. This often lessened as they became more familiar with the illness, its treatment, and the prognosis. However, a change in the child's health, such as an acute chest infection, inevitably produced increased distress as well as a heavier workload.

Siblings were sad that the child was dying and that they were losing a playmate and sibling. They were also angry because the child was dying, and angry or upset that their parents and others focused most of their attention on the child. One sibling feared that her parents would separate. On the positive side, a couple of siblings were self-sufficient, confident, empathetic, and adaptable to changing circumstances. The siblings were generally viewed as less demanding than other children of their age. In addition, some siblings had reasoning abilities that would be expected of an older child.

Parents reported a range of onset patterns for the child's illness. For many, the beginning had come when a parent, usually the mother, noticed the child exhibiting some unusual behavior or symptom. The process of diagnosis was often long and drawn out and was usually accompanied by severe emotional distress. A major component of the distress was uncertainty and fear about the diagnosis, yet most parents were relieved once the diagnosis had been made. Although the children were diagnosed with NLTIs that would lead to their eventual death, the families remained uncertain about how the child would respond to medical treatments, how long the child could be expected to live, and how their ability to manage would be altered as the child's disease progressed. The uncertain course of the illness caused enormous stress for families and contributed to increased intrusiveness in their lives. They were taken on a roller-coaster ride over which they had little control.

### Illness Trajectory

*Navigating uncharted territory* was a continuous process set in motion by the initial precipitating event. Over time, families shifted their priorities, found meaning in the situation, and settled into a pe-

**FIGURE A7-1** **Navigating uncharted territory. (Adapted with permission from Steel, R. G. Trajectory of certain death at an unknown time: Children with neurodegenerative life-threatening illnesses. *Canadian Journal of Nursing Research, 32*[3], 49–67.)**

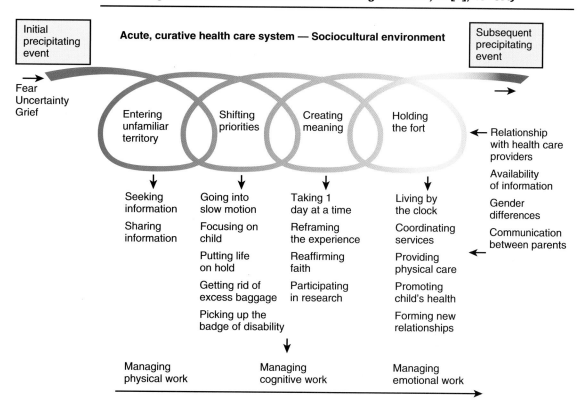

riod of relative stability. Although families explored their new territory and found ways of managing their new world, that world did not stay the same for long. Subsequent precipitating events, such as a decline in the child's physical health or a need for new medical equipment, sent families into unfamiliar territory once again and impacted on the other dimensions of the process. Families described these times as *dropping off the plateau* (see Figure A7–2).

Families adjusted their lives every time their child's condition changed. In most families, changes occurred most rapidly at the beginning of the illness, eventually slowing down. However, there was no predictable pattern. Occasionally a child's condition improved slightly for a period, yet parents knew that the child was on a downward trajectory towards inevitable death.

The trajectory, however, was not a steady decline. Instead, families lived their lives on plateaus of relative stability, waiting for the next crisis or a sudden decline in their child's condition. While on a plateau, parents tended to keep their thoughts about the illness and prognosis in the background. When the child became really sick, their thoughts about the illness and prognosis moved to the forefront. During each crisis, families dropped off the current plateau and fell until they reached the next plateau:

*She will go along on a plateau of doing things. Well, say for instance, like right now she is going along seeing things and then all of a sudden she will drop off not seeing anything.*

The extent of the drop depended on both the severity of the precipitating event and the corrective options available. In the beginning, families were often faced with short plateaus accompanied by sharp drops as the child lost abilities. Then, as the child's condition worsened and there was little more to lose, the drops would become less severe. Treatments could shorten the drop, but treatment options became more limited as the illness progressed.

**FIGURE A7-2**    **Dropping off the plateau. (Adapted with permission from Steel, R. G. Trajectory of certain death at an unknown time: Children with neurodegenerative life-threatening illnesses. *Canadian Journal of Nursing Research, 32*[3], 49–67.)**

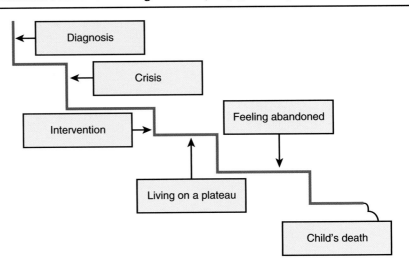

Families worked hard to extend the length of the plateaus. They expended much time and energy promoting the child's health in order to prevent the deterioration that would push them off the plateau. The primary goal for many families was to keep the child as healthy as possible, for two reasons: to make the child live longer, and to lessen disruptions to family life. Parents worked hard to keep the child safe, prevent the child from becoming ill, and provide the child with good nutrition. They continually monitored the child to identify potential health threats. Families lived in fear of the child developing pneumonia or another illness that might hasten death. They developed strategies to limit contact with those who might be infectious. If the child attended school and other students were ill, the child was kept home until the perceived danger was over. In one case nurses and other workers in the home had "strict instructions that if they have, if they think they are even coming down with anything, don't bother setting foot in the door." A parent with even a minor illness such as a cold did not, wherever possible, provide care to the child. Either the other parent assumed full responsibility for care or, as in one case, "You wear rubber gloves. You don't breathe anywhere near her trying to keep your face away. You wash your hands 500 million times in a day."

Families spent most of their lives on plateaus. Living on a plateau was easier than dealing with crises:

*Right now we are at a stage where he's reached a plateau. Although he is still deteriorating, we can cope because he is moving at a really slow pace.*

Yet many families also felt frightened and alone on the plateaus, abandoned by the health-care system. Although parents emphasized the importance of an ongoing relationship with a few key individuals in the health-care system, they often interacted with and received help from the system only when they were in crisis. In many cases, consequently, professionals failed to see the whole picture. Some professionals made decisions based on intermittent, crises-induced interactions, decisions that were irrelevant to the families' everyday lives. For example, a dietitian insisted that a child needed a gastrostomy tube because of his low weight, even though the weight loss had been caused by an episode of pneumonia. The child's father said:

*They're looking at this situation right now, right here, right now. But . . .right here, right now is diddly on the overall perspective [The nutritionist] only sees him when he's sick, so she wants a [feeding]tube in him. She's never seen him when he's in good health. Or on a good day.*

Professionals seldom recognized a family's need for ongoing support when the child's condition was relatively stable, thus families often struggled in isolation. One mother urged passionately:

*When people like us end up in your world, don't leave us alone. Just don't shove us out of the door and leave us alone . . .once we left [the hospital], that was it. That was IT. It was like they were throwing us to the wolves.*

*Dropping off the plateau* affected all other dimensions of the process. There was an increase in either fear, uncertainty, or grief, depending on the particular precipitating event. Each time families fell to the next plateau, they found themselves once again in new territory. Consequently, they needed to once again learn about the new area and find ways to manage their world. Families continued moving through the process of *navigating uncharted territory* as they encountered further precipitating events. The process would eventually end with the child's death.

## DISCUSSION

Life with a child who has an NLTI cannot be reduced to simply identifying the coping strategies used by individual family members, or even the family as a whole, when faced with acute or chronic stressors. The family's full biography and illness trajectory must be taken into account. The families in this study experienced an incredible workload because of the child's illness. They had to manage the physical, cognitive, and emotional work generated by the situation, while also continuing with daily life. Managing the work required a great deal of effort and extensive maintenance. Professionals, extended family, and friends seldom recognized the effort involved as families navigated this uncharted territory.

The work of chronic illness has been well documented by Corbin and Strauss (1988, 1991). While their framework was developed with adults only, many of its areas are relevant for exploring the experiences of families with a child who has an NLTI. This current study extends Corbin and Strauss's theoretical formulations to include such families. Corbin and Strauss describe the management of a chronic illness as a complex process, and this was found to be true in the present study, as families managed the long-term illness of their child.

A significant finding of this study is the importance of understanding that the work faced by families caring for a child with NLTIs does not consist simply of a list of tasks. Often with little outside support for extended periods of time, the families carried out this work while grieving the losses associated with the child's diagnosis, prognosis, and deterioration. Moreover, the demands of each task were not static. Family members could not relax once they had learned one task: over time, the demand for a particular task changed or other tasks became necessary as families moved through the illness trajectory.

Corbin and Strauss (1988, 1991) used the term *trajectory* to encompass not only the course of the illness, but also the organizational work involved and the impact on those who carry it out. These authors view the illness trajectory as a way of recognizing the active role that people take in changing the course of an illness, and as a way of capturing experiences involving time, work, non-medical features, and the interplay of patients, spouses, and health-care providers. In the present study, families were a critical component in all aspects of the child's illness trajectory. They played a vital role in changing the course of the illness, did most of the organizational work, and suffered the impact of that labor. These findings provide evidence that the work of Corbin and Strauss could be extended to include families.

For the families of children with NLTIs, the experiences of navigating uncharted territory were found to be unrelated to steady decline in the child's health. Families lived their lives on plateaus of relative stability, waiting for the next crisis or sudden decline in the child's condition. With each crisis, the family dropped off the current plateau and fell until they reached the next one. Ground that was lost could seldom be regained. Families therefore faced frequent losses and held out little hope for rehabilitation. They concentrated on making the best of the abilities their child still had and worked hard to prevent further losses. While initially some decline could be slowed down medically if an appropriate treatment was available, most of the credit for preventing deterioration belonged with families. Their management skills in health promotion and illness prevention were key in extending the length of the plateaus. Health-care professionals may not always recognize the expertise of families, yet it was this expertise that kept the child as healthy as possible. The skills and knowledge developed by families may be an invaluable resource for professionals.

The uneven and stair-like trajectory of certain death at an unknown time has not been previously documented in pediatric research. However, Rolland (1994) notes that progressive illnesses are often characterized by a stepwise or progressive deterioration, either rapid or slow. He suggests that patients and caregivers receive minimal relief from symptoms during progressive illness, as they have to constantly adapt and adjust to role changes. The idea of plateaus and drop-offs is also partially supported by research with parents of chronically ill children that identified critical times in a child's illness when the family faces increased needs or changes in the support structure (Clements, Copeland, & Loftus, 1990; Whyte, 1992). Family researchers also support the concept of plateaus during illness experiences, though indirectly (Clements et al.; Whyte, 1992). They describe families as living in a state of equilibrium when emotional and physical support is available to meet their needs.

The present study found that relationships with health-care professionals were very important, both in the home and in tertiary settings. Although the families spent most of their lives at home, the inevitable crises in the child's life brought them into intermittent contact with the system of acute health care. Relationships with key individuals in tertiary care were important to families as these individuals could function as entry points to the system (e.g., physicians) or as ongoing resources (e.g., nurses, social workers). In addition, families wanted to have someone in the system who knew the family history and could facilitate access to relevant information, resources, and professional and non-professional assistance. The potential for these relationships to make a family's journey smoother and less stressful should not be underestimated.

Researchers have identified feelings of isolation and loneliness among those living on plateaus (Davies, 1996; Diehl, Moffitt, & Wade, 1991; Walker, Epstein, Taylor, Crocker, & Tuttle, 1989; Woolley, 1991; Woolley, Stein, Forrest, & Baum, 1991). When families have little contact with health-care providers in hospital, they often feel lost and alone. Many families have advocated for an ongoing relationship with one person who will coordinate care, provide guidance, and develop a close and trusting relationship with them (Chambers, Oakhill, Cornish, & Curnick, 1989; Davies, 1996; Diehl et al., 1991; James & Johnson, 1997; Stein & Woolley, 1990; Woolley, 1991; Woolley et al., 1991). Research on the effectiveness of such contact, however, is limited. One group of researchers (Burke, Handley-Derry, Costello, Kauffmann, & Dillon, 1997) used a two-group, pretest-posttest design to determine the efficacy of a community-based, stress-point nursing intervention with families of chronically ill children. A research nurse worked with parents in the experimental group to identify their stresses and to develop coping strategies. She maintained contact with families by telephone, mail, and face-to-face meetings. Results showed improved coping and family functioning when the families received the intervention. It appears that contact with the tertiary system, even if minimal, may provide a sense of comfort or a safety net for families who are largely managing on their own.

## RESEARCH AND PRACTICE IMPLICATIONS

A variety of both qualitative and quantitative research methods and data-analysis techniques need to be developed and tested for their usefulness at the family level. Neither qualitative nor quantitative research alone seems sufficient to capture the complexity of family life. There is a need to examine the links between qualitative and quantitative research. Practitioners need to know both the processes by which families manage the experience and the outcomes associated with different subjective perceptions and management approaches.

There is little available research that examines the link or interface between families and the health-care system. Yet the present study found that relationships within the system played an important role. Further research, using both qualitative and quantitative methods, might examine family interactions with the health-care system so that practitioners can gain a better understanding of the types of intervention that are most appropriate for families.

The families in the present study clearly valued ongoing contact with one person in the health-care system. An intervention study could be designed to evaluate interactions between a coordinator and a family. Outcomes could include families' satisfaction with care and their perception of the degree of fragmentation in the system before and after the intervention.

There is little research examining the trajectory of certain death at an unknown time. Copp (1996, cited in Copp, 1998) appears to be the only researcher to have explored this trajectory. Apart from her study, the nature of the form, shape, and duration of this death trajectory has not been articulated in any depth. This current study adds to the available knowledge about the trajectory of certain death at an unknown time, but further research, to determine similarities and differences across varying populations, is warranted. While it may be possible to extend Corbin and Strauss's (1988, 1991) conceptualization of chronic illness to include families of children with NLTIs, further research is required to validate this suggestion.

Clinicians may believe they lack the knowledge to help the families of a child with an NLTI. However, if they resolve to move beyond the medical diagnosis and think in terms of illness trajectory and its implications, clinicians may find that the knowledge they have accumulated in practice can be applied in many ways. Clinicians should also be honest about areas in which they lack knowledge and make an effort to educate themselves. A willingness to learn from families and collaborate with them may result in positive relationships and the sharing of valuable knowledge.

Two specific suggestions arise from this study: recognizing the work that families undertake; and identifying and sharing strategies that families can use to mitigate their work. Clinicians can then work with families to identify interventions that might lessen their workload. Telling a family that they are doing a great job in caring for their child is an intervention that takes little time and costs no money, yet is very important in helping them feel appreciated.

Ongoing contact with a professional who provides information and coordinates care may alleviate a family's anxiety and sense of isolation. Having one person who knows the family and can provide continuity of care may prevent problems and, when necessary, facilitate movement through the health-care system. Advocacy and support are extremely helpful as families learn how to provide the best care for their child. Information may help reduce fear and uncertainty. Written rather than verbal information is often the most useful, as families can read it repeatedly as needed. Anticipatory guidance on an ongoing basis and raising possibilities for the future as changes occur may help families manage plateau drop-offs.

Finally, providing care to the whole family is extremely important. It requires that professionals develop skills in family-level care, yet education of health professionals has primarily focused on the ill individual as the unit of care. Learning about a family's biography and providing family-level care require time and specialized skills. These are not abundant in the current system. However, professionals can learn ways of providing family-level care in basic and continuing-education courses. Collaboration with colleagues and professional support groups can also be used to improve one's expertise.

## References

Ashby, M., Kosky, R., Laver, H., & Sims, E. (1991). An enquiry into death and dying at the Adelaide Children's Hospital: A useful model? *Medical Journal of Australia, 154,* 165–170.

Birenbaum, L.K., & Clarke-Steffen, L. (1992). Terminal care costs in childhood cancer. *Pediatric Nursing, 18*(3), 285–288.

Bluebond-Langner, M. (1996). *In the shadow of illness: Parents and siblings of the chronically ill child.* Princeton, NJ: Princeton University Press.

Broome, M. (1998). *Children and families in health and illness.* Thousand Oaks, CA: Sage.

Burke, S.O., Handley-Derry, M.H., Costello, E.A., Kauffmann, E., & Dillon, M.C. (1997). Stress-point intervention for parents of repeatedly hospitalized children with chronic conditions. *Research in Nursing and Health, 20*(6), 475–485.

Burne, S.R., Dominica, F., & Baum, J.D. (1984). Helen House—A hospice for children: Analysis of the first year. *British Medical Journal, 289*(6459), 1665–1668.

Caring Institute of the Foundation for Hospice and Home Care. (1987). *The crisis of chronically ill children in America: Triumph of technology—Failure of public policy.* Washington: Author.

Chambers, E., Oakhill, A., Cornish, J., & Curnick, S. (1989). Terminal care at home for children with cancer. *British Medical Journal, 298,* 937–940.

Clarke-Steffen, L. (1997). Reconstructing reality: Family strategies for managing childhood cancer. *Journal of Pediatric Nursing, 12*(5), 278–287.

Clements, D.B., Copeland, L.G., & Loftus, M. (1990). Critical times for families with a chronically ill child. *Pediatric Nursing, 16*(2), 156–161, 224.

Copp, G. (1996). *Facing impending death: The experiences of patients and their nurses in a hospice setting.* Unpublished doctoral dissertation, Oxford Brookes, Oxford, UK.

Copp, G. (1998). A review of current theories of death and dying. *Journal of Advanced Nursing, 28*(2), 382–290.

Corbin, J., & Strauss, A. (1988). *Unending work and care: Managing chronic illness at home.* San Francisco: Jossey-Bass.

Corbin, J., & Strauss, A. (1991). A nursing model for chronic illness management based upon the Trajectory Framework. *Scholarly Inquiry and Nursing Practice, 5*(3), 155–174.

Davies, B. (1992). *Final report: Assessment of need for a children's hospice facility in British Columbia.* Submitted to the Board of the HUGS Children's Hospice Society. Vancouver: Author.

Davies, B., & Howell, D. (1998). Special services for children. In D. Doyle, G. Hanks, & N. MacDonald (Eds.), *Oxford textbook of palliative medicine, 2nd ed.* (pp. 1077–1084). Oxford: Oxford University Press.

Davies, H. (1996). Living with dying: Families coping with a child who has a neurodegenerative genetic disorder. *Axon, 18*(2), 38–44.

Diehl, S.F., Moffitt, K.A., & Wade, S.M. (1991). Focus group interview with parents of children with medically complex needs: An intimate look at their perceptions and feelings. *Children's Health Care, 20*(3), 170–178.

Glaser, B., & Strauss, A. (1967). *The discovery of grounded theory: Strategies for qualitative research.* Hawthorne, NY: Aldine.

Goldman, A. (1996). Home care of the dying child. *Journal of Palliative Care, 12*(3), 16–19.

Goldman, A. (1998). Life threatening illnesses and symptom control in children. In D. Doyle, G. Hanks, & N. MacDonald (Eds.), *Oxford textbook of palliative medicine, 2nd ed.* (pp. 1033–1043). Oxford: Oxford University Press.

Gravelle, A.M. (1997). Caring for a child with a progressive illness during the complex chronic phase: Parents' experience of facing adversity. *Journal of Advanced Nursing, 25*(4), 738–745.

Hunt, A., & Burne, R. (1995). Medical and nursing problems of children with neurodegenerative disease. *Palliative Medicine, 9*(1), 19–26.

James, L., & Johnson, B. (1997). The needs of parents of pediatric oncology patients during the palliative care phase. *Journal of Pediatric Oncology Nursing, 14*(2), 83–95.

Leonard, B.J., Johnson, A.L., & Brust, J.B. (1993). Caregivers of children with disabilities: A comparison of those managing "OK" and those needing more help. *Children's Health Care, 22*(2), 93–105.

Martinson, I.M. (1993). Hospice care for children: Past, present, and future. *Journal of Pediatric Oncology Nursing, 10*(3), 93–98.

Parker, M. (1996). Families caring for chronically ill children with tuberous sclerosis complex. *Family and Community Health, 19*(3), 73–84.

Rolland, J. (1994). *Families, illness and disability: An integrative treatment model.* New York: Basic Books.

Steele, R. (1999). *Navigating uncharted territory: Experiences of families when a child has a neurodegenerative life threatening illness.* Unpublished doctoral dissertation, University of British Columbia, Vancouver, BC.

Stein, A., Forrest, G.C., Woolley, H., & Baum, J.D. (1989). Life threatening illness and hospice care [see comments]. *Archives of Disease in Childhood, 64*(5), 697–702.

Stein, A., & Woolley, H. (1990). An evaluation of hospice care for children. In J. Baum, F. Dominica, & R. Woodward (Eds.), *Listen: My child has a lot of living to do* (pp. 66–90). New York: Oxford University Press.

Stevens, M. (1998). Care of the dying child and adolescent: Family adjustment and support. In D. Doyle, G. Hanks, & N. MacDonald (Eds.), *Oxford textbook of palliative medicine, 2nd ed.* (pp. 1057–1075). Oxford: Oxford University Press.

Stewart, M.J., Ritchie, J.A., McGrath, P., Thompson, D., & Bruce, B. (1994). Mothers of children with chronic conditions: Supportive and stressful interactions with partners and professionals regarding caregiving burdens. *Canadian Journal of Nursing Research, 26*(4), 61–82.

Strauss, A., & Corbin, J. (1990). *Basics of qualitative research: Grounded theory procedures and techniques.* Newbury Park, CA: Sage.

Walker, D.K., Epstein, S.G., Taylor, A.B., Crocker, A.C., & Tuttle, G.A. (1989). Perceived needs of families with children who have chronic health conditions. *Children's Health Care, 18*(4), 196–201.

Whyte, D.A. (1992). A family nursing approach to the care of a child with a chronic illness. *Journal of Advanced Nursing, 17*(3), 317–327.

Wiener, L., Theut, S., Steinberg, S.M., Riekert, K.A., & Pizzo, P.A. (1994). The HIV-infected child: Parental responses and psychosocial implications. *American Journal of Orthopsychiatry, 64*(3), 485–492.

Woolley, H. (1991). Cornerstone carers for family support. *Nursing Times, 87*(43), 56.

Woolley, H., Stein, A., Forrest, G.C., & Baum, J.D. (1991). Cornerstone care for families of children with life-threatening illness. *Developmental Medicine and Child Neurology, 33*(3), 216–224.

# Distress and Growth Outcomes in Mothers of Medically Fragile Infants

Margaret Shandor Miles, Dian Holditch-Davis,
Peg Burchinal, Deborah Nelson

***Background:*** *With recent advances in medical and nursing care, many high-risk infants are surviving the neonatal period with severe, life-threatening chronic illnesses, resulting in extended hospitalizations and/or frequent rehospitalizations and long periods of dependence on technology for survival.*

***Objective:*** *To describe the factors predicting maternal adjustment in mothers caring for medically fragile infants.*

***Method:*** *Subjects were mothers (n = 67) whose infants had a serious life-threatening illness requiring hospitalization and technology for survival. Data for this longitudinal study were collected at enrollment and hospital discharge, and at 6, 12, and 16 months after birth. Distress was measured as depressive symptoms using the Center for Epidemiologic Studies Depression Scale, and growth was assessed using a personal developmental impact rating scale. Data about personal characteristics, parental role attainment, infant-illness characteristics, and maternal illness distress were collected.*

***Results:*** *Mothers of medically fragile infants experience distress and growth as a result of their child's illness. Mean scores on the depression scale at both time points were moderately high and a high percentage of mothers scored at risk for depressive symptoms. Maternal development impact ratings at 6 months were neutral to slightly negative and at 16 months were be-tween neutral and positive. While the mean depressive symptom scores and maternal developmental ratings were lower at the later time points, these differences were not significant. Maternal depressive symptoms and developmental impact ratings were moderately but negatively correlated at 6 and 16 months, indicating that higher depressive symptoms were related to more negative developmental impact ratings. Distress was influenced by maternal characteristics, hospital environmental stress, and worry about the child's health. Growth was influenced by characteristics of the child's illness, hospital environmental stress, concern about the child's health, and level of maternal role attainment.*

***Conclusions:*** *Nurses should consider personal characteristics and level of parental role attainment as well as characteristics of the child and illness-related distress in their approaches to intervention with mothers of critically ill infants.*

With recent advances in medical and nursing care, many high-risk infants are surviving the neonatal period with severe, life-threatening chronic illnesses such as bronchopulmonary dysplasia, severe gastrointestinal malformations, neurological anomalies, complex congenital heart disease, and multisystem syndromes. These medically fragile infants experience extended hospitalizations and/or frequent rehospitalizations and long periods of dependence on technology for survival (Miles & D'Auria, 1994). Most of these infants are discharged home with chronic health problems that require continued dependence on technology and medical surveillance for months or years (Leonberg et al., 1998; Piecuch, Leonard, Cooper, & Sehring, 1997; Singer et al., 1989; Singer, Yamashito, Lilien, Collins, & Baley, 1997).

During hospitalization, parents of medically fragile infants are distressed at seeing their infant in a critical care unit surrounded by technology and are concerned about whether the infant will survive (Gennaro, York, & Brooten, 1990; Meyer et al., 1995; Miles, Funk, & Kasper, 1992). These parents also face challenges in assuming the parental role while their infant is too sick to hold or feed and others have the major responsibility for the infant's care (Miles & Frauman, 1993; Odom & Chandler, 1990).

After hospital discharge, parents must give care to a sick child who has needs beyond those of a normal developing infant (Fleming et al., 1994; Leonard, Brust, & Nelson, 1993; Patterson, Leonard, & Titus, 1992; Sterling, Jones, Johnson, & Bowen, 1996; Young, Creighton, & Sauve, 1988). Caring for the child's complex medical needs places a significant burden on parents (Diehl, Moffitt, & Wade, 1991; Deatrick & Knafl, 1990; Goldberg, Morris, Simmons, Fowler, & Levison, 1990), particularly mothers who assume the major role in caregiving (Anderson & Elfert, 1989). Caregiving of medically fragile infants includes specialized, time-consuming, illness-related care and advocating on behalf of the child with healthcare professionals, school personnel, and family (Leonard et al., 1993; Miles, D'Auria, Hart, Sedlack, & Watral, 1993; Patterson et al., 1992; Ray & Ritchie, 1993; Sterling et al., 1996; Young et al., 1988). Aspects of the infant's behavior and atypical responses to parental interactions may also complicate parenting (Goldberg et al., 1990; Holaday, 1981; Lobo, 1992; Pridham, Martin, Sondel, & Tluczek, 1989; Singer & Farkas, 1989).

Thus, caring for chronically ill children may place mothers at risk for emotional distress (Cadman, Rosenbaum, Boyle, & Offord, 1991; Jessop, Riessman, & Stein, 1988; Kronenberger & Thompson, 1992; Wallander, Varni, Babani, Banis, & Wilcox, 1989), particularly depressive symptoms (Bristol, Gallagher, & Schopler, 1988). However, mothers may respond with resilience and adaptive functioning (Van Riper, Ryff, & Pridham, 1992). A number of maternal, family, and child-illness factors have been found to be associated with maternal psychological outcomes. More stressful family life events, lack of family support, and lower levels of marital satisfaction were related to higher levels of distress in several studies with mothers of chronically ill children (Bristol et al., 1988; Jessop et al., 1988; Mullins et al., 1991; Ray & Ritchie, 1993; Wallender,

Varni, Babani, DeHaan, et al., 1989). Conversely, several investigators found higher levels of social support associated with more maternal distress (Hauenstein, 1990; Kazak, Reber, & Carter, 1988). Characteristics of the child's illness, such as acuity level or amount of disability, also influenced psychological adaptation of mothers in some studies (Cowen et al., 1986; Jessop et al., 1988), but not in others (Mullins et al., 1991; Thompson, Gil, Burbach, Keith, & Kinney, 1993; Thompson, Gustafson, Hamlett, & Spock, 1992; Wallender, Varni, Babani, Banis, et al., 1989).

Much of the literature that is focused on the impact of chronic illness on caregivers was conducted from a negative or *burden* perspective. Recently, the concept of burden has been challenged, and researchers have been urged to examine the experience of caregiving from a broader perspective that encompasses both distress and positive outcomes (Folkman, 1997; O'Neill & Ross, 1991; Park, Cohen, & Murch, 1996). The study of caregiving from a broader perspective is particularly important for parents of children with chronic health problems. Because caring for a seriously ill child involves both challenges and opportunities for growth, it is possible that distress and growth may occur simultaneously (Affleck & Tennen, 1993; Van Riper et al., 1992).

The adjustment of mothers to the care of medically fragile infants should be examined as a process that occurs over time from birth and hospitalization to the period of home care management (Odom & Chandler, 1990; Patterson et al., 1992; Svavarsdottir & McCubbin, 1996). However, few studies of mothers of chronically ill infants have been longitudinal and no studies have included the degree to which the mother has attained the parental role as a factor influencing maternal outcomes in infancy and early childhood. Parental role attainment encompasses the level of maternal identity as parent of the child, the amount of parental presence with the child, and the mother's competence in interacting with the child (Mercer, 1995; Miles, 1998; Rubin, 1984). Measuring maternal role attainment provides an indication of the extent to which the mother has been able to assume her normal caregiving role within the context of parenting a sick child. Because the child's illness and long hospitalization reduces the ability of mothers of medically fragile children to assume the usual maternal role, this loss of the expected maternal role may affect maternal distress and growth.

The purpose of this study was to examine the extent to which attributes of the mother, the mother's level of parental role attainment with the child, characteristics of the child's illness, and maternal illness-related distress influence adjustment in mothers caring for medically fragile infants. This study was based on a transactional model of stress (Folkman,

1997; Lazarus & Folkman, 1984; Pearlin, Mullan, Semple, & Skaff, 1990; Schaeffer & Moos, 1992) and growth (Antonovsky, 1987; Janoff-Bulman, 1992; Tedeschi & Calhoun, 1995). In this model, adjustment is conceptualized as both distress (depressive symptoms) and growth (positive or negative personal developmental impact). Adjustment is thought to be influenced by selected characteristics of the mother, by her level of maternal role attainment with the child, and by factors related to the child's illness and the mother's illness-related distress.

The research questions for the study were: (a) How do attributes of the mother, the level of maternal role attainment with the child, characteristics of the child's illness, and maternal illness-related distress influence maternal distress (depressive symptoms) at the infant's hospital discharge and at 12 months of age? and (b) How do attributes of the mother, the level of maternal role attainment with the child, characteristics of the child's illness, and maternal illness-related distress affect maternal growth (positive or negative developmental impact) at 6 and 16 months of age?

## METHOD
### Subjects
Participants were 67 mothers of medically fragile infants who were part of a longitudinal study of parental role attainment (Miles, 1998). Infants met the enrollment criteria if they had a life-threatening illness that required technology for survival, were likely to remain hospitalized for several weeks or months, and were likely to be discharged with one or more chronic health problems. Mothers were included if the infant remained in the larger study at hospital discharge or at the 16-month data collection point. Reasons for maternal loss ($n = 8$) to the study over time included child death, geographic relocation, withdrawal from the study, change of child custody, and missing data.

The mean age of the mothers was 27 years (range = 16 to 41). The mean educational level was 13 years (range = 8 to 18). Most (55%) were married; 54% were White, 34% were Black, and the rest were Asian, Native American, and Hispanic (12%).

The infants were 58% males. About two-thirds were premature (67%). The mean birthweight was 2,040 grams (range = 510 to 4,120). The mean chronological age at enrollment was 11 weeks, and the mean gestational age was 33 weeks. The mean number of days hospitalized at enrollment was 52 (range = 5 to 200). The primary diagnoses of the infants included: bronchopulmonary dysplasia ($n = 18$), severe gastrointestinal problems ($n = 15$), severe congenital heart disease ($n = 12$), congenital abnormalities of the airway ($n = 8$), neurological disorder ($n = 6$), and other chronic diseases ($n = 8$).

### Data Collection Methods
Methodological triangulation was used in data collection for this study (Hinds, 1989). Data included self-report questionnaires, semi-structured interviews, behavioral observations of mother-child interaction, and research team ratings of mothers.

### Outcome Variables
The maternal adjustment outcomes were distress (depressive symptoms) and growth (positive or negative developmental impact).

*Distress.* The Center for Epidemiologic Studies Depression Scale (CES-D) was developed to measure depressive symptoms experienced in the past week by a general population (Radloff, 1977). This 20-item scale assesses the frequency of the occurrence of feelings or behaviors such as the blues, loneliness, and sadness; not feeling as good as others or thinking one's life was a failure; difficulty concentrating; and sleep and appetite problems. Items are rated on a 4-point rating scale ranging from 0 (rarely) to 3 (frequently); the range of scores is 0 to 60. It has been suggested that a score of 16 indicates risk for experiencing depression (Radloff, 1977). A modest relationship has been found between self-reported symptoms of depression using the CES-D cutoff score of 16 and the diagnosis of depression (Myers & Weissman, 1980; Roberts & Vernon, 1983). The CES-D has repeatedly demonstrated high internal consistency with Cronbach's alphas ranging from .86 to .90 (Ensel, 1985). Cronbach's alpha in this sample was .90 at hospital discharge and .88 at 12 months.

*Growth.* To capture the overall parental experiences over the course of this longitudinal study, a developmental impact rating scale was developed by the investigators. Developmental impact was assessed with a single rating on a 7-point scale ranging from negative impact to positive impact (growth):

1. severely negative experience with parent dysfunctional because of mental or emotional problems;
2. definite negative experience with signs of severe distress with interference with personal and family functioning;
3. moderately negative with signs of moderate personal distress and mild interference with personal or family functioning;
4. slightly negative with parent showing mild distress not interfering with personal or family functioning;
5. neutral with positive effects and costs generally equal;
6. somewhat positive with positive effects greater than distress; and
7. generally positive with the signs of personal growth and minimal distress.

A higher score indicates more growth and a lower score indicates a negative impact.

The ratings were based on field notes, interviews, questionnaire data, data about the child's illness, and observational data of parent-child interaction up to the 6- and 16-month data collection points. The rating scale was developed, used with several cases, and then revised to be clearer. Ratings were done independently by the two members of the research team who had the most contact with the parents. These researchers reviewed all of the data for each case before making the rating. Four members of the research team and the principal investigator then met as a group; each rating was discussed individually. When there were differences between the raters, discussion among the whole team ensued, and a consensus was reached regarding the final rating. At 6 months, there was 85% agreement, and at 16 months there was 83% agreement within 1 point.

### Predictor Variables

*Maternal attributes.* Data about four personal attributes—educational level, marital status, personal control, and satisfaction with family—were collected. A personal demographic data sheet was used on entry into the study to collect standard descriptive demographic data including educational level and marital status.

The Sense of Mastery Scale (SOM) was used to assess the caregiver's general sense of control over problems, life, the future, and change (Pearlin, Lieberman, Menagham, & Mullan, 1981). Respondents were asked to indicate the degree of their agreement with 7 items on a 4-point scale ranging from 'strongly agree' to 'strongly disagree.' A higher score indicates higher levels of mastery. A factor analysis resulted in one factor with loadings from .47 to .76. Cronbach's alpha on our sample was .68 on enrollment and .70 at 12 months. The mean score on the SOM at enrollment was 3.1 ($SD = .52$) and at 12 months was 3.2 ($SD = .52$).

The Family Apgar was used to measure parents' level of satisfaction with various areas of family life (Smilkstein, Ashworth, & Montano, 1982). Respondents rate 5 items on a 5-point scale ranging from 'always' to 'never.' A lower score indicates a higher perception of one's family. Moderate to high correlations have been found between the Family Apgar and other family tools as well as therapist ratings of families. Cronbach's alpha for our sample was .86 at enrollment and at 12 months. The mean Family Apgar score at enrollment was 1.8 ($SD = .71$) and at 12 months was 2.1 ($SD = .73$).

*Maternal role attainment.* Based on the work of Mercer (1995), Rubin (1984), and Walker et al. (1986), maternal role attainment was defined as the process by which a mother or father achieves an identity as a parent, establishes their presence with the child, and becomes competent in parental caregiving. These three constructs were used as predictor variables.

Maternal identity (the degree to which the mother reports feeling like she is a mother to her infant) was assessed using only a self-report measure because it is an internal feeling state. It was assessed on enrollment because identity was thought to be a process that occurred early in the parenting experience. Data were collected using the Maternal Identity Scale: Critically Ill Infant (MIS; Miles, 1998) The MIS was adapted from the Fogel Inventory of Maternal Identity (Fogel, 1992). On the MIS, parents are asked to respond to questions using a 4-point Likert scale ranging from 'strongly agree' to 'strongly disagree.' A higher score reflects higher identity. Cronbach's alpha for the MIS was .85. The mean score on enrollment was 1.5 ($SD = .29$).

Maternal presence and maternal competence were assessed using a triangulation of approaches because, as complex phenomena, these constructs could not be adequately measured with a single approach. Thus, ratings of maternal interviews (a type of self-report) and data from behavioral observations of mother-infant interactions were used to develop composite scores for these constructs. Different ratings and behaviors were used for the two measures; the variables to be used for each construct were hypothesized a priori based on the conceptualizations of maternal role attainment (Miles, 1998). Maternal presence and competence were assessed at three time points—at enrollment, at 6 months, and at 16 months—because they were conceptualized as maternal behaviors that evolve over time. Higher scores on maternal presence and competence reflect a higher level of maternal role attainment.

Maternal presence (the amount of physical closeness with the infant) is a composite score that incorporated ratings of the degree to which the mother reported engaging in three types of activities with the child during interviews (amount of interaction, general caregiving, and illness caregiving), and the amount of four mother interactive behaviors from naturalistic observations (the percent of time the mother was observed holding, having close body contact, and interacting with the infant, and the percent of time she was not involved with the child—reversed). Interviewer ratings were done by trained research assistants using a preset coding system. Percent agreements on the individual interviewer ratings ranged from 67.8% to 100%; the average was 88%. The observations involved recording mother and child behaviors during a 60-minute observation when the infant was being fed (for younger ages) or playing with the mother (for older ages; for methodological details see Holditch-Davis, Tesh, Burchinal, & Miles, 1999). Observations done in the hospital and home used a coding system developed by Holditch-Davis, Sandelowski, and Harris (1998) and Tesh and Holditch-Davis (1997) from a schema developed by Holditch-Davis and Thoman (1988) and Thoman, Becker, and Freese (1978). The coding system is capable of recording the occurrence of 97 infant, mother, and mother-infant behaviors and locations. Observations were done by trained research assistants who achieved ongoing interrater reliabilities (kappas) ranging from .51 to .96. Cronbach's alphas for the maternal presence composite scores were .61, .78, and .51 for enrollment, 6 months, and 16 months, respectively.

Parental competence, the quality and effectiveness of parenting, was a composite score that included four interview rating items, the amount of four mother-child interaction items from the naturalistic observations, and 6 subscale scores from the Home Observation for Measurement of the Environment (HOME). HOME (0–3 year version) is a standardized instrument designed to identify children at risk for developmental delay because their home environment fails to provide appropriate stimulation for learning (Bradley, 1989; Caldwell & Bradley, 1984). It has been successfully used with children with disabilities (Bradley, Rock, Caldwell, & Brisby, 1989). The 45 binary items are organized into 6 subscales: (a) responsivity; (b) acceptance; (c) organization of the environment; (d) involvement; (e) play materials; and (f) variety of daily activities. It is scored using a combination of semistructured mother interview, observation of mother-child relationship, and assessment of kinds of play materials available to the child. HOME was administered by three observers who were trained by an experienced HOME tester until they had a minimum interrater reliability of 95%. Interrater reliabilities for the data collectors averaged 97%. Internal consistency of HOME for this sample, calculated using Kuder-Richardson 20, was .86 at 6 months and .80 at 16 months.

The composite scores for maternal competence included whether the mother reported in interviews that she observed and understood behavioral cues from her child, advocated for and supported her child, and provided stimulation to the child during visits; the percent of the 1-hour naturalistic observation that the mother was talking with, making positive comments to, and playing with the child; the percent of the child's awake time during the observation that the mother was interacting with the child; and the 6 subscales from the HOME. Cronbach's alphas for the maternal competence composite scores were .63, .81, and .79 at enrollment, 6 months, and 16 months, respectively.

*Child-illness characteristics.* The three child illness-related variables used were: whether the child had a multisystem diagnosis; level of technology dependence; and level of mental development. Data about the child's health were collected weekly from the medical record while hospitalized and after hospital discharge by interview with the parent. Four masters-prepared pediatric nurses collected the medical record data. The data collection procedures were developed by one nurse in consultation with the nurse investigators who checked the system for inclusiveness and clarity. Medical record data collected by the first nurse was checked by a second nurse for accuracy until they reached full agreement. The other nurses were trained and checked for accuracy in data collection procedures using the first nurse as the standard. Data from the medical record were used to determine the principal and additional diagnoses; all diagnoses from the progress notes were recorded. Infants with multiple major diagnoses or with a diagnosis involving more than one physiological system (such as Di-George Syndrome or Downs Syndrome with duodenal atresia) were identified as having multisystem diagnoses by the research team using a consensus process. Thirty-six percent of the children had a multisystem diagnosis at enrollment. At 16 months, 34% of the remaining children had a multisystem diagnosis.

A technology dependence score was developed to capture the different technologies a child was using at each data collection point as a measure of acuity and burden of caregiving (Miles, 1998). The Office of Technological Assistance (1987) classifications for technology-dependent children was used as a starting guide for the list of technologies. However, the categorical approach used in this tool did not have enough variance and, further, the items were not comprehensive enough for the medically fragile children in our study due to the complexity of their treatments and the new technologies developed since 1987. Thus, technologies relevant to medically fragile infants were added to the tool after a medical record review of the first several children enrolled in the study. These technologies were then clustered into similar types of procedures and a count of technologies used in caring for the child at each data collection point were used to reflect the acuity of the child's illness. Technologies included parenteral and intravenous lines, monitoring equipment, oxygen, oxygen monitoring, respiratory support, tracheostomy, respiratory toiletry, chest tube, gastrointestinal/feeding equipment, total parenteral nutrition, elimination technology, neurological devices, orthopedic devices, physical therapy, transplantation, thermoregulation, transfusions, and ten categories of medications. Transplantation was included because it is a biological technology and requires constant monitoring of the child due to possible rejection and side effects of immunosuppression drugs. The possible range of scores was from 0 to 27. The mean at enrollment was 5.7 ($SD = 2.8$) and at 16 months was 2.0 ($SD = 1.8$).

The Mental Development Index (MDI) of the Bayley II Scale (Bayley, 1993) was used to measure aspects of infant cognitive abilities and visual/fine motor coordination at 16 months adjusted age. The Bayley was standardized on a national representative random sample of 1,700 children; the reliability coefficient was .88. In very low birthweight, premature infants, the 12-month MDI had a correlation of .48 with preschool year IQ and .50 with early school age IQ (Lawson, Koller, Rose, & McCarton, 1996). The Bayley exams were done by masters-prepared registered nurses trained by a child psychologist reliable in conducting the Bayley exam and experienced in training. To standardize the exam, a table and two chairs were taken into each child's home, along with the standard equipment needed for the examination. All exams were videotaped. The nurses' reliability was established prior to data collection and were checked periodically by the child psychologist who evaluated selected videotapes of the exams for each nurse. Additionally, two nurse examiners participated in each exam, one assisting and one conducting the exam. The staff member assisting observed the examiner, took notes regarding her evaluation, and provided immediate feedback to the examiner upon conclusion of the examination. The mean Bayley score for our sample was 80 ($SD = 16.7$).

*Maternal illness-related distress.* Maternal distress related to the child's illness and hospitalization was assessed using the Parental Stressor Scale: Infant Hospitalization (PSS) and the Child Health Worry Scale. The PSS was used to assess perceived hospital environmental stress related to the sights and sounds of the hospital unit, to the infant's behavior and appearance, and to changes in the parental role at enrollment (Miles, 1998). The PSS was adapted from the Parental Stressor Scale: Neonatal Intensive Care Unit developed by Miles, Funk, and Carlson (1993). Items from the original scale were altered to reflect the experiences of parents with hospitalized infants of varying ages who might be hospitalized on any unit of the hospital. On the 22-item PSS, mothers rated their stress on a 5-point scale. A higher score indicated more stress. Cronbach's alpha for the total score was .87. Mean scores at enrollment were 3.8 ($SD = .64$).

The Child Health Worry Scale was used to assess distress related to worry about the child's health (Miles, 1998). Mothers were asked to rate the degree to which they worry about the child's medical problem; about whether the child will be normal, might die, or will always be sick; and about when the parent will be able to take the baby home. In the home version of the tool, the latter item was changed to worry about whether the baby might have to go back to the hospital. Mothers rated their degree of worry on 5 items using a 5-point scale ranging from 1 'not at all' to 5 'very much.' A higher score indicated more worry. Cronbach's alpha was .71 at hospital enrollment and .90 and .85 at 12 and 16 months. The mean score at enrollment was 3.8 ($SD = .87$), and at 12 and 16 months was 2.7 ($SD = 1.2$).

## Data Collection

Infants and parents were recruited from the pediatric and neonatal intensive care units of a tertiary care university medical center. Nurses and physicians helped identify potential infants who met the criteria for enrollment. Parents were then told about the study and what was involved, and those who participated signed an Institutional Review Board-approved consent form.

Data were collected at enrollment in the hospital, at hospital discharge, and when the infants were 6, 12, and 16 months of age, corrected for prematurity if necessary. Table A8–1 displays the variables for the study and the data collection points.

## Data Analysis

All data were entered into a SAS (SAS Institute, Cary, NC) data set and double-checked for accuracy. Multiple regression procedures were used to examine the relationship of predictor variables to maternal depressive symptoms at hospital discharge and maternal developmental impact ratings at 6 months. General linear mixed model analyses were used to examine longitudinally the relationship of predictor variables to depressive symptoms through 12 months and personal developmental impact ratings through 16 months.

Predictor variables for the two multiple regression analyses (depressive symptoms and developmental impact) were identical; all data were collected at enrollment. The variables were: personal characteristics (education, marital status, SOM, and Family Apgar); parental role attainment (MIS and composite scores measuring presence and competence); child illness-related variables of multisystem diagnosis and level of technology dependence during hospitalization; and maternal illness-related distress (PSS and Child Health Worry Scale).

General linear mixed model analyses (hierarchical linear models) were used to examine the relationship of predictor variables to depressive symptoms through 12 months and personal developmental impact ratings through 16 months to include time-varying longitudinal predictors in the analysis. This mixed model analysis allowed us to examine the relationships among dependent and predictor variables, and the way in which these relationships varied

### TABLE A8-1　Data Collection Variables and Times Data Was Obtained

|  | Enrollment | Discharge | 6-months* | 12-months* | 16-months* |
|---|---|---|---|---|---|
| Outcome Variables |  |  |  |  |  |
| CES-D |  | × |  | × |  |
| Personal impact rating |  |  | × |  | × |
| Predictor Variables |  |  |  |  |  |
| *Personal Characteristics* |  |  |  |  |  |
| Demographics** | × |  |  |  |  |
| Sense of mastery | × |  |  | × |  |
| Family Apgar | × |  |  | × |  |
| *Maternal Role Attainment* |  |  |  |  |  |
| Maternal Identity Scale | × |  |  |  |  |
| Maternal presence | × |  | × |  | × |
| Maternal competence | × |  | × |  | × |
| *Infant Illness Characteristics* |  |  |  |  |  |
| Medical record data*** | × |  |  |  |  |
| Technology | × |  |  |  | × |
| Bayley |  |  |  |  | × |
| *Maternal Illness-related Distress* |  |  |  |  |  |
| Parental Stressor Scale | × |  |  |  |  |
| Child health worry | × |  |  | × | × |

*Child age adjusted for prematurity.
**Demographic data were updated at each contact.
***Medical record data were collected weekly during hospitalization, which could have included the 6- and 12-month data collection point for selected children.

over time. The general linear mixed model accounts for irregular timing (unequal time intervals between data points) and/or inconsistent timing (different schedules for different families) of data collection (Andrade & Helms, 1986; Bryk & Raudenbush, 1987; Burchinal, Bailey, & Snyder, 1994; Fairclough & Helms, 1986; Holditch-Davis, Edwards, & Helms, 1998). Time-invariant variables were two personal characteristics (educational level and marital status), MIS at enrollment, presence of a multisystem diagnosis, and the Bayley score at 16 months. Longitudinal (time-varying) variables were SOM, Family Apgar, Maternal Presence and Competence, Child Health Worry Scale, and level of technological dependence. These were similar predictor variables used in the regression with the exception that one additional child illness-related variable was entered—the child's Bayley MDI at 16 months—as an assessment of the child's development, and the PSS

was dropped because it was not thought to be a timely variable. Because of the longitudinal analysis, we added a time effect to determine whether the distress and growth variables differed between the two time points and we added the interactions between time and the longitudinal predictor variables to test whether any of the predictors had a different effect at different time points. No overall statistic can be calculated when a mixed model is computed because there is more than one source of random variability (variability among individual differences in intercepts and slope and due to error). Therefore, only the significance of the individual predictors is reported.

All analyses were conducted by first fitting the whole model; this included all interactions between each predictor and each time point in the mixed model. We used a stepwise backward elimination model based on the size of the p-value to increase interpretability of regression coefficients. Overlap in variance among predictors and interaction terms deflates coefficients, masking associations contributed to the variance accounted for by the model. We first deleted nonsignificant interactions (for the mixed model only) and then iteratively deleted other predictors, starting with the largest p-values, as long as they weren't part of a significant interaction. Decisions about which variables to delete next were based on the results of the most recent model. Time points were always retained in the mixed model to represent the repeated assessment, even if it was nonsignificant.

## RESULTS

### Descriptive Statistics

The mothers' mean CES-D score at hospital discharge was 15.4 ($SD = 12$, range $= 0–52$). The mean at 12 months was 13.6 ($SD = 10$, range $= 0–41$). Forty-five percent of mothers at discharge and 36% at 12 months had CES-D scores above the cutoff score of 16, indicating risk for depression. The mean personal developmental impact rating at 6 months was 4.5 ($SD = 1.3$) which indicated an outcome between neutral and slightly negative. At 16 months, the mean was 5.3 ($SD = 1.3$) which indicated that the average personal developmental impact outcome was between somewhat positive and neutral. At 16 months, only 3 of the 59 mothers were rated at the lowest levels (1 or 2) indicating a definite negative experience, while 31 were rated as having a somewhat or generally positive outcome (6 or 7). The CES-D and personal developmental impact rating were moderately but significantly correlated at the early data collection point ($r = -.39$, $p < .01$) and the final point ($r = -.52$, $p < .001$). Negative personal developmental outcomes were related to more depressive symptoms.

### Relationship of Predictors to Maternal Depression

The regression analysis examining the relationship of predictor variables to depressive symptoms at hospital discharge revealed that only two variables were significant in the full model—mastery and hospital environmental stress. In the reduced model, these variables predicted 25% of the variance (Table A8–2). Lower mastery and higher hospital environmental stress related to more depressive symptoms.

---

**TABLE A8-2** Regression Analysis of Predictors of Depressive Symptoms at Hospital Discharge for 59 Mothers

| | Full Model | | Final Model | |
|---|---|---|---|---|
| | *Beta* | *SE* | *Beta* | *SE* |
| Intercept | 16.00 | 21.0 | 4.77 | 12.2 |
| Maternal education | −0.99 | 0.7 | | |
| Marital status | 0.57 | 3.8 | | |
| Mastery | −6.71* | 3.1 | −6.34* | 2.8 |
| Satisfaction with family | 3.10 | 2.1 | | |
| Parental identity | −2.96 | 6.5 | | |
| Parental presence | 3.22 | 3.1 | | |
| Parental competence | −0.69 | 4.4 | | |
| Multisystem diagnosis | −4.84 | 3.1 | | |
| Technology dependence | 0.38 | 0.5 | | |
| Hospital environmental stress | 6.40* | 2.8 | 7.89** | 2.1 |
| Worry about child's health | 1.62 | 1.9 | | |
| $R^2$ | | | 25% | |

SE = standard error.
*$p < .05$; **$p < .001$.

In the longitudinal analysis of depressive symptoms from hospital discharge to 16 months using general linear mixed models, mastery, satisfaction with family, and worry about the child's health were the only significant predictors in the full model; maternal education was marginally significant. In the reduced model, these four variables were retained and were significant (Table A8–3). The lower the educational level, the lower the mastery, the higher the satisfaction with family, and the more worry about the child's health, the more depressive symptoms reported. There were no significant changes in depressive symptoms over time.

### Relationship of Predictors to Developmental Impact Ratings

In the regression analysis of the personal developmental impact ratings at 6 months, parental presence, multisystem diagnosis, and hospital environmental stress (PSS) were significant in the full model; level of worry about the child's health was marginal. In the reduced model, these four variables were retained. All four variables were significant and predicted 31% of the variance (Table A8–4). Higher levels of parental presence, having a child with a multisystem diagnosis, higher levels of environmental stress, and more worry about the child's health related to a more negative maternal developmental impact.

In the longitudinal analysis of personal developmental impact using general linear mixed models, technology dependence by time, mental development of the child (Bayley scores), and worry about the child's health were significant in the full model. In the reduced model, these same variables were retained plus parental identity and technology dependence which became significant as the model was reduced. Parental identity, mental development, the technology by time interaction, and worry about the child's health were significant. Higher parental identity in the early months of life, lower mental development of the child, and more worry about the child's health were related to a more negative maternal developmental impact. In addition, mothers with infants who were more technology dependent at an early age had a more negative maternal developmental impact. There were no significant changes in maternal developmental impact ratings over time (Table A8–5).

### DISCUSSION

Findings indicate that mothers of medically fragile infants experience both distress and growth as a result of their child's illness. Mean scores on the depression scale at both time points were moderately high and a high percentage of mothers had scores placing them at risk for depressive symptoms. Maternal developmental impact ratings at 6 months were neutral to slightly negative and at 16 months were between neutral and positive. Maternal depressive symptoms and developmental impact ratings were moderately but negatively correlated at 6 and 16 months indicating that higher depressive symptoms were related to more negative developmental impact ratings. While the mean depressive symptom scores and maternal developmental ratings were lower at the later time

---

**TABLE A8-3** Hierarchical Linear Regression of Predictors of Depressive Symptoms at 12 Months on 57 Mothers

| | Final Model | |
| --- | --- | --- |
| | **Beta** | **SE** |
| Intercept | 26.56** | 8.7 |
| Time | 1.52 | 1.8 |
| Maternal education | −0.72* | 0.3 |
| Mastery | −5.72** | 1.7 |
| Satisfaction with family | 2.32* | 1.1 |
| Worry about child's health | 3.15*** | 0.8 |

SE = standard error.
*$p < .05$; **$p < .01$; ***$p < .001$.

TABLE **A8-4** Regression Analysis of Predictors of Maternal Developmental Impact at 6 Months on 67 Mothers

| | Full Model | | Final Model | |
|---|---|---|---|---|
| | *Beta* | *SE* | *Beta* | *SE* |
| Intercept | 9.39*** | 2.0 | 9.01**** | 1.1 |
| Maternal education | −0.08 | 0.1 | | |
| Marital status | 0.08 | 0.4 | | |
| Mastery | 0.08 | 0.3 | | |
| Satisfaction with family | 0.28 | 0.2 | | |
| Parental identity | 0.38 | 0.6 | | |
| Parental presence | 0.64* | 0.3 | 0.60* | 0.3 |
| Parental competence | −0.15 | 0.4 | | |
| Multisystem diagnosis | 0.85* | 0.3 | 0.82** | 0.3 |
| Technology dependence | 0.15 | 0.6 | | |
| Hospital environmental stress | 0.68* | 0.3 | 0.65* | 0.2 |
| Worry about child's health | 0.38† | 0.2 | 0.43* | 0.2 |
| $R^2$ | | | 31% | |

$*p < .05; **p < .01; ***p < .001; ****p < .0001; †p = .07$

TABLE **A8-5** Hierarchical Linear Regression of Predictors of Parental Developmental Impact at 16 Months in 59 Mothers

| | Final Model | |
|---|---|---|
| | *Beta* | *SE* |
| Intercept | 5.84*** | 1.1 |
| Time | 0.37 | 0.4 |
| Parental identity | 1.03* | 0.4 |
| Technology dependence | 0.01 | 0.1 |
| Bayley | 0.03** | 0.0 |
| Worry about child's health | 0.48*** | 0.1 |
| Technology by time | −0.26* | 0.1 |

$*p < .05; **p < .01; ***p < .001.$

points, these differences were not significant. The lower means at later ages may reflect mothers lost to the study whose children were sicker and who subsequently died or mothers who were unduly distressed and withdrew from the study because of interpersonal problems and/or lost custody of the child.

While most mothers had positive outcomes, there was a group of mothers with negative outcomes at 12 to 16 months. Almost half of the mothers at discharge (45%) and about a third of the mothers at 12 months (36%) had CES-D scores at or above the risk score for serious depression. In addition, 3 mothers were rated on the personal developmental impact scale as having a definite negative developmental change. This supports previous research that found mothers of chronically ill children at risk for emotional distress (Bristol et al., 1988; Cadman et al., 1991; Jessop et al., 1988; Kronenberger & Thompson, 1992; Wallander, Varni, Babani, Banis et al., 1989).

The finding of developmental growth in mothers, despite the distress associated with caring for a medically fragile infant, supports the view that personal growth may be the outcome of struggling with a serious life event such as illness. Antonovsky (1987) suggests that positive outcomes help to make stressors more understandable and meaningful. Tedeschi and Calhoun (1995) propose that personal growth frequently results from significant trauma as a result of the process of rumination and positive revision of one's schemas. Janoff-Bulman (1992) also suggests that tragedy shatters one's basic schemas about life and, as they are rebuilt over time, they often include increased wisdom and empathy. Recently, Folkman (1997) reported that positive mood states occur in caregivers of gay males with AIDS.

While depressive symptoms and personal developmental impacts were moderately correlated, these outcomes had different patterns of predictors. Distress was influenced by maternal characteristics personal sense of mastery, maternal education, satisfaction with family, and maternal illness-related distress; hospital environmental stress; and worry about the child's health. Growth was influenced by characteristics of the child's illness multisystem diagnosis, cognitive development, and technology; maternal illness-related distress—hospital environmental stress and worry about the child's health; and level of maternal role attainment, identity, and competence. These findings support the transactional model of stress that suggests that personal, family, and situational factors influence outcomes in a stressful situation (Lazarus & Folkman, 1984; Schaefer & Moos, 1992).

It is not surprising that lower mastery and higher education were related to depressive symptoms at both time periods. Other investigators have found an association between mastery and educational level and depressive symptoms (Ensel, 1985; Myers & Weissman, 1980; Pearlin et al., 1981; Roberts & Vernon, 1983). In contrast, higher satisfaction with family predicted depressive symptoms at 12 months. It is not known whether families of mothers who were more depressed provided more satisfactory support as a result or whether there is something about family support that contributes to depressive symptoms in these mothers.

It is interesting that distress associated with the child's hospitalization was related to more depressive symptoms at hospital discharge and more negative personal developmental impact ratings at 6 months. Distress associated with worry about the child's health was also associated with depressive symptoms at 12 months and more negative maternal developmental impact ratings at 6 and 16 months. This suggests that mothers may experience sequelae from the distress associated with their infant's illness and hospitalization following hospital discharge. These findings are similar to those of other investigators who found that mothers of prematurely born children continue to recall distressful aspects of their infant's illness for many months and years afterward (Affleck, Tennen, Rowe, & Higgins, 1990; Wereszczak, Miles, & Holditch-Davis, 1997). The severity of the child's ongoing health problems also affected maternal growth. Mothers who had infants with a multisystem diagnosis had more negative developmental impacts at 6 months, and mothers whose children had lower mental development and more technology at an early age had more negative developmental impact ratings at 16 months. These findings support those of other investigators who found that characteristics of the child's chronic illness affected maternal outcomes (Cowen et al., 1986; Jessop et al., 1988).

Maternal role attainment had no impact on depressive symptoms, but maternal presence and maternal identity had an impact on maternal developmental impact. Maternal identity in early infancy predicted maternal developmental impact at 16 months, and maternal presence predicted maternal developmental impact at 16 months. However, parental competence did not have an impact on outcomes. Thus, it appears that some mothers can be competent but do so at a personal cost, whereas other mothers can be competent and have a growth experience.

The triangulation of data collection methods used in this study is important when studying complex phenomena such as parenting a seriously ill child. The study was unique in measuring both distress and growth as aspects of adjustment in mothers of medically fragile infants. However, there were limitations in using only one measure of distress and one of growth. Measuring only depressive symptoms as a measure of distress may not capture other aspects of distress that are important. In addition, while the measure of growth was assessed as objectively as possible by the research team based on their extensive observations of and interviews with the mothers over time, there still likely was some bias in the ratings. It is recommended that future studies use additional measures of distress such as measures of anxiety and mood disturbance, and also use a valid and reliable self-report measure of growth in order to assess the mothers' own perspective about her developmental impact. It is also recommended that distress and growth variables be measured longitudinally as in this study. Results of this study need to be considered with caution due to the relatively small sample size; chance associations with a small sample can limit the generalizability of findings. Thus, replication of this study with another larger sample is recommended.

Findings from this study support the need to develop interventions to help mothers of critically ill infants during hospitalization and following the hospital discharge when mothers are caring for the sick child. During hospitalization, mothers need interventions that reduce the stress they experience related to seeing their sick child undergoing treatment, changes in the expected maternal role and the overall sights and sounds of the hospital environment, and interventions that help them achieve their identity as the mother of the child. After discharge, mothers may continue to need help through reflective debriefing regarding their recall of these stressful experiences. Both during hospitalization and after discharge, mothers should be encouraged to share their worries about their sick child and should be given information and hope that realistically reduces worry about their child's health. Additionally, mothers with less education and lower levels of perceived control (mastery) should be assessed for depressive symptoms. These mothers may need additional support from nurses and other healthcare professionals throughout their child's illness to reduce their distress. Additionally, mothers of children who are more technology dependent particularly during the early months of life, children who have multisystem health problems, and/or children showing cognitive delays need nursing interventions to help them cope with the ongoing care of their child while also meeting their own personal needs.

## References

Affleck, G., & Tennen, H. (1993). Cognitive adaptation to adversity: Insights from parents of medically fragile children. In A. P. Turnbull et al. (Eds.), *Cognitive coping, families and disability* (pp. 135–150). Baltimore, MD: Brookes.

Affleck, G., Tennen, H., Rowe, J., & Higgins, P. (1990). Mothers' remembrances of newborn intensive care: A predictive study. *Journal of Pediatric Psychology, 15,* 67–81.

Anderson, J. M., & Elfert, H. (1989). Managing chronic illness in the family: Women as caretakers. *Journal of Advanced Nursing, 14,* 735–743.

Andrade, D. A., & Helms, R. W. (1986). ML estimation and LR tests for the multivariate normal distribution with general linear model mean and linear-structure covariance matrix: K-population, complete data case. *Communications in Statistics-Theory and Methods, 13,* 89–108.

Antonovsky, A. (1987). *Unraveling the mystery of health: How people manage stress and stay well.* San Francisco, CA: Jossey-Bass.

Bayley, N. (1993). *Manual for the Bayley Scales of Infant Development* (2nd ed). San Antonio: Psychological Corporation.

Bradley, R. (1989). The HOME Inventory: A review of the first 15 years. In N. J. Anastasiow, W. K. Frankenburg, & A. Fandel (Eds.), *Identifying the developmentally delayed child.* Baltimore, MD: University Park.

Bradley, R. H., Rock, S. L., Caldwell, B. M., & Brisby, J. A. (1989). Uses of the HOME Inventory for families with handicapped children. *American Journal of Mental Retardation, 94,* 313–330.

Bristol, M. M., Gallagher, J. J., & Schopler, E. (1988). Mothers and fathers of young developmentally disabled and nondisabled boys: Adaptation and spousal support. *Developmental Psychology, 24,* 441–451.

Bryk, A. S., & Raudenbush, S. W. (1987). Application of hierarchical linear models to assessing change. *Psychological Bulletin, 101,* 147–158.

Burchinal, M. R., Bailey, D. B., & Snyder, P. (1994). Using growth curve analysis to evaluate child change in longitudinal investigations. *Journal of Early Intervention, 18,* 403–423.

Cadman, D., Rosenbaum, P., Boyle, M., & Offord, D. R. (1991). Children with chronic illness: Family and parent demographic characteristics and psychosocial adjustment. *Pediatrics, 87,* 884–889.

Caldwell, B., & Bradley, R. (1984). *Home observation for measurement of the environment.* Little Rock, AR: University of Arkansas at Little Rock.

Cowen, L., Mok, J., Corey, M., McMillan, H., Simmons, R., & Levinson, H. (1986). Psychologic adjustment of the family with a member who has cystic fibrosis. *Pediatrics, 77,* 745–753.

Deatrick, J. A., & Knafl, K. A. (1990). Management behaviors: Day-to-day adjustments to childhood chronic conditions. *Journal of Pediatric Nursing, 5,* 15–22.

Diehl, S. F., Moffitt, K. A., & Wade, S. M. (1991). Focus group interview with parents of children with medically complex needs: An intimate look at their perceptions and feelings. *Children's Health Care, 20,* 170–178.

Ensel, W. M. (1985). Sex differences in the epidemiology of depression and physical illness: A sociological perspective. In A. Dean (Ed.), *Depression in multidisciplinary perspective* (pp. 83–102). New York, NY: Brunner/Mazel.

Fairclough, D. L., & Helms, R. W. (1986). A mixed linear model with linear covariance structure: A sensitivity analysis of the maximum likelihood estimators. *Journal of Statistical Computation and Simulation, 25,* 205–236.

Fleming, J., Challela, M., Eland, J., Hornick, R., Johnson, P., Martinson, I., Nativio, D., Nokes, K., Riddle, I., Steele, N., Sudela, K., Thomas, R., Turner, Q., Wheller, B., & Young, A. (1994). Impact on the family of children who are technology dependent and cared for in the home. *Pediatric Nursing, 20,* 379–388.

Fogel, C. (1992). *Fogel inventory of maternal identity.* Unpublished instrument manual.

Folkman, S. (1997). Positive psychological states and coping with severe stress. *Social Science and Medicine, 45,* 1207–1221.

Gennaro, S., York, R., & Brooten, D. (1990). Anxiety and depression in mothers of low birthweight and very low birth-weight infants: Birth through 5 months. *Issues in Comprehensive Pediatric Nursing, 13,* 97–109.

Goldberg, S., Morris, P., Simmons, R. J., Fowler, R. S., & Levison, H. (1990). Chronic illness in infancy and parenting stress: A comparison of three groups of parents. *Journal of Pediatric Psychology, 15,* 347–358.

Hauenstein, E. J. (1990). The experience of distress in parents of chronically ill children: Potential or likely outcome? *Journal of Clinical Child Psychology, 19,* 356–364.

Hinds, P. S. (1989). Method triangulation to index change in clinical phenomena. *Western Journal of Nursing Research, 11,* 440–447.

Holaday, B. (1981). Maternal response to their chronically ill infants' attachment behavior of crying. *Nursing Research, 30,* 343–348.

Holditch-Davis, D., & Thoman, E. B. (1988). The early social environment of premature and full-term infants. *Early Human Development, 17,* 221–232.

Holditch-Davis, D., Sandelowski, M., & Harris, B. G. (1998). Infertility and early parent-infant interactions. *Journal of Advanced Nursing, 27,* 99–101.

Holditch-Davis, D., Edwards, L. J., & Helms, R. W. (1998). Modeling development of sleep-wake behaviors: I. Using the mixed general linear model. *Physiology and Behavior, 63,* 311–318.

Holditch-Davis, D., Tesh, E. M., Burchinal, M., & Miles, M. S. (1999). Early interactions between mothers and their medically fragile infants. *Applied Developmental Science, 3,* 155–167.

Janoff-Bulman, R. (1992). *Shattered assumptions: Towards a new psychology of trauma.* New York: Free Press.

Jessop, D. J., Riessman, C. K., & Stein, R. E. K. (1988). Chronic childhood illness and maternal mental health. *Journal of Developmental and Behavioral Pediatrics, 9,* 147–155.

Kazak, A. E., Reber, M., & Carter, A. (1988). Structural and qualitative aspects of social networks in families with young chronically ill children. *Journal of Pediatric Psychology, 13,* 171–182.

Kronenberger, W. G., & Thompson, R. J., Jr. (1992). Medical stress, appraised stress, and the psychological adjustment of mothers of children with myelomeningocele. *Journal of Developmental and Behavioral Pediatrics, 13,* 405–411.

Lawson, K. R., Koller, H., Rose, S. A., & McCarton, C. (1996, April). Relationships between early assessments and outcome for extremely low birthweight infants. Poster presented at the tenth biennial International

Conference on Infant Studies, Providence, RI. (Abstract published in *Infant Behavior and Development,* Special ICIS Issue, 19, 564).

Lazarus, R. S., & Folkman, S. (1984). *Stress, appraisal, and coping.* New York: Springer.

Leonard, B. J., Brust, J. D., & Nelson, R. P. (1993). Parental distress: Caring for medically fragile children at home. *Journal of Pediatric Nursing, 8,* 22–30.

Leonberg, G. L., Chuang, E., Eicher, P., Tershakovec, A. M., Leonard, L., & Stallings, V. A. (1998). Long-term growth and development in children after home parental nutrition. *Journal of Pediatrics, 132,* 461–466.

Lobo, M. L. (1992). Parent-infant interaction during feeding when the infant has congenital heart disease. *Journal of Pediatric Nursing, 7,* 97–105.

Mercer, R. T. (1995). *Becoming a mother: Research on maternal identity from Rubin to the present.* New York: Springer.

Meyer, E. C., Garcia Coll, C. T., Seifer, R., Ramos, A., Kilis, E., & Oh, W. (1995). Psychological distress in mothers of preterm infants. *Journal of Developmental and Behavioral Pediatrics, 16,* 412–417.

Miles, M. S., & Frauman, A. (1993). Barriers and bridges: Nurses' and parents' negotiations of caregiving roles for medically fragile infants. In S. G. Funk, E. M. Tornquist, M. T. Champagne, & R. A. Weise (Eds.), *Key aspects of caring for the chronically ill: Hospital and home* (pp. 239–249). New York: Springer.

Miles, M. S. (1998). *Parental role attainment with medically fragile infants.* Grant Report to the National Institute of Nursing Research, National Institute of Health.

Miles, M. S., Funk, S. G., & Carlson, J. (1993). Parental Stressor Scale: Neonatal Intensive Care Unit. *Nursing Research, 42,* 148–152.

Miles, M. S., & D'Auria, J. (1994). Parenting the medically fragile infant. *Capsules & Comments in Pediatric Nursing, 1,* 2–6.

Miles, M. S., D'Auria, J., Hart, E. M., Sedlack, D. A., & Watral, M. A. (1993). Parental role alterations experienced by mothers of children with a life-threatening chronic illness. In S. Funk, E. M. Tornquist, M. T. Champagne, & R. A. Wiese (Eds.), *Key aspects of caring for the chronically ill: Home and hospital* (pp. 281–289). New York: Springer.

Miles, M. S., Funk, S. G., & Kasper, M. A. (1992). The stress response of mothers and fathers of preterm infants. *Research in Nursing and Health, 15,* 261–269.

Mullins, L. L., Olson, R. A., Reyes, S., Bernardy, N., Huszti, H. C., & Volk, R. J. (1991). Risk and resistance factors in the adaptation of mothers of children with cystic fibrosis. *Journal of Pediatric Psychology, 16,* 701–715.

Myers, J. K., & Weissman, M. M. (1980). Use of a self-report symptom scale to detect depression in a community sample. *American Journal of Psychiatry, 137,* 1081–1084.

O'Neill, G., & Ross, M. M. (1991). Burden of care: An important concept for nurses. *Health Care for Women International, 12,* 111–121.

Odom, S. L., & Chandler, L. (1990). Transition to parenthood for parents of technology-assisted infants. *Topics in Early Childhood Special Education, 9*(4), 43–54.

Office of Technology Assessment. (1987). *Technology-dependent children: Hospital vs. home care* (OTA-TM-H-38). Washington DC: U.S. Government Printing Office.

Park, C. L., Cohen, L. H., & Murch, R. L. (1996). Assessment and prediction of stress-related growth. *Journal of Personality, 64,* 71–105.

Patterson, J. M., Leonard, B. J., & Titus, J. C. (1992). Home care for medically fragile children: Impact on family health and well-being. *Journal of Developmental and Behavioral Pediatrics, 13,* 248–255.

Pearlin, L. I., Lieberman, M. A., Menaghan, E. G., & Mullan, J. T. (1981). The stress process. *Journal of Health and Social Behavior, 22,* 337–356.

Pearlin, L. I., Mullan, J. T., Semple, S. J., & Skaff, M. M. (1990). Caregiving and the stress process: An overview of concepts and their measures. *Gerontologist, 30,* 583–594.

Piecuch, R. E., Leonard, C. H., Cooper, B. A., & Sehring, S. A. (1997). Outcome of extremely low birth weight infants (500 to 999 grams) over a 12-year period. *Pediatrics, 100,* 633–639.

Pridham, K. F., Martin, R., Sondel, S., & Tluczek, A. (1989). Parental issues in feeding young children with bronchopulmonary dysplasia. *Journal of Pediatric Nursing, 4,* 177–185.

Radloff, L. S. (1977). The CES-D Scale: A self-report depression scale for research in the general population. *Applied Psychological Measurement, 1,* 385–401.

Ray, L. D., & Ritchie, J. A. (1993). Caring for chronically ill children at home: Factors that influence parents' coping. *Journal of Pediatric Nursing, 8,* 217–225.

Roberts, R. E., & Vernon, S. W. (1983). The Center for Epidemiologic Studies Depression Scale: Its use in a community sample. *American Journal of Psychiatry, 140,* 41–46.

Rubin, R. (1984). *Maternal identity and the maternal experience.* New York: Springer.

Schaeffer, J., & Moos, R. (1992). Life crises and personal growth. In B. N. Carpenter (Ed.), *Personal coping: Theory, research, and application* (pp. 159–170). Westport, CT: Praeger.

Singer, L. T., Kercsmar, C., Legris, G., Orlowski, J. P., Hill, B. P., & Doershuk, C. (1989). Developmental sequelae of long-term infant tracheostomy. *Developmental Medicine and Child Neurology, 31,* 224–230.

Singer, L., & Farkas, K. J. (1989). The impact of infant disability on maternal perception of stress. *Family Relations, 38,* 444–449.

Singer, L., Yamashita, T., Lilien, L., Collin, M., & Baley, J. (1997). A longitudinal study of developmental outcome of infants with bronchopulmonary dysplasia and very low birth weight. *Pediatrics, 100,* 987–993.

Smilkstein, G., Ashworth, C., & Montano, D. (1982). Validity and reliability of the family APGAR as a test of family function. *Journal of Family Practice, 15,* 303–311.

Sterling, Y. M., Jones, L. C., Johnson, D. H., & Bowen, M. R. (1996). Parents' resources and home management of the care of chronically ill infants. *Journal of the Society of Pediatric Nurses, 1,* 103–109.

Svavarsdottir, E. K., & McCubbin, M. (1996). Parenthood transition for parents of an infant diagnosed with a congenital heart condition. *Journal of Pediatric Nursing, 11,* 207–216.

Tedeschi, R. G., & Calhoun, L. G. (1995). *Trauma and transformation: Growing in the aftermath of suffering.* Thousand Oaks, CA: Sage.

Tesh, E. M., & Holditch-Davis, D. (1997). HOME Inventory and NCATS: Relation to mother and child behaviors during naturalistic observation. *Research in Nursing and Health, 20,* 295–307.

Thoman, E. B., Becker, P. T., & Freese, M. P. (1978). Individual patterns of mother-infant interactions. In G. P. Sackett (Ed.), *Observing behavior, Vol I: Theory and applications in mental retardation* (pp. 95–114). Baltimore, MD: University Park Press.

Thompson, R. J., Jr., Gil, K. M., Burbach, D. J., Keith, B. R., & Kinney, T. R. (1993). Psychological adjustment of mothers of children and adolescents with sickle cell disease: The role of stress, coping methods, and family functioning. *Journal of Pediatric Psychology, 18,* 549–559.

Thompson, R. J., Gustafson, K. E., Hamlett, K. W., & Spock, A. (1992). Stress, coping, and family functioning in the psychological adjustment of mothers of children and adolescents with cystic fibrosis. *Journal of Pediatric Psychology, 17,* 573–585.

Van Riper, M., Ryff, C., & Pridham, K. (1992). Parental and family well-being in families of children with Down syndrome: A comparative study. *Research in Nursing and Health, 15,* 227–235.

Wallander, J. L., Varni, J. W., Babani, L., Banis, H. T., & Wilcox, K. T. (1989). Family resources as resistance factors for psychological maladjustment in chronically ill and handicapped children. *Journal of Pediatric Psychology, 14,* 157–173.

Wallander, J. L., Varni, J. W., Babani, L., DeHaan, C. B., Wilcox, K. T., & Banis, H. T. (1989). The social environment and the adaptation of mothers of physically handicapped children. *Journal of Pediatric Psychology, 14,* 371–387.

Walker, L. O., Crain, H., & Thompson, E. (1986). Mothering behavior and maternal role attainment during the postpartum period. *Nursing Research, 35,* 352–355.

Wereszczak, J., Miles, M. S., & Holditch-Davis, D. (1997). Maternal recall of the neonatal intensive care unit. *Neonatal Networks, 16*(4), 33–40.

Young, L. Y., Creighton, D. E., & Sauve, R. S. (1988). The needs of families of infants discharged home with continuous oxygen therapy. *Journal of Obstetric, Gynecologic, and Neonatal Nursing, 17,* 187–193.

# Exercise in Heart Failure: A Synthesis of Current Research

**Cynthia D. Adams, Susan Bennett**

## ABSTRACT

*(1) Exercise intolerance, as a hallmark symptom in patients with heart failure, has been the focus of numerous research initiatives in recent years. The purpose of this review is to synthesize the current literature in order to provide the clinician with an understanding of the state of knowledge regarding the role of exercise in treatment of heart failure. Many studies speak to the effect of exercise training in this population. While sample sizes have been small and restricted predominantly to male subjects with ischemic cardiomyopathies, strong support has been documented in favor of beneficial effects of exercise in heart failure. Future research should target more representative subject pools (i.e., families, non-ischemic cardiomyopathies, cultural minorities, frail elderly, and NYHA class IV), evaluation of impact on quality of life outcomes, exploration of different types and intensity of exercise, and formulation of specific activity prescription tools which can guide practitioners in making activity and/or exercise recommendations to those patients who have no access, or limited access, to cardiac rehabilitation programs.*

## STATEMENT OF THE PRACTICE PROBLEM

(2) Exercise intolerance is a major limiting factor in terms of functional status and quality of life for patients with heart failure and presents a frustrating and complicated problem for practitioners managing their care. Pharmacologic treatment is most often the focus in the large, well-funded research initiatives, which determine state of the art treatment of heart failure. Advances in pharmacologic treatment over the past decade have shown significant improvements in survival and quality of life in heart failure. Nonpharmacologic treatments such as activity recommendations and patient education, on the other hand, often continue to reflect the beliefs of the early models of heart failure, and their potential additive effect on survival and quality of life are too often overlooked. The importance of the role of nursing in advancing knowledge and research in this area cannot be overstated.

(3) Over the past decades, there have been major changes in the philosophy underlying treatment and management of heart failure (CHF). In a recent synopsis of the philosophical and physiological evolution of the conceptual model of heart failure over the past 50 years, Packer (1993 [45]) highlights the paradigm shifts, which have taken place with regard to the pathological processes and treatments associated with the heart failure syndrome. In the early years, management of CHF was designed to rid the body of excess water and attempt to strengthen the heartbeat by use of digitalis and diuretics. Bed rest was often prescribed to allow rest for the heart, and to promote

*The Online Journal of Knowledge Synthesis for Nursing, Volume 7, February 9, 2000, Document Number 5*

diuresis in fluid overloaded patients (Sullivan & Hawthorne, 1996 [48]). As hemodynamic measurement became more accessible, attention shifted to reducing preload and afterload to optimize cardiac output. The use of vasodilators and inotropic agents emerged during this period. In the late 1980s and early 90s, the theory of neurohormonal activation has been introduced, as the mortality and morbidity reduction resulting from ACE inhibition and beta blockade have been discovered (Packer, 1993 [45]). As a result of this evolutionary shift, other major advances have come to light which clarify the role of biochemical compensatory mechanisms resulting in increased norepinephrine levels, altered gene expression, down-regulation of sympathetic receptor sites, impairment of oxidative capacity of skeletal muscle cells, and vascular remodeling (Balady & Pina, 1997 [5]; Sullivan & Hawthorne, 1996 [48]; Hosenpud & Greenbert, 1994 [22]; Patterson & Adams, 1996 [46]).

(4) Recent advances have made it possible to better understand the etiology and pathophysiology which results in reduced exercise capacity and potential benefits of maximizing physical activity, and even aerobic training. The purpose of this paper is to review the literature related to the role of exercise in heart failure, synthesize the findings to identify implications for further research, and determine the degree of clinical applicability which exists in the conclusions drawn.

## SUMMARY OF RESEARCH
### Pathophysiology of Exercise Intolerance in CHF

(5) Exercise intolerance is a well-known component of the syndrome of heart failure. Historically, excessive muscle fatigue and breathlessness were felt to be a result of inadequate perfusion of skeletal muscle and end organs due to impaired cardiac output. Recent studies have revealed intrinsic changes in skeletal muscle fibers which may be responsible for impaired metabolism and result in early muscle fatigue. These changes include reduced mitochondrial density, reduction in lipolytic oxidative enzymes, and fiber atrophy (Coats, 1993 [11]; Mancini et al., 1992 [33]; Minotti & Massie, 1992 [42]; Wilson, Mancini, & Dunkman, 1993 [51]). In addition to these intrinsic changes, underperfusion secondary to impaired regional blood flow in CHF may be a contributing factor (Braith & Mills, 1994 [8]). A differential shunting of cardiac output in CHF results in reduction in maximal skeletal-muscle flow during exercise. Long-term ACE inhibitor and vasodilator therapy are believed to increase peripheral perfusion and have a favorable effect on skeletal muscle blood flow (Braith & Mills, 1994 [8]).

(6) While deconditioning of peripheral musculature due to inactivity may play a role in exercise intolerance, there have been key differences noted at the cellular level between muscle cells of deconditioned "healthy" subjects, and those of patients with CHF (Minotti & Massie, 1992 [42]). Some of these changes include cellular atrophy restricted to type II fibers in CHF, which is in contrast to the generalized changes in all fiber types in disuse (Massie & Camacho, 1995 [34]), and specific mitochondrial changes (Minotti & Massie, 1992 [42]).

### Exercise Testing and Interpretation of Data

(7) The historically accepted measure of cardiorespiratory endurance is the direct measure of peak oxygen uptake (VO2max) during performance of exercise of increasing intensity (American College of Sports Medicine [ACSM], 1995 [3]). Studies have shown a strong correlation between systemic VO2max and survival in CHF (Braith & Mills, 1994 [8]). In addition to serving as a measure of functional status, VO2max is utilized as an indicator for the appropriateness and timing of cardiac transplantation (Cahalin, 1996 [10]). Peak oxygen consumption is the maximum amount of oxygen a subject uses while performing dynamic exercise involving a large portion of the total muscle mass (ACSM, 1995 [3]; Fletcher, Froelicher, Hartley, Haskell, & Pollock, 1990 [18]). For reporting purposes, VO2max values are generally expressed relative to body weight in units of ml/kg/min. For clinically interpretive purposes, a VO2max of less than or equal to 14 ml/kg/min is a predictor of poor survival, and the point at which cardiac transplantation, if other candidacy criteria are met, becomes a considerable option (Mehra, Lavie, & Milani, 1996 [37]).

(8) Oxygen uptake depends on diffusion capacity in the lung, transportation via circulation, peripheral perfusion and diffusion, and mitochondrial function in the cells (Moran, 1996 [43]). Factors which affect VO2max are age, gender, physical condition, heredity, and cardiovascular disease (Fletcher et al., 1996 [17]). Women have a lower VO2max than men, and there is an estimated decrease of 5–9% per decade of life. It is estimated that VO2max decreases approximately 25% after 3 weeks of bed rest in healthy men (Fletcher et al., 1990 [18]).

(9) In exercise testing and cardiac rehabilitation arenas, oxygen uptake is also commonly expressed in terms of metabolic equivalents, or METs. One MET is the average estimate of sitting, resting oxygen uptake (VO2 equal to 3.5 ml/kg/min). Two and four METs correspond with oxygen uptake at two and four miles per hour, respectively. Maximal oxygen uptake of less than five METs at peak exercise is as-

sociated with poor prognosis, and is equivalent to the activities of daily living. Ten METs is associated with prognosis similar to coronary bypass surgery. Thirteen METs at peak exercise is associated with excellent prognosis. METs of 18–20 are seen in elite and world class athletes (Fletcher et al., 1990 [18]).

(10) Direct measurement of peak oxygen consumption requires use of maximal exercise testing. This testing requires use of specialized equipment such as a treadmill or stationary bike. Continuous ECG monitoring is performed, as well as respiratory gas analysis to determine the oxygen consumption. This testing can be costly in terms of equipment as well as personnel resources (ACSM, 1995 [3]). There has been substantial support in the literature to suggest that the six-minute walk test may be useful in estimating functional capacity, as well as short-term survival, at a much lower cost, and can place much less strain on the patient (Cahalin et al., 1996 [9]; Faggiano, D'Aloia, Gualeni, Lavatelli & Giordano, 1997 [16]; Mehra et al., 1996 [37]; Milligan, Havey, & Dossa, 1997 [41]; Peters & Mets, 1996 [47]). The six-minute walk test is a self-paced, submaximal corridor walk during which duration of time and distance walked are measured, as well as the perceived exertion (Guyatt et al., 1985 [19]). Patients walk at their own pace, and stop for rest periods as needed throughout the test. This test has not been shown to correlate closely with maximal testing, but appears to be a better indicator of functional capacity with regard to activities of daily living (Cahalin et al., 1996 [9]; Mehra et al., 1996 [37]). Additionally, it has been suggested that abnormalities contributing to performance of maximal exercise may differ from those affecting submaximal performance (Balady & Pina, 1997 [5]).

(11) It has been repeatedly shown throughout the literature that ejection fraction has not been found to be a reliable predictor of functional capacity or survival (Braith & Mills, 1994 [8]; Mayou, Blackwood, Bryant, & Garnham, 1991 [35]; Moran, 1996 [43]). Rather, exercise capacity is the result of complex physiological interactions which eludes measurement by any single resting parameter (Balady & Pina, 1997 [5]).

## Exercise Training in Heart Failure

(12) Many studies have been published which demonstrate the benefit of exercise training in heart failure patients. This review targets research published within the past five years. However, the early hallmark studies which first suggested benefit from exercise in heart failure are widely cited throughout these studies, and therefore, were included in this discussion. Details of each of the selected studies are summarized in Table A9–1.

(13) Early studies from Duke University demonstrated improvement in exercise capacity in 12 patients with ejection fractions of 13–25%, New York Heart Association (NYHA) classification I–III, after 4–6 months of exercise conditioning (Sullivan, Higginbotham, & Cobb, 1988 [49]). Patients were trained at 75% of VO2max 60 minutes per session, 3–5 times weekly. The VO2max increased from 16.8 +/- 3.7 ml/kg/min to 20.6 +/- 4.7 ml/kg/min ($p < 0.01$) and functional class improved from NYHA class 2.4 +/- 0.6 to 1.3 +/- 0.7. Additionally, there were no reported exercise-related complications. Cardiac output showed no change at submaximal exercise, but did increase at maximal exercise. Heart rate was reduced at rest and submaximal exercise, but did not change at maximal exercise. There were no significant changes found in measurable cardiac function or size after training. Additional findings included increased blood flow and oxygen delivery to the leg, measured by thermodilution, reduction in arterial and venous lactate production, and an increase in exercise time at the fixed submaximal work rate (Sullivan et al., 1988 [49]).

(14) Coats and associates (1992 [12]) studied 17 men with stable moderate to severe CHF in the first prospective, controlled study of exercise in heart failure. A controlled crossover design was utilized and subjects were randomly assigned to begin in either the exercise or activity restriction phases. Findings demonstrated significant increases in exercise tolerance and peak oxygen consumption compared to control condition. There was an increase in cardiac output at submaximal and peak exercise, as well as a reduction in systemic vascular resistance. An important finding in this study was the demonstrated empirical support for enhancement of vagal tone, and reduction in sympathetic activity after training in these individuals (Coats et al., 1992 [12]).

(15) Meyer et al. published three random order crossover trials which support the benefit of interval training and associated short-term effects in 18 male patients. Significant improvements in VO2max were documented. An important observation in Meyer's studies was a rapid detraining effect which occurred in the restricted group after crossover from the training phase. These studies support the potential value of interval training as an alternative to a continuous aerobic training program. It is suggested that interval training, referring to short bouts of intense exercise alternating with frequent rest periods, may provide desired training effects with less strain on the heart than prolonged aerobic regimens (Meyer, Görnandt, et al., 1997 [38]; Meyer, Samek, et al., 1997 [39]; Meyer, Schwaibold, et al., 1996 [40]).

(16) Adamopoulos et al. performed a controlled, random order crossover study involving 12 patients

**TABLE A9-1** Clinical Trials of Exercise in Heart Failure

| Study | N | Design/ Pt. Selection | Training Program | Duration | Findings/Comments |
|---|---|---|---|---|---|
| Sullivan et al. (1988 [49]) | 12 | Non-randomized, no control group; EF 9–33% | Cycle, walking, jogging, stair climbing 60 min 3–5×/week | 16–24 weeks | Peak VO2 increased 23% |
| Jugdutt et al. (1988 [24]) | 46 | Non-randomized, control group; EF 36–63% | 11 min/day calisthenics and stationary run | 12 weeks | Increased total work; Increased LV asynergy; LVEF decreased from 43% to 30% |
| Arvan (1988 [4]) | 25 | Non-randomized, no control group; 12 week post MI EF<40% | Cycle, treadmill, arm ergometer 30–45 min 3×/week; 75–85% of peak VO2 | 12 weeks | Exercise time increased; No significant increase in peak VO2 |
| Jette et al. (1991 [23]) | 39 | Randomized, controlled; 10 weeks post MI; no prior | In hospital program; jog, calisthenics, relaxation, cycling; 70–80% peak; 30–60 min b.i.d. | 4 weeks | No change in EF Increase in peak VO2 |
| Koch et al. (1992 [29]) | 25 | Randomized, controlled; EF approx. 26%; NYHA II-III | 40 1 1/2 hour sessions isolating small muscle groups; graded exercise regimen | 3 months | All functional parameters improved; No adverse events; No change EF; Quality of life scores improved 52–63% |
| Coats et al. (1992 [12]) | 17 | Randomized, crossover, controlled; ischemic | Home-based; bicycle 20 minutes (50 rpms) 5×/week; 60–80% peak heart rate | 8 weeks | Exercise time increased, peak VO2 increased by 2.4 ml/min/kg; Improved symptoms; Reduced sympathetic tone |
| Adamopoulos et al. (1993 [1]) | 12 | Randomized, crossover, controlled | Home-based, bicycle 20 minutes 5×/week; 70–80% peak heart rate | 8 weeks | Correction of impaired skeletal muscle oxidative capacity |

**TABLE A9-1** Clinical Trials of Exercise in Heart Failure (Continued)

| Study | N | Design/ Pt. Selection | Training Program | Duration | Findings/Comments |
|---|---|---|---|---|---|
| Kataoka et al. (1994 [25]) | 1 | Case study; continuous dobutamine infusion | Treadmill, cycle, rowing, arm ergometer, stairs 42 min 3×/week; supervised regimen | 32 weeks | Absolute peak VO2 increased 19%; Resting HR decreased 10 bpm; Norepinephrine level decreased; Enabled discontinuance of infusion |
| Mancini et al. (1995 [32]) | 14 | Non-randomized, no control group; EF approx. 23%; NYHA I-IV | Specified respiratory muscle training regimen | 12 weeks | Submaximal and maximal exercise capacity improved; 6-minute walk test and peak VO2 improved; Dyspnea subjectively improved |
| Hambrecht et al. (1995 [20]) | 10 | Randomized, controlled; EF 12–35% | Ambulatory training | 26 weeks | 31% improvement in peak VO2; Improved ventilatory threshold; Improved cellular metabolism |
| Belardinelli et al. (1995 [7]) | 27 | Matched groups by clinical and functional status; mild CHF | 30 min cycle at 40% peak VO2; 3×/week | 8 weeks | 17% increase in peak VO2; Improved lactic acid threshold; Improved peak work load; Decreased norepinephrine levels; Improved oxidative capacity; No serious adverse events |
| Kiilavuori et al. (1996 [28]) | 27 | Randomized, controlled; NYHA II-III EF<40% | 30 min 3×/week, cycle; 50–60% peak VO2 | 12 weeks supervised; 12 weeks at home | NYHA 2.4 to 1.9 at 12 weeks; 12% increase in peak VO2 (NS); Increased maximal achieved work load (p<0.05); Symptom improvement; Improvement in submaximal endurance |

**TABLE A9-1** Clinical Trials of Exercise in Heart Failure (Continued)

| Study | N | Design/<br>Pt. Selection | Training Program | Duration | Findings/Comments |
|---|---|---|---|---|---|
| Keteyian et al. (1996 [27]) | 40 | Randomized, controlled; all male subjects | 33 min aerobic with various equipment; 3×/week; 60–80% peak VO2 | 24 weeks | 16.3% increase in absolute peak VO2; 46% improved peak VO2 due to increased peak heart rate; 85% of improvement occurred by week 12; Reversal of chrono-tropic incompetence |
| Kavanagh et al. (1996 [26]) | 21 | Non-randomized; control with initial 9-week period; NYHA II–III | Progressive aerobic walking through formal cardiac rehabilitation program; 50–60% peak VO2 | 52 weeks | Improvement in peak VO2, peak heart rate, anaerobic threshold, and peak power output; Gains plateaued at 16–26 weeks; 10–15% improvement in 6-minute walk test; Improved quality of life |
| Cohen-Solal et al. (1996 [13]) | 4 | Case studies | Graded exercise testing | NA | Decreased VO2 may result from hemody-namic disturbances during exercise; likely due to lowered cardiac output |
| Wilson et al. (1996 [50]) | 32 | Non-randomized; no control group; EF 15–31% | Standard cardiac rehabilitation program; 15 min warm-up, 45 min training with treadmill, stairs, cycle; 60–70% maximal heart rate | 12 weeks | Patients with normal cardiac output response to exercise responded signifi-cantly better than those with abnormal exercise response; only one patient with abnormal cardiac output response improved |

**TABLE A9-1** Clinical Trials of Exercise in Heart Failure (Continued)

| Study | N | Design/ Pt. Selection | Training Program | Duration | Findings/Comments |
|---|---|---|---|---|---|
| Meyer et al. (1996 [40]) | 18 | Random order crossover trial; hospitalized patients; EF 20–22%; all male subjects | Interval training program; cycle and treadmill walking at varied work/rest intervals; supervised program | 3 weeks at each phase | Peak VO2 increased 23.7%; Decreases in aerobic capacity during the restricted phase occurs as quickly as training effect in the active phase |
| Meyer, Görnandt et al. (1997 [38]) | 18 | Random order crossover trial; all male subjects | Interval training program; cycle and treadmill walking at varied intervals; 50% steep ramp max | 3 weeks at each phase | Significant increase in peak VO2; Steep ramp test measures effect; No changes in heart rate, blood pressure, or Borg ratings |
| Meyer, Samek et al. (1997 [39]) | 18 | Random order crossover trial; all male subjects | Interval training program; cycle and treadmill walking at varied intervals; exercises to enhance strength, flexibility | 3 weeks at each phase | Three parameters accounted for 85% variance in peak VO2: -VO2 at ventilatory threshold -Decreased dead space to tidal volume ratio -Heart rate at ventilatory threshold |
| Demopoulos et al. (1997 [15]) | 16 | Non-randomized, no control group; NYHA II-IV | Low intensity cycle; <50% peak VO2; 1 hr/day 4×/week | 12 weeks | 22–30% increase in peak VO2; Study group includes NYHA IV; Lower wall stress than more intense training regimens |
| Belardinelli et al. (1999 [6]) | 110 | Randomized, controlled; stable CHF | Moderate intensity (60% peak); 3/week × 8 weeks then 2/week × 1 year | 12 months | Improved peak VO2 and thallium activity; Improved quality of life and functional status |

with stable ischemic cardiomyopathy with NYHA class II–III. The training phase included an 8-week, home-based cycling exercise program. The control group consisted of 15 healthy male subjects. The objective of the study was to determine the effects of training on skeletal muscle metabolism in patients with heart failure. Their findings suggested correction of impaired oxidative capacity of skeletal muscle as evidenced by the lack of a significant difference of measured cell metabolic components between treatment and control conditions after training. The authors concluded that further research is needed to identify the impact of these muscular changes on exercise performance (Adamopoulos et al., 1993 [3]).

(17) Six randomized, controlled studies were found which lend support to the benefits of exercise in heart failure in the process of this review. Jette et al. randomized 39 male patients who had suffered large anterior myocardial infarctions in the prior 20-week period with resultant ejection fractions of less than 50% to either the exercise or control. The two groups were further divided into ejection fraction <30% or 31–50%. There was a significant improvement in VO2max in the training/<30% ejection fraction group, but also a significant increase in pulmonary wedge pressure in this group. The authors purport that this finding could suggest that patients were able to gain higher levels of exercise intensity, but at the cost of some overload of ventricular function. Ejection fraction was improved in both the training and control groups, but was not associated with increase in work capacity. The authors concluded that training effects in patients with left ventricular dysfunction are likely to be due to corrected impaired vasodilation, due to the lack of effect on hemodynamic measurements (Jette, Heller, Landry, & Blumchen, 1991 [23]).

(18) Koch et al. randomized 25 patients with either ischemic or idiopathic cardiomyopathy to either graded exercise training or control. The training program consisted of 40 sessions, each 11/2 hours, over a 90-day period. Emphasis was placed on building up of small numbers of muscle groups at a time in attempt to avoid excessive pressure on the heart. The load for each patient was determined individually based upon the testing results at baseline and at intervals throughout the program. Findings included a 34% improvement in exercise performance, and a 63% improvement in perceived quality of life (Koch, Douard, & Broustet, 1992 [29]).

(19) Hambrecht et al. randomized 10 patients with ejection fractions of 12–35% to 6 months of ambulatory training versus control. A 31% improvement in VO2max was reported. Additionally, measurement of cardiac outputs at baseline and at the end of the study period reflected no change in submaximal cardiac output after exercise training (Hambrecht, Niebauer, & Fiehn, 1995 [20]).

(20) Keteyian et al. randomized 40 male subjects to 24 weeks of aerobic exercise versus control. The sample included both ischemic and dilated cardiomyopathy patients. The authors reported a 16.3% increase in absolute VO2max (15.6% increase in VO2max relative to body mass). They observed greater benefit in terms of VO2max in the idiopathic dilated cardiomyopathy group compared to the ischemic group, but this observation did not reach statistical significance ($p = 0.07$). Additionally, a significant increase in peak heart rate in the treatment group was found. An interesting outcome of the data analysis in this study was the conclusion that 46% of the improvement in VO2max could be attributed to the increase in peak heart rate, as a result of reversal of chronotropic incompetence. Additionally, it was noted that 85% of the improvement occurred by the twelfth week (Keteyian et al., 1996 [27]).

(21) Kiilavuori et al. designed a randomized, controlled study to determine the effect of low intensity exercise on VO2max in heart failure patients. They randomized 27 subjects to treatment versus control. The treatment consisted of a 12-week, supervised training program during which the treatment group performed cycle training at 50–60% of VO2max, followed by 12 weeks of home-based exercise at the same intensity. There was a 12% increase in the VO2max which was not statistically significant. The authors conclude that the submaximal level of training in this study may have led to benefits which are underestimated by use of VO2max. They suggest that increase in submaximal exercise endurance observed (88% improvement) represents clinically significant data, as submaximal exercise capacity correlates better with changes in quality of life scores due to general well-being of patients who are more able to achieve activities of daily living. Furthermore, the authors conclude that their findings suggest that periodic moderate level training between lower intensity exercise which is in excess of normal daily activity may be sufficient to improve the exercise capacity in CHF (Kiilavuori, Sovijarvi, Naveri, Ikonen, & Leinonen, 1996 [28]).

(22) Kostis et al. randomly assigned 20 patients to one of three study groups including: combined nonpharmacologic treatment; digoxin titrated to achieve a blood level between 0.8 and 2.0 ng/ml; and double blind placebo. Subjects were CHF patients with NYHA class II–III, and ejection fraction less than 40%. The nonpharmacological treatment arm consisted of exercise, diet counseling, and cognitive therapies. The exercise component was a formal cardiac rehabilitation program and consisted of walking, cycling, rowing, and stair climbing for 1 hour 3–5 times

weekly for a 3-week period. The authors concluded that the nonpharmacologic therapy treatment group demonstrated significantly improved functional capacity, body weight, and mood state at the conclusion of the study period (Kostis, Rosen, Cosgrove, Shindler, & Wilson, 1994 [30]). Because of the combined intervention, it is not possible to isolate the exercise component in this study, which renders the findings of questionable utility with regard to the specific question of exercise.

(23) While the above studies lend strong support to the benefits of exercise in heart failure, there have been published studies which report no improvement, or present evidence of worsening cardiac function associated with exercise training. Arvan et al. reported no improvement in exercise tolerance with training in patients with recent myocardial infarction, left ventricular dysfunction, and symptomatic ischemia with initial exercise testing (Arvan, 1988 [4]). Additionally, Jugdutt et al. report worsened anterior wall motion and deterioration in ejection fraction in patients who had experienced myocardial infarction 12 weeks earlier with anterior wall akinesis greater than 18% (Jugdutt, Michorowski, & Kappagoda, 1988 [24]). Cohen-Solal et al. outlined four case studies of subjects in whom transient diminished or plateaued VO2max occurred during exercise testing in conjunction with observed cardiac abnormalities. These included: atrial fibrillation in the presence of severe mitral stenosis; hypotension secondary to acute worsening of mitral regurgitation due to papillary muscle dysfunction; probably atrial tachycardia with widening of existing bundle branch block; and worsening of 2nd degree AV block from 2:1 to 3:1 with resultant bradycardia lasting for approximately 8 minutes, after which heart rate and VO2max increased. The fall in VO2max was believed to be due to lowered cardiac output with impaired compensatory reserve. The authors conclude that these findings illuminate the interdependence of VO2max and pulmonary blood flow during exercise (Cohen-Solal, Aupetit, Page, Geneves, & Gourgon, 1996 [13]).

(24) In addition to Kiilavuori et al., two further, nonrandomized studies utilizing low intensity exercise regimens have been conducted. Demopoulos et al. exercised 16 patients with NYHA class II–IV at low intensity (<50% peak VO2max) for periods of 1 hour per day, 4 times weekly for 12 weeks. They documented a 22% increase in VO2max at 6 weeks and a 30% increase at 12 weeks. Peak reactive hyperemia in the calf was significantly increased after training compared with that in the forearm, suggesting that the improvement in VO2max may result from maximum vasodilation in the trained limb (Demopoulos, Bijou, Fergus, Jones, Strom, & LeJemtel, 1997 [15]). This study is important because it extends the studied

population to NYHA class IV patients. Belardinelli et al. studied 27 patients with mild heart failure. They assigned the patients to one of two groups: training and nontraining. They trained at 40% VO2max in 30-minute intervals 3 times weekly for 8 weeks. They observed a 17% increase in VO2max in the trained group, as well as increased lactic acid threshold, and peak work load. Additionally, they documented lower norepinephrine levels in the trained group and an increase in the cross sectional area of type I and type II fibers and an increase in mitochondrial density. These findings support potential gains in exercise training effect and reversal of impaired oxidative capacity from low intensity exercise (Belardinelli, Georgiou, Scocco, Barstow, & Purcaro, 1995 [7]).

(25) Mancini et al. conducted a study which involved selective respiratory muscle training and resultant exercise capacity in 14 patients with CHF. The training program consisted of 3 weekly training sessions including isocapnic hyperpnea at maximal ventilatory capacity, resistive breathing, and strength training, for a study duration of three months. The authors noted a significant increase in submaximal and maximal exercise capacity as measured by a 33% +/− 15% improvement in the six-minute walk test and an increased maximal VO2 measurement of 1.8 +/− 1.7 ml/kg/min. Subjective dyspnea ratings improved as well. The lack of change in resting heart rate and VO2 at anaerobic threshold suggested that the improvements were independent of systemic training effect (Mancini, Henson, LaManca, Donchez, & Levine, 1995 [32]).

(26) Kavanagh et al. conducted a study which contributed evidence of improvement over the course of a longer study period (52 weeks). The study was non-randomized but did include a control group for comparative purposes over the first 9-week period. They found both submaximal and maximal exercise capacity improvements as well as a marked improvement in quality of life, as measured by the Chronic Heart Failure Questionnaire and the Standard Gamble measure. They also noted that the gains achieved plateaued at 16–26 weeks into the training program. This longer study period enabled the time course with regard to outcomes to be tracked (Kavanagh, Myers, Baigrie, Mertens, Sawyer, & Shephard, 1996 [26]).

(27) Wilson et al. studied 32 patients undergoing a 3-month cardiac rehabilitation program. Patients were subdivided for the purpose of analysis by hemodynamic response to baseline maximal treadmill exercise. All of the 21 patients with normal hemodynamic response to exercise were able to complete the 3-month training period. Nine patients (43%) responded with a >10% improvement in VO2max and anaerobic threshold. Of the 11 patients who showed abnormal hemodynamic response to exercise, 3

patients discontinued the training due to exhaustion, and only 1 patient (9%) was able to achieve the desired effect. The authors suggest that these findings support the hypothesis that response to exercise training is affected by the level of circulatory dysfunction. With regard to findings in other studies, the authors caution that the reported mean results are often skewed due to a great improvement of a relatively few patients (Wilson, Groves, & Rayos, 1996 [50]).

(28) Kataoka et al. report a single case study of a 53-year-old patient who required continuous infusion of dobutamine for the 10-month period preceding the study, and had failed attempts to wean and discontinue the infusion. The etiology of heart failure was idiopathic dilated cardiomyopathy, and the estimated ejection fraction was 15%. The patient was exercised for 42 minutes (including a 33-minute aerobic phase) 3 times weekly for 32 weeks. The program utilized treadmill, cycle, rowing, arm ergometer, and stair climbing exercises. Findings included an absolute VO2max increase of 19.4%, and a relative increase of 14.8%, with a reduction in resting heart rate from 88 to 78, and a measured decrease in norepinephrine levels. In addition to the measured improvements, the patient was able to wean from dobutamine and Lasix at 24 weeks. Eight weeks after the infusion was discontinued, the effects were maintained. The patient continued unsupervised exercise at home for 4 weeks, and then underwent cardiac transplantation (Kataoka, Keteyian, Marks, Fedel, Levine, & Levine, 1994 [25]).

(29) A recent trial published by Belardinelli et al. randomized 110 patients with stable CHF to exercise at 60% of their peak VO2 3 times weekly for 8 weeks, then twice weekly for 1 year, versus control (no exercise). They found significant improvements in peak VO2 and myocardial perfusion measured by a thallium activity score, and parallel improvements in quality of life with exercise. The treatment arm also experienced a lower incidence of mortality and hospital admission (Belardinelli, Georgiou, Cianci, & Purcaro, 1999 [6]). This study not only provides further support for moderate level exercise training in stable CHF patients, but also identifies peak VO2 and myocardial perfusion (thallium uptake) at baseline as important independent predictors of improvement in functional capacity after exercise training. Additionally, the study supported sustained improvements at 1 year with exercise as infrequently as twice weekly (after the initial 8 weeks), which may be favorable in terms of long term compliance.

(30) In a recent abstract Oka et al. (1998 [44]) reported 3 of 4 domains of quality of life improved by a 12-week, in-home moderate intensity walking and resistance training program. The study reported significant improvements in fatigue, mastery, and emotional function, and clinical improvement which did not reach statistical significance in the dyspnea subscale.

(31) In contrast, an abstract of the EXERT trial (Randomized Controlled Trial of Exercise Training in Patients With Congestive Heart Failure) reported no significant change in quality of life at 3 and 12 months of exercise training in spite of a 10% increase in VO2 and a 15% increase in strength. It was noted that there were no further improvements noted at 12 months in comparison to the 3-month data. The conclusions reached by the authors were that exercise training appears to be safe in heart failure, and does improve functional capacity, but that this improvement does not result in improved quality of life. There were no details of the frequency or intensity of the exercise regimen, or the quality of life measure reported in the abstract (McKelvie et al., 1998 [36]).

## PRACTICE IMPLICATIONS

### Current Recommendations for Exercise in CHF

(32) The Agency for Health Care Policy and Research *Clinical Practice Guidelines for Cardiac Rehabilitation as Secondary Prevention* grade the strength of evidence supporting the value of exercise training in heart failure as "A," meaning that "scientific evidence from well-designed and well-conducted controlled trials (randomized and non-randomized) provides statistically significant results that consistently support the guidelines statement" (U.S. Department of Health and Human Services 1995 [2]). Therefore, cardiac rehabilitation exercise training is recommended to maintain functional capacity and alleviate symptoms. It is interesting to note that the American College of Cardiology/American Heart Association's 1995 "Guidelines for the Evaluation and Management of Heart Failure" do not address the role of exercise therapy as a treatment modality for heart failure.

(33) The American College of Sports Medicine has outlined signs and symptoms below which the exercise intensity should be limited. These include:

1. Onset of angina or other symptoms of cardiovascular disease
2. Plateau or decrease in systolic blood pressure, systolic blood pressure >240 mm Hg, or diastolic blood pressure >110 mm Hg
3. >1mm ST segment depression, horizontal or downsloping
4. Radionuclide evidence of LV dysfunction or onset of moderate to severe wall motion abnormalities during exertion
5. Increased frequency of ventricular arrhythmias
6. Other significant ECG disturbances

7. Other signs/symptoms of intolerance to exercise (ACSM, 1995 [3]).

(34) A specific program design which will best fit the heart failure patient with regard to the modality and intensity is yet unknown (Balady & Pina, 1997 [5]). Braith and Mills recommend screening of patients with ejection fraction of less than 30% for ischemia prior to implementing a training program. They also suggest that a baseline monitored graded exercise test is required. Further recommendations suggest that patients can exercise at 60–80% of their maximum heart rate or 50–70% of VO2 max if stable during the exercise test (Braith & Mills, 1994 [8]; LeJemtel, Demopulos, Jondeau, Testa, & Fanelli, 1997 [31]). It is also suggested that weight training and hyperthermia be avoided. Walking, flexibility exercises, calisthenics, cycling, and stair climbing are all acceptable forms of exercise training. As suggested by Meyer et al., interval training is thought to be well suited for this population (Braith & Mills, 1994 [8]; Hanson, 1994 [21]). Hanson recommends beginning exercise training at 60–65% VO2max for 10–15 minutes duration beginning with 2–4 minutes of exercise separated by 1-minute periods of rest. The exercise interval can be gradually increased according to patient tolerance by 1–2 minutes. The eventual goal is 30–40 minutes of training. Also recommended is a 10-minute warm-up phase to achieve optimal vasodilation. The frequency of exercise should be tailored to the needs of the patient, but should be 3–5 times weekly (Hanson, 1994 [21]). At the very minimum, patients with heart failure should be encouraged to remain as active as possible and abandon any belief that physical activity should be restricted or avoided completely. Home walking programs are often desirable for these patients, and can be encouraged with little concern regarding adverse events. Patients should be instructed to adjust their program if they experience excessive fatigue on the day following exercise, as this is evidence of overexertion (Dracup et al., 1994 [14]).

## Compliance Related Issues

(35) Many barriers to compliance exist which threaten the integrity of the planned treatment regimen for the patient with heart failure. The majority of patients diagnosed with CHF are elderly people. These patients carry with them a unique challenge in terms of age-related needs. Many patients experience orthostatic hypotension related to vascular dysfunction which may or may not be pharmacologically induced. This may predispose them to falling, or unstable gait, which impacts the ability to perform physical activities. Additionally, elderly patients often live alone, or lack resources for transportation to suitable exercise facilities. During inclement weather, activities outside the home are of particular concern due to the recommended avoidance of temperature extremes, and the possible lack of transportation to an exercise facility. Physical activity must be tailored to address these potential barriers to compliance with the prescribed regimen. Reasonable, achievable goals must be identified and serve as a foundation for building the exercise prescription.

## RESEARCH NEEDED

(36) The study findings reviewed lend strong support to the potential benefits of exercise in heart failure. However, the need for a large, randomized longitudinal trial persists. The number of subjects included in these studies was small, and few were randomized and controlled. As individual differences vary substantially, it becomes important to obtain larger study groups to avoid skewed mean values (Jette et al., 1991 [23]; Wilson et al., 1996 [50]). Furthermore, many of the studies involve subjects who were primarily, if not exclusively, male, and often tend to study patients with ischemic as opposed to idiopathic cardiomyopathy. Further study is required to clarify the value and mechanisms involved with submaximal versus maximal testing and the impact of these interventions on morbidity and mortality in heart failure, and the issues surrounding capability of performing activities of daily living and quality of life. More study is required in severely debilitated patients (NYHA IV), to determine potential gains, as well as feasible exercise programs, for patients who are unable to perform maximal training. As further findings support specific exercise regimens, practical guidelines for clinicians should be developed which delineate appropriate candidates for exercise training, levels of intensity and specific exercises (such as interval training, strength training, graded protocols, or programs which isolate small muscle groups) and goals to be achieved. As more data become available correlating exercise training with morbidity and mortality in CHF, the findings should be compared with the results of clinical trials conducted for the purpose of gaining FDA approval for new pharmacological agents, with regard to cost–benefit analyses.

(37) The studies reviewed were devoid of discussion of cultural or compliance issues related to prescription of exercise in the heart failure population. These areas, as well as further exploration of the impact on quality of life and translating research findings into practice guidelines, are fertile areas for future nursing research.

## SEARCH STRATEGIES

(38) The search undertaken for this review was conducted via electronic search of the health care literature through MEDLINE and CINAHL. The search

period was restricted to 1995–1999 and materials were restricted to those published in the English language. Additional studies were identified through manual search of reference lists, clinical resource materials, and textbooks.

(39) Keywords utilized for the search included: heart failure; congestive heart failure; exercise; functional capacity. Studies were excluded from review if exercise was not included as an intervention, if the target population was restricted to transplant patients, and if the main objective was to evaluate pharmacologic therapy.

## References

1. Adamopoulos, S., Coats, A.J.S., Brunotte, F., Arnolda, L., Meyer, T., Thompson, C.H., Dunn, J.F., Stratton, J., Kemp, G., Radda, G., & Rajagopalan, B. (1993). Physical training improves skeletal muscle metabolism in patients with chronic heart failure. *Journal of the American College of Cardiology, 21*, 1101–1106.
2. Agency for Health Care Policy and Research. (1995). *Cardiac rehabilitation as secondary prevention: Clinical practice guideline.* Rockville, MD: U.S. Department of Health and Human Services.
3. American College of Sports Medicine. (1995). *ACSM's guidelines for exercise testing and prescription.* Baltimore, MD: Williams & Wilkins.
4. Arvan, S. (1988). Exercise performance of the high risk acute myocardial infarction patient after cardiac rehabilitation. *American Journal of Cardiology, 62*, 197–201. [MEDLINE]
5. Balady, G.J. & Pina, I.L. (1997). *Exercise and heart failure.* American Heart Association Monograph Series. New York: Futura Publishing Company, Inc.
6. Belardinelli, R., Georgiou, D., Cianci, G., & Purcaro, A. (1999). Randomized, controlled trial of long-term moderate exercise training in chronic heart failure: Effects on functional capacity, quality of life, and clinical outcome. *Circulation, 99*, 1173–1182. [MEDLINE]
7. Belardinelli, R., Georgiou, D., Scocco, V., Barstow, T.J., & Purcaro, A. (1995). Low intensity exercise training in patients with chronic heart failure. *Journal of the American College of Cardiology, 26*(4), 975–982. [MEDLINE]
8. Braith, R.W. & Mills, R.M. (1994). Exercise training in patients with congestive heart failure: How to achieve benefits safely. *Postgraduate Medicine, 96*(2), 119–130. [MEDLINE]
9. Cahalin, L.P., Mathier, M.A., Semigran, M.J., Dec, W., & Disalvo, T.G. (1996). The six-minute walk test predicts peak oxygen uptake and survival in patients with advanced heart failure. *Chest, 110*(2), 325–332. [MEDLINE]
10. Cahalin, L.P. (1996). Heart failure. Special series: Cardiopulmonary physical therapy. *Physical Therapy, 76*(5), 516.
11. Coats, A.J.S. (1993). Exercise rehabilitation in chronic heart failure. *Journal of the American College of Cardiology, 22*(4), 172A–177A. [MEDLINE]
12. Coats, A.J.S., Adamopoulos, S., Radaelli, A., McCance, A., Meyer, T.E., Bernardi, L., Solda, P.L., Davey, P., Ormerod, O., Forfar, C., Conway, J., & Sleight, P.

(1992). Controlled trial of physical training in chronic heart failure: Exercise performance, hemodynamics, ventilation, and autonomic function. *Circulation, 85*(6), 2119–2131. [MEDLINE]
13. Cohen-Solal, A., Aupetit, J.F., Page, E., Geneves, J., & Gourgon, R. (1996). Transient fall in oxygen intake during exercise in congestive heart failure. *Chest, 110*, 841–844.
14. Dracup, K., Baker, D.W., Dunbar, S.B., Dacey, R.A., Brooks, N.H., Johnson, J.C., Oken, C., & Massie, B.M. (1994). Management of heart failure: Counseling, education, and lifestyle modifications. *Journal of the American Medical Association, 272*(18), 1442–1446. [MEDLINE]
15. Demopoulos, L., Bijou, R., Fergus, I., Jones, M., Strom, J., & LeJemtel, T.H. (1997). Exercise training in patients with severe congestive heart failure: Enhancing peak aerobic capacity while minimizing the increase in ventricular wall stress. *Journal of the American College of Cardiology, 29*(3), 597–603. [MEDLINE]
16. Faggiano, P., D'Aloia, A., Gualeni, A., Lavatelli, A., & Giordano, A. (1997). Assessment of oxygen uptake during the 6-minute walk test in patients with heart failure: Preliminary experience with a portable device. *American Heart Journal, 134*, 203–206. [MEDLINE]
17. Fletcher, G.F., Balady, G., Blair, S.N., Blumenthal, J., Casperson, C., Chaitman, B., Epstein, S., Froelicher, E.S.S., Froelicher, V.F., Pina, I.L., & Pollick, M.L. (1996). Statement on exercise: Benefits and recommendations for physical activity programs for all Americans. *Circulation, 94*(4), 857–862. [MEDLINE]
18. Fletcher, G.F., Froelicher, V.F., Hartley, L.H., Haskell, W.L., & Pollock, M.L. (1990). Exercise standards: A statement for health professionals from the American Heart Association. Special Report, *Circulation, 82*(6), 2286–2322. [MEDLINE]
19. Guyatt, G.H., Sullivan, M.J., Thompson, P.J., Fallen, E.L., Pugsley, S.O., Taylor, D.W., & Berman, L.B. (1985). The 6-minute walk: A new measure of exercise capacity in patients with chronic heart failure. *Canadian Medical Association Journal, 132*(8), 919–923. [MEDLINE]
20. Hambrecht, R., Niebauer, J., & Fiehn, E. (1995). Physical training in patients with stable chronic heart failure: Effects on cardiorespiratory fitness and ultrastructural abnormalities of leg muscles. *Journal of the American College of Cardiology, 25*, 1239–1249. [MEDLINE]
21. Hanson, P. (1994). Exercise testing and training in patients with chronic heart failure. *Medicine and Science in Sports and Exercise, 26*(5), 527–537. [MEDLINE]
22. Hosenpud, J.D. & Greenbert, B.H. (1994). Congestive heart failure: Pathophysiology, diagnosis, and comprehensive approach to management. New York: Springer-Verlag.
23. Jette, M., Heller, R., Landry, F., & Blumchen, G. (1991). Randomized 4-week exercise program in patients with impaired left ventricular function. *Circulation, 84*(4), 1561–1567. [MEDLINE]
24. Jugdutt, B.I., Michorowski, B.L., & Kappagoda, C.T. (1988). Exercise training after anterior Q wave myocardial infarction: Importance of regional left ventricular function and topography. *Journal of the American College of Cardiology, 12*, 362–372. [MEDLINE]

25. Kataoka, T., Keteyian, S.J., Marks, C.R.C., Fedel, F.J., Levine, A.B., & Levine, T.B. (1994). Exercise training in a patient with congestive heart failure on continuous dobutamine. *Medicine and Science in Sports and Exercise, 26*(6), 678–681. [MEDLINE]

26. Kavanagh, T., Myers, M.G., Baigrie, R.S., Mertens, D.J., Sawyer, P., & Shephard, R.J. (1996). Quality of life and cardiorespiratory function in chronic heart failure: Effects of 12 months' aerobic training. *Heart, 76,* 42–49. [MEDLINE]

27. Keteyian, S.J., Levine, A.B., Brawner, C.A., Kataoka, T., Rogers, F.J., Shairer, J.R., Stein, P.D., Levine, T.B., & Goldstein, S. (1996). Exercise training in patients with heart failure: A randomized, controlled trial. *Annals of Internal Medicine, 124,* 1051–1057. [MEDLINE]

28. Kiilavuori, K., Sovijarvi, A., Naveri, H., Ikonen, T., & Leinonen, H. (1996). Effect of physical training on exercise capacity and gas exchange in patients with chronic heart failure. *Chest, 110,* 985–991. [MEDLINE]

29. Koch, M., Douard, H., & Broustet, J.P. (1992). The benefit of graded physical exercise in chronic heart failure. *Chest, 101*(5), 231S–235S. [MEDLINE]

30. Kostis, J.B., Rosen, R.C., Cosgrove, N.M., Shindler, D.M., & Wilson, A. (1994). Nonpharmacologic therapy improves functional and emotional status in congestive heart failure. *Chest, 106*(4), 996–1001. [MEDLINE]

31. LeJemtel, T.H., Demopoulos, L., Jondeau, G., Testa, M., & Fanelli, R. (1997). Exercise training for patients with congestive heart failure. *Contemporary Internal Medicine, 9*(7), 23–28.

32. Mancini, D.M., Henson, D., LaManca, J., Donchez, L., & Levine S. (1995). Benefit of selective respiratory muscle training on exercise capacity in patients with chronic congestive heart failure. *Circulation, 91,* 320–329. [MEDLINE]

33. Mancini, D.M., Walter, G., Reichek, N., Lenkinski, R., McCully, K.K., Mullen, J.L., & Wilson, J. (1992). Contribution of skeletal muscle atrophy to exercise intolerance and altered muscle metabolism in heart failure. *Circulation, 85*(4), 1364–1373. [MEDLINE]

34. Massie, B.M. & Camacho, S.S. (1995). *Cahners scientific meeting reports: Heart failure review.* Belle Mead, NJ: Excerpta Medica.

35. Mayou, R., Blackwood, R., Bryant, B., & Garnham, J. (1991). Cardiac failure: Symptoms and functional status. *Journal of Psychosomatic Research, 35*(4/5), 399–407. [MEDLINE]

36. McKelvie, R.S., Teo, K.K., McCartney R.S., Roberts, R.S., Costantini, L.A., Montague, T.J., Humen, D.P., Guyatt, G.H., & Yusuf, S. (1998). Randomized controlled trial of exercise training in patients with congestive heart failure (EXERT). *Journal of the American College of Cardiology, 31*(suppl. A), 1226–1231.

37. Mehra, M.R., Lavie, C.J., & Milani, R.V. (1996). Predicting prognosis in advanced heart failure: Use of exercise indices. *Chest, 110*(2), 310. [MEDLINE]

38. Meyer, K., Görnandt, L., Schwaibold, M., Westbrook, S., Hajric, R., Peters, K., Beneke, R., Schnellbacher, K., & Roskamm, H. (1997). Predictors of response to exer-

cise training in severe chronic congestive heart failure. *American Journal of Cardiology, 80,* 56–60. [MEDLINE]

39. Meyer, K., Samek, L., Schwaibold, M., Westbrook, S., Hajric, R., Beneke, R., Lehmann, M., & Roskamm, H. (1997). Interval training in patients with severe chronic heart failure: Analysis and recommendations for exercise procedures. *Medicine and Science in Sports and Exercise, 29*(3), 306–312. [MEDLINE]

40. Meyer, K., Schwaibold, M., Westbrook, S., Beneke, R., Hajric, R., Görnandt, L., Lehmann, M., & Roskamm, H. (1996). Effects of short-term exercise training and activity restriction on functional capacity in patients with severe chronic congestive heart failure. *American Journal of Cardiology, 78,* 1017–1022. [MEDLINE]

41. Milligan, N.P., Havey, J., & Dossa, A. (1997). Using a 6-minute walk test to predict outcomes in patients with left ventricular dysfunction. *Rehabilitation Nursing 22*(4), 177–181. [MEDLINE]

42. Minotti, J.R. & Massie, B.M. (1992). Exercise training in heart failure patients: Does reversing the peripheral abnormalities protect the heart? *Circulation, 85*(6) 2323–2325. [MEDLINE]

43. Moran, J.F. (1996). Exercise in heart failure and exercise prescription, Lecture text, Midwest Heart Specialists Heart Failure Tutorial, Oak Brook, IL.

44. Oka, R.K., De Marco, T., Bolen, K., Botvinick, E., Dae, M., Woodley, S., Haskell, W.L., & Chatterjee, K. (1998). Impact of a home-based exercise program on quality of life in patients with class II–III chronic heart failure. *Journal of the American College of Cardiology, 31* (suppl. A), 1226–1229.

45. Packer, M. (1993). How should physicians view heart failure? The philosophical and physiological evolution of three conceptual models of the disease. *American Journal of Cardiology, 71,* 3C–11C. [MEDLINE]

46. Patterson, J.H. & Adams, K.F. (1996). Pathophysiology of heart failure: Changing perceptions. *Pharmacotherapy, 16*(2), 27S–36S. [MEDLINE]

47. Peters, P. & Mets, T. (1996). The 6-minute walk as an appropriate exercise test in elderly patients with chronic heart failure. *Journal of Gerontology: Medical Sciences, 51A*(4), M147–M151.

48. Sullivan, M.J. & Hawthorne, M.H. (1996). Non-pharmacologic interventions in the treatment of heart failure. *Journal of Cardiovascular Nursing 10*(2), 47–57. [MEDLINE]

49. Sullivan, M.J., Higginbotham, M.B., & Cobb, F.R. (1988). Exercise training in patients with severe left ventricular dysfunction: Hemodynamic and metabolic effects. *Circulation, 78,* 506–515. [MEDLINE]

50. Wilson, J.R., Groves, J., & Rayos, G. (1996). Circulatory status and response to cardiac rehabilitation in patients with heart failure. *Circulation, 94*(7), 1567–1572. [MEDLINE]

51. Wilson, J.R., Mancini, D.M., & Dunkman, W.B. (1993). Exertional fatigue due to skeletal muscle dysfunction in patients with heart failure. *Circulation, 87*(2), 470–475. [MEDLINE]

APPENDIX

**A-10**

# Effect of Positioning on $S\bar{v}O_2$ in the Critically Ill Patient With a Low Ejection Fraction

**Anna Gawlinski, Kathleen Dracup**

***Background:*** *Critically ill patients with a low ejection fraction may be vulnerable to decreased mixed venous oxygen saturation ($S\bar{v}O_2$) resulting from position change.*

***Objectives:*** *The objectives of this study were to describe the effects of changes in positioning on $S\bar{v}O_2$ in critically ill patients with a low ejection fraction ($\leq 30\%$) and to describe the contribution of variables of oxygen delivery ($DO_2$) and oxygen consumption ($VO_2$) to the variance in $S\bar{v}O_2$.*

***Method:*** *An experimental two-group repeated-measures design was used to study 42 critically ill patients with an ejection fraction of less than or equal to 30% ($M = 19.5\%$). Patients were assigned randomly to one of two position sequences: supine, right lateral, left lateral; or supine, left lateral, right lateral. Data on $S\bar{v}O_2$ were collected at baseline, each minute after position change for 5 minutes, and at 15 and 25 minutes.*

***Results:*** *Repeated-measures multivariate analysis of variance showed a difference in $S\bar{v}O_2$ among the three positions across time ($p < .0001$), with the greatest differences occurring within the first 4 minutes and in the left lateral position. Stepwise multiple regression showed that $VO_2$ accounted for a greater proportion of the variance in $S\bar{v}O_2$ with position change than did $DO_2$ (54% [$p = .001$] vs. 31% [$p = .001$]).*

***Conclusions:*** *Changes in $S\bar{v}O_2$ occur with positioning in critically ill patients with a low ejection fraction. These changes are transient and are the result of changes in $VO_2$ rather than changes in $DO_2$.*

Positioning can have adverse effects in critically ill patients. Dysrhythmia, hypotension, low cardiac output, and hypoxemia have reportedly occurred during positioning (Gillespie & Rehder, 1987; Remolina, Khan, Santiago, & Edelman, 1981; Rivara, Artucio, Arcos, & Hiriart, 1984; Winslow, Clark, White, & Tyler, 1990). Positioning can also improve oxygenation by improved ventilation-perfusion matching and prevention of complications such as atelectasis, pneumonia, and pooling of secretions (Brunner & Suddarth, 1988; Kersten, 1989). Thus, positioning a critically ill patient may initiate a dangerous or beneficial sequence of events depending on its effects on oxygen delivery ($DO_2$) and oxygen consumption ($VO_2$) (Winslow et al.). To date, the effects of positioning on cardiopulmonary function, $DO_2$, and $VO_2$ are still unknown.

In healthy subjects, oxygen supply is sufficient to meet demand (Shively & Clark, 1986). If oxygen demand increases, $VO_2$ normally will increase through one of the following: (a) an increased extraction of oxygen from arterial blood as it traverses the capillary bed (i.e., an increase in arterial mixed venous oxygen content difference [C(a-v)O$_2$]) or (b) an increase in blood flow (i.e., via vasodilatation and an increase in cardiac output [CO]). Both oxygen extraction and CO may increase by approximately threefold in healthy subjects when oxygen demand increases (Nelson, 1986).

Increasing CO is one of the most important compensatory mechanisms used to maintain and increase DO$_2$ to tissues. For example, if oxygen saturation (SO$_2$) falls to a value of 50%, a patient can maintain DO$_2$ by doubling CO. Many critically ill patients, however, have reduced ventricular performance because of some degree of myocardial failure. These critically ill patients may not be able to compensate for increases in VO$_2$ that are caused by various procedures such as turning, bathing, and obtaining a bedscale weight.

In the intensive care unit, nurses can calculate DO$_2$ and VO$_2$ at the bedside using various hemodynamic values (i.e., CO), oxygen transport values (i.e., partial pressure of oxygen in arterial blood [PaO$_2$] and arterial oxygen saturation [SaO$_2$]), and constants (0.0033, 10, 1.34). DO$_2$ and VO$_2$ can then be used to calculate the oxygen extraction ratio, which reflects the balance between DO$_2$ and VO$_2$. More recently, however, clinicians are using S$\bar{v}$O$_2$ values (normal range 60%–80%) as an indicator for the balance between DO$_2$ and metabolic demand of the tissue (Epstein & Henning, 1993; Varon, 1994). Similar to the oxygen extract ratio, variables such as CO, hemoglobin, and SaO$_2$ are important determinants for S$\bar{v}$O$_2$ as well as VO$_2$. S$\bar{v}$O$_2$ values can be monitored continuously in patients with a pulmonary artery fiberoptic catheter, and therefore changes in a patient's oxygenation status in response to various nursing care procedures can be evaluated.

The purpose of the present research was to determine the effect on S$\bar{v}$O$_2$ of right and left lateral position changes from supine in patients with a cardiac ejection fraction of less than or equal to 30% and to identify the contribution of DO$_2$ and VO$_2$ to the variance in S$\bar{v}$O$_2$ with positioning.

## RELEVANT LITERATURE

Although many researchers have examined the effect of position on oxygenation, only four studies have examined the effect of position on S$\bar{v}$O$_2$ (Peña, 1989; Shively, 1988; Tidwell, Ryan, Osguthorpe, Paull, & Smith, 1990; Winslow et al., 1990). Shively studied the effect of four positions (right lateral with the head of bed [HOB] elevated at 20°, supine with HOB elevated 40°, left lateral with HOB elevated 20°, and supine with HOB elevated 20°) on S$\bar{v}$O$_2$ in 30 patients following coronary artery bypass graft surgery. There was no significant difference ($p = .13$) in S$\bar{v}$O$_2$ among the four positions, but there was a significant difference ($p = .001$) in S$\bar{v}$O$_2$ among the times that it was measured for each position. For example, most of the patients studied had an 8% to 11% decrease in S$\bar{v}$O$_2$ immediately after each position change; however, within 5 minutes S$\bar{v}$O$_2$ returned to baseline values. Shively concluded that the early decrease in S$\bar{v}$O$_2$ after positioning was related to an increase in VO$_2$ versus a change in DO$_2$. Unfortunately, VO$_2$ and the variables that affect DO$_2$ (CO, hemoglobin, and SaO$_2$) were not measured.

Peña (1989) measured the effect on S$\bar{v}$O$_2$ in 12 mechanically ventilated bypass cardiac surgery patients. Patients were turned every 2 hours for a total of two turns. An 8.5% decrease and 12.3% decrease in S$\bar{v}$O$_2$ values were documented immediately after the first and second position turns. S$\bar{v}$O$_2$ returned to baseline within 3.7 minutes after turning and remained at baseline 20 minutes after the turning episode. Peña concluded that the sudden drop in S$\bar{v}$O$_2$ could be explained by the increase in muscular activity that occurs with positioning. VO$_2$, however, was not a measured variable, and the sequence of positioning was not randomized in this study.

Winslow et al. (1990) studied the effect of lateral positioning on S$\bar{v}$O$_2$ in 174 critically ill patients. The direction of the turn was determined by the placement of the tip of the pulmonary artery catheter; for example, if the catheter tip was in the right pulmonary artery, the patient was turned toward the right side. Eighty-five percent of subjects studied were turned to the right side and 15% were turned to the left side. There was a significant decrease in mean S$\bar{v}$O$_2$ from baseline immediately after turning ($p < .0001$). Mean S$\bar{v}$O$_2$ decreased from a baseline of 67% ±8% (range 49%–89%) to 61% ±10% (range 38%–89%). S$\bar{v}$O$_2$ gradually returned to baseline within 4 minutes. These statistically significant changes were not clinically significant for most patients.

---

# BOX A10–1

S$\bar{v}$O$_2$ = oxygen saturation

DO$_2$ = oxygen delivery

VO$_2$ = oxygen consumption

CO = cardiac output

SaO$_2$ = arterial oxygen saturation

CaO$_2$ = arterial oxygen content

PaO$_2$ = partial pressure of oxygen in arterial blood

PCWP = pulmonary capillary wedge pressure

Tidwell et al. (1990) studied the effect of lateral position in 34 patients who had undergone cardiac surgery. The initial position change for all subjects was from supine to HOB elevation of 30°. After a return to supine, subjects were turned to the right or left lateral position and back to supine. A significant decrease in $S\bar{v}O_2$ measurements was found in all the position changes ($p < .01$). The greatest difference in mean $S\bar{v}O_2$ values from baseline to 1 minute after positioning was with the supine to right lateral position change, which was associated with a 6.1% decrease in $S\bar{v}O_2$ values from baseline values. The change from supine to left lateral position resulted in a similar difference in $S\bar{v}O_2$ (5.6%). The decrease in $S\bar{v}O_2$ translated to a change in $S\bar{v}O_2$ of 8% to 9%. Although the mean $S\bar{v}O_2$ decreased acutely with a change in position, it did not drop below 60% and the decrease was not sustained beyond 5 minutes. The investigators concluded that most subjects were able to tolerate position changes with no clinically significant change in $S\bar{v}O_2$. Because CO, stroke volume, and heart rate were not reported, it was difficult to determine if any of these patients had limited cardiac reserve.

Limitations of the studies regarding the effect of position change on continuous $S\bar{v}O_2$ values included small sample size, heterogenous population with normal CO values, and lack of randomization of position order. Despite these limitations, investigators have demonstrated a consistent decrease in $S\bar{v}O_2$ of 8% to 11% immediately after positioning and a return to baseline within 5 minutes. Because most studies (Peña, 1989; Shively, 1988; Tidwell et al., 1990; Winslow et al., 1990) were conducted with patients who had normal cardiopulmonary function, the effect of an abnormally low cardiac ejection fraction on oxygenation secondary to position change remains unknown.

## METHOD

An experimental two-group repeated-measures design was used.

### Sample

A convenience sample of 42 patients admitted to the cardiac care unit or cardiac observation unit of a university tertiary care center was screened for participation in the study. Patients who met the sample selection criteria and who agreed to participate were enrolled and randomly assigned to one of two groups with two different position sequences. Sample inclusion criteria were as follows: (a) 18 to 80 years of age, (b) an ejection fraction of less than 30% documented by two-dimensional echocardiography or radionuclide ventriculography, and (c) an existing fiberoptic pulmonary artery catheter in place. Patients with the diagnosis of septic shock documented in the medical record were excluded

from the study. Patients were not excluded on the basis of low CO or $S\bar{v}O_2$ values.

The mean age of the subjects was 54 years. Seventy-six percent of the sample were men, 24% were women. The majority of the patients had dilated (50%) or ischemic cardiomyopathy (46%). Twenty-eight patients did not receive any medications up to 6 hours prior to and during the study protocol. Fourteen patients did receive medications during the protocol. To control for the effect of medications, doses were not titrated 30 minutes prior to data collection and remained constant throughout the data collection period.

### Instruments

*Mixed venous oxygenation saturation.* $S\bar{v}O_2$ was measured with a two-wavelength pulmonary artery fiberoptic catheter connected to a SAT-2 oximeter (Baxter Healthcare Corp., Santa Ana, CA). The system had three basic components: the catheter, the optical module, and the processor. The two light-emitting diodes in the optical module sent alternating pulses of two different wavelengths down one fiberoptic channel in the catheter. The blood was then illuminated by the two different wavelengths of light. The light was absorbed and refracted by the hemoglobin constituents and reflected down another fiberoptic channel in the catheter. Thus, the relative amounts of oxygenated hemoglobin and deoxygenated hemoglobin were determined by measuring the absorption of light at the selected wavelengths.

The accuracy of the SAT-2 oximeter has been reported with a correlation coefficient of .92 compared to standard laboratory co-oximetry over a saturation range of 39% to 96% (Baxter Healthcare Corporation, 1991). The reliability of the system is reported to be ±3.5% oxygen saturation over the range of 40% to 92% saturation (Pond, Blessios, Bowlin, McCawley, & Lappas, 1992). The SAT-2 oximeter was calibrated before data collection according to the manufacturer's instructions.

*Thermodilution cardiac output.* CO is the amount of blood ejected from the heart in liters per minute (normal range 4–8 l/min). All CO values were measured by a closed-system ice thermodilution technique using the Hewlett Packard Model 7855 and M1012A (Hewlett Packard, Andover, MA). Measurements of CO were performed according to the intensive care unit standard protocol (i.e., 10 ml iced injectate, triplicate injectate method with the three values averaged, injected within 4 seconds at end-expiration, assess CO curve). Each CO curve was assessed, and the value was discarded if it varied from the median value by more than 10%. The transducer was calibrated according to the manufacturer's specifications before data collection. Construct validity of CO determinations by the thermodilution method, compared with CO obtained by the direct Fick and dye dilution methods, has been established by a variety of investigators with correlations of .88 to .99 (Forrester et al., 1972; Kadota, 1986). Stetz and colleagues (Stetz, Miller, Kelly, & Raffin, 1982) calculated the standard error of the mean percentage for all studies previously published in which triplicate CO measurements were used and determined the reliability of the thermodilution method to be acceptable.

*Oxygen consumption.* Measurement of $VO_2$ was mathematically derived using the Fick equation, which allows an approximate measurement of $VO_2$ (Liggett, St. John, & Lefrak, 1987; Pomes Iparraguirre, Giniger, Garber, Quiroga, & Jorge, 1988). Investigators have reported significantly high correlations between calculated and measured $VO_2$ ($r = .84$, $p < .001$) (Pomes Iparraguirre et al.). Validity of the calculated $VO_2$ versus measured $VO_2$ was determined in a subgroup of 5 patients from the current sample of 42 patients. $VO_2$ was measured via an open-circuit, exhaled gas analysis technique using the MedGraphics Critical Care Management System (St. Paul, MN) and compared with the mathematically derived value. The correlation coefficient for the measured versus calculated $VO_2$ was $r = .87$ ($p < .05$).

*Oxygen delivery.* As mentioned previously, $DO_2$ is the amount of oxygen delivered to the tissues. It was calculated using CO, hemoglobin, and $SaO_2$. CO and $SaO_2$ were measured at baseline and 3 minutes after positioning. Hemoglobin was measured at baseline. Arterial oxygen content was derived from the following formula:

$$DO_2 = \text{arterial oxygen content } (CaO_2) \times CO \times 10$$
$$CaO_2 = (1.34 \times \text{hemoglobin} \times SaO_2) + (0.0031 \times PaO_2)$$

However, $PaO_2$ was not used in the equation because the contribution of $PaO_2$ to the total arterial oxygen content is small ($< .3\%$) and the $PaO_2$ value (.0031) is often omitted from the calculation of $CaO_2$ (Vierheller, 1993).

## Procedure

Seventeen patients randomly assigned to group 1 were placed first in the supine position, followed by the right lateral and then the left lateral positions. Twenty-five patients in group 2 were placed first in the supine position, followed by the left lateral and then right lateral positions. To test the randomization process, independent $t$ tests and chi-square statistics were used to examine potential group differences at baseline. There were no significant differences be-

tween the groups first positioned right lateral versus left lateral on a variety of baseline clinical characteristics. Only the pulmonary capillary wedge pressure (PCWP) was significantly higher in group 1 than in group 2 ($p = .03$) (Table A10–1).

Data were collected at baseline, at each minute after positioning for the first 5 minutes, and once at 15 minutes and 25 minutes. Patients were in each position for 25 minutes. On the basis of previous studies, a stabilization period of 15 minutes in the supine position occurred before data collection and between lateral position change (Doering & Dracup, 1988; Eggers, DeGroot, Tanner, & Lenard, 1963; McCarthy, 1968). S⊽O₂ data were collected from baseline to 25 minutes after positioning. Values for CO were determined with use of the closed-system 10-ml iced injection technique at baseline and at 3-minute intervals after positioning. Only one postpositioning measurement of CO in each position (at the 3-minute interval after positioning) was performed to minimize the risk of fluid overload and to be consistent with the standard of nursing practice in the unit. The 3-minute time period was selected because other researchers have reported that this period corresponds to the greatest change in S⊽O₂ after positioning (Peña, 1989; Shively, 1988; Tidwell et al., 1990; Winslow et al., 1990). The study was conducted within 24 hours of catheter insertion in all subjects, with the exception of one subject for whom measurements were determined 4 days after catheter insertion.

Data were also collected on variables affecting CO: right atrial pressure (RA), pulmonary artery pressure (PAP), PCWP, and heart rate (HR). The purpose for collecting these data was to characterize the sample. In addition, data were collected on the variables known to affect S⊽O₂ (i.e., CO, $SaO_2$, and $VO_2$) at baseline and 3 minutes after positioning. These variables were continuously (S⊽O₂, $SaO_2$, HR, PAP) or intermittently (CO, RA, PCWP) monitored and were recorded from the bedside monitor at each data collection point.

## Data Analysis

The sample size of 42 allowed detection of a moderate to large order effect of approximately .63 with power of .80 and alpha of .05 (based on a two-tailed $t$ test). For assessing the difference between the supine (baseline) position and the lateral position at any given time within either group, the sample size allowed the detection of a moderate effect of approximately .44 with power of .80 and alpha of .05, assuming a correlation between positions of .50. The correlation was based on a two-tailed paired $t$ test comparison, which was similar to the planned comparison required within the repeated-measures analysis of variance for testing the same hypothesis.

**TABLE A10-1** Clinical Characteristics of the Two Study Groups

| Variable | Group 1 ($n = 23$) | | Group 2 ($n = 19$) | | $t^a$ | df | p |
|---|---|---|---|---|---|---|---|
| | M | SD | M | SD | | | |
| EF (%) | 19.43 | 6.42 | 19.58 | 4.32 | −.08 | 40 | .93 |
| Mean arterial pressure (mm Hg) | 81.21 | 13.36 | 83.65 | 14.29 | −.57 | 40 | .57 |
| RA (mm Hg) | 12.13 | 6.48 | 12.79 | 6.58 | −.32 | 40 | .57 |
| PCWP (mm Hg) | 21.57 | 7.82 | 27.79 | 9.38 | −2.28 | 38 | .03* |
| CO (l/min) | 3.90 | 1.39 | 3.84 | 1.52 | .12 | 40 | .91 |
| CI (l/min/m²) | 2.64 | 3.12 | 2.07 | .74 | .86 | 25 | .40 |
| SVR (dynes/s/cm$^{-5}$) | 1556.14 | 528.60 | 1652.87 | 591.66 | −.56 | 40 | .58 |
| S$\bar{v}$O$_2$ (%) | 59.48 | 12.70 | 58.37 | 11.47 | .29 | 40 | .77 |
| Hemoglobin (gm/dl) | 12.96 | 1.96 | 12.52 | 1.41 | .83 | 40 | .41 |
| Hematocrit (%) | 38.77 | 5.81 | 37.45 | 4.24 | .82 | 40 | .42 |
| SaO$_2$ (%) | 96.30 | 3.15 | 96.10 | 2.02 | .24 | 40 | .81 |
| DO$_2$ (mL/min) | 654.64 | 266.53 | 599.80 | 185.74 | .76 | 40 | .45 |
| VO$_2$ (mL/min) | 226.87 | 65.09 | 222.39 | 58.33 | .23 | 40 | .82 |

EF = ejection fraction; RA = right arterial pressure; PCWP = pulmonary capillary wedge pressure; CO = cardiac output; CI = cardiac index; SVR = systemic vascular resistance; S$\bar{v}$O$_2$ = mixed venous oxygen saturation; SaO$_2$ = arterial oxygen saturation; DO$_2$ = oxygen delivery; VO$_2$ = oxygen consumption.
$^a$t test, comparisons between group 1 and group 2.
*$p < .05$.

With the use of a two-group experimental design, data were measured in all of the three possible positions (supine, right lateral, and left lateral). The numeric value of each variable at each data collection time was entered into the data analysis program. Missing data points were coded as missing rather than substituting mean values. Statistical analysis was performed using the SAS statistical package (SAS Institute, Cary, NC).

The first objective of the study concerned the main effect of the within-subject differences in S$\bar{v}$O$_2$ between supine and lateral positions. This effect was tested using a repeated-measures multivariate analysis of variance that included one between-group factor and two within-group factors. The between-group factor was position order (supine, right lateral; or supine, left lateral). The within-subject factors were position (supine, right lateral, or left lateral) and timing of measurement. A multivariate analysis of variance with repeated measures was performed to rule out alternative explanations, such as order and specific lateral position effects. For the second objective, a stepwise regression was performed with S$\bar{v}$O$_2$ as the dependent variable and variables of DO$_2$ (CO, hemoglobin, SaO$_2$) and VO$_2$ as the independent variables. The stepwise regression included data from the 3-minute postposition change. A p value of $\leq .05$ was used in all analyses as the criterion for significance.

**Results**

A significant difference occurred in S$\bar{v}$O$_2$ among the three positions across time, ($F(7,266) = 26.27$; $p = .0001$). Figure A10–1 illustrates the mean S$\bar{v}$O$_2$ values for each position. When patients were turned laterally, there was a decrease in S$\bar{v}$O$_2$ at 1 minute in both the right lateral and left lateral positions. The decrease in S$\bar{v}$O$_2$ at 1 minute after positioning represents a percent change of 8.5% from baseline in the right lateral position and 11.3% from baseline in the

**FIGURE A10-1**    **Changes in mixed venous oxygenation saturation ($S\bar{v}O_2$) over time by position. Subjects were positioned in the right or left lateral position immediately after baseline measurements at time 0. Values are *M* $\pm$ *SEM* and represent actual decreases in $S\bar{v}O_2$ (%) from baseline values. Circle, supine position; triangle, right lateral position; square, left lateral position. (Adapted with permission from Gawlinski, A., & Dracup, K. [1998, Sept./Oct.]. Effect of positioning on $S\bar{v}O_2$ in the critically ill patient with a low ejection fraction. *Nursing Research, 47*[5], 293–299.)**

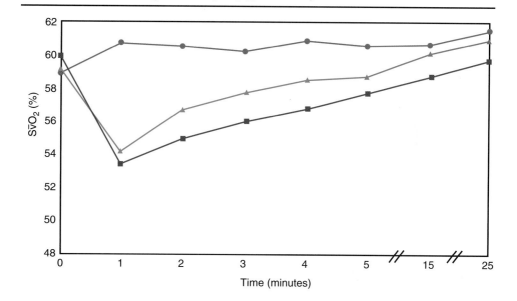

left lateral position. $S\bar{v}O_2$ gradually returned to baseline within 5 minutes.

Comparisons were made across time (each time compared with baseline) and within each position. Because multiple comparisons were made, a level of significance at $p < .002$ was chosen on the basis of the Bonferroni inequality. There was a significant difference ($p < .002$) between baseline and 1 minute to 2 minutes after positioning in the right lateral position. There was a significant difference ($p < .002$) between baseline and 1 minute to 4 minutes after positioning in the left lateral position. Most patients had a decrease in $S\bar{v}O_2$ at 1 minute after each turn and usually returned to their baseline within 5 minutes. $S\bar{v}O_2$ values at 15 minutes and 25 minutes were not statistically different from baseline in either position.

Comparisons of position (supine to right lateral and supine to left lateral) were made at each time period. There were significant differences in $S\bar{v}O_2$ between supine and right lateral positions at 1 minute and 2 minutes after positioning ($p < .002$). There were statistically significant differences in $S\bar{v}O_2$ between supine and left lateral positions from 1 minute to 4 minutes after positioning ($p < .002$). There were no significant differences in $S\bar{v}O_2$ between supine and

right lateral at 3, 4, 5, 15, and 25 minutes after positioning. There were no significant differences in $S\bar{v}O_2$ between supine and left lateral at 5, 15, and 25 minutes after positioning.

To describe the contribution of variables of $DO_2$ and $VO_2$ to the variance in $S\bar{v}O_2$ in the critically ill patient with a low ejection fraction, two sets of analyses were done. A stepwise multiple regression analysis was conducted with $S\bar{v}O_2$ as the dependent variable and $DO_2$ and $VO_2$ as the predictor variables. The first variable entered into the equation was $DO_2$. $DO_2$ had a significant direct relationship with $S\bar{v}O_2$ and accounted for 31% of the variance of the dependent variable ($p = .0001$). $VO_2$ was entered into the equation next and contributed an additional 54% to the variance of the dependent variable ($p = .0001$) (Table A10–2).

In the second analysis, stepwise multiple regression was conducted using the difference in $S\bar{v}O_2$ from baseline to 3 minutes after positioning as the dependent variable. The differences in the predictor variables $DO_2$ and $VO_2$ from baseline to 3 minutes after positioning were the independent variables. The first variable entered into the equation was $VO_2$. $VO_2$ had a statistically significant relationship with $S\bar{v}O_2$ and

---

**TABLE A10-2 Results of Stepwise Multiple Regression Analysis**

| Step | Order Variable Entered | Increase in $R^2$ | Coefficient | SE | F |
|------|------------------------|-------------------|-------------|-----|---|
| | Contribution of oxygen delivery ($DO_2$) and oxygen consumption ($VO_2$) to mixed venous oxygen saturation ($S\bar{v}O_2$) in the left lateral position 3 minutes after position change ($N = 42$) | | | | |
| 1 | $DO_2$ | .31 | 1.08 | .004 | 18.03* |
| 2 | $VO_2$ | .54 | −.90 | .013 | 141.86* |
| | Contribution of oxygen consumption ($VO_2$) and oxygen delivery ($DO_2$) to the change in mixed venous oxygen saturation ($S\bar{v}O_2$) from baseline to 3 minutes ($N = 42$) | | | | |
| 1 | $VO_2$ | .46 | −.84 | .014 | 33.55* |
| 2 | $DO_2$ | .02 | .22 | .003 | 1.52 |

*$p < .05$.

---

accounted for 46% of the variance ($p = .0001$). $DO_2$ was entered into the equation in the next step and contributed an additional 2% to the variance in the dependent variable ($p = .2254$) (Table A10–2).

## DISCUSSION

There was a significant change in $S\bar{v}O_2$ after positioning in critically ill patients with a low ejection fraction. There were no significant differences in $S\bar{v}O_2$ in patients turned first from supine to the right lateral position versus from supine to the left lateral position. The finding of an 8.5% to 11.3% decrease in $S\bar{v}O_2$ and return to baseline within 5 minutes is comparable to results from other investigators (Peña, 1989; Shively, 1988; Tidwell et al., 1990; Winslow et al., 1990). Three mechanisms can be postulated for the rapid $S\bar{v}O_2$ decrease with position change. These mechanisms are altered ventilation-perfusion matching in the lungs, altered CO, and increased $VO_2$.

Gravity is a major factor affecting ventilation-perfusion matching. In this study, most patients had left ventricular failure evidenced by high PCWP values and low CO. Left ventricular failure leads to increased pulmonary congestion and can reduce ventilation relative to perfusion. $SaO_2$ levels can be used to assess ventilation-perfusion balance owing to the relationship between $PaO_2$ and $SaO_2$ levels. There was no significant difference in $SaO_2$ levels from baseline to 3 minutes after positioning. Therefore, it is unlikely that decreases in $S\bar{v}O_2$ after positioning were due to ventilation-perfusion imbalance.

Another potential mechanism for the decrease in $S\bar{v}O_2$ after positioning is a change in $DO_2$ due to a change in CO. In the current study of patients with low ejection fraction, there was no significant difference in CO measurements from baseline to 3 minutes after positioning. Therefore, it is unlikely that CO played a role in the observed changes.

The most probable mechanism for the observed rapid decrease in $S\bar{v}O_2$ is increased peripheral use of oxygen due to muscular activity. The muscle movement required for position change increases $VO_2$ (Shively, 1988; Weissman et al., 1984; Winslow et al., 1990), with a consequent decrease in $S\bar{v}O_2$. Other factors known to reduce $S\bar{v}O_2$ are $SaO_2$ and hemoglobin level. $SaO_2$ levels were constant for all patients. Because there was no evidence of bleeding in this sample, hemoglobin levels probably also remained constant. Thus, an increase in $VO_2$ is the most likely cause of the documented decrease in $S\bar{v}O_2$.

The return of S⊽O$_2$ to baseline within 5 minutes indicates that most patients are able to compensate for the increase in VO$_2$ that occurs with position change. Group means tend to mask individual differences, however, especially when moderate to large standard deviations exist, as they did in this study (Winslow et al., 1990). Tests of statistical significance do not provide information about the clinical importance of research findings (Barlow, 1981; LeFort, 1993). A change in S⊽O$_2$ is clinically significant if S⊽O$_2$ is outside the 60–80% normal range and/or the S⊽O$_2$ changes ±5–10% for longer than 5 minutes (Hoyt, Sottile, Durkin, Swain, & McLachlan, 1983). Thus, in this study, S⊽O$_2$ decreases were clinically important in 38% of patients turned to the right lateral position and 48% of patients turned to the left lateral position. For example, one patient had a decrease in S⊽O$_2$ from 54% baseline to 41% when turned to the left lateral position, a change of 24% in S⊽O$_2$. The S⊽O$_2$ increased only to 45% 25 minutes after baseline. The patient's S⊽O$_2$ remained low at 48% after the 15-minute equalization period in the supine position and decreased to 38%, a change of 21% in S⊽O$_2$, at 1 minute after right lateral positioning. Clearly, the change in S⊽O$_2$ was clinically significant for this patient.

In terms of the effect of positioning, nurses should expect an immediate decrease in S⊽O$_2$ of approximately 9% on the average from baseline after positioning and a return to baseline within 4 or 5 minutes. If the S⊽O$_2$ decrease is substantially more than 10% or if the S⊽O$_2$ fails to return gradually to baseline, the patient should be placed in the supine position and the determinants of DO$_2$ and VO$_2$ should be assessed carefully to identify appropriate interventions (Peña, 1989; Winslow et al., 1990).

VO$_2$ accounted for the greatest proportion of the variance in S⊽O$_2$ from baseline to 3 minutes after positioning ($r = .54$). This finding substantiates the hypothesis that the change in S⊽O$_2$ after positioning is primarily due to changes in VO$_2$. Data from the current study indicate that VO$_2$ accounts for the greater proportion of the variance in S⊽O$_2$ after positioning than does DO$_2$.

## References

Barlow, D. H. (1981). On the relation of clinical research to clinical practice: Current issues, new directions. *Journal of Consulting and Clinical Psychology, 49* (2), 147–155.

Baxter Healthcare Corporation. (1991). *Model SAT-2 oximeter/cardiac output operations manual.* Software Version 7.12.

Brunner, L. S., & Suddarth, D. S. (1988). *Textbook of medical nursing* (6th ed.). Philadelphia: Lippincott.

Doering, L., & Dracup, K. (1988). Comparisons of cardiac output in supine and lateral positions. *Nursing Research, 37,* 114–118.

Eggers, G. W. N., DeGroot, W. J., Tanner, C. R., & Lenard, J. J. (1963). Hemodynamic changes associated with various surgical positions. *JAMA, 185,* 81–85.

Epstein, C. D., & Henning, R. J. (1993). Oxygen transport variables in the identification and treatment of tissue hypoxia. *Heart and Lung, 22,* 328–345.

Forrester, J. S., Ganz, W., Diamond, G., McHugh, T., Chonette, D. W., & Swan, H. J. C. (1972). Thermodilution cardiac output determination with a single flow-directed catheter. *American Heart Journal, 83,* 306–311.

Gillespie, D. J., & Rehder, K. (1987). Body position and ventilation-perfusion relationships in unilateral pulmonary disease. *Chest, 91,* 75–79.

Hoyt, J. V., Sottile, F. D., Durkin, C. G., Swain, R. F., & McLachlan, H. D. (1983). Continuous S⊽O$_2$ as predictor of changes in cardiac output: Clinical observations. In J. F. Schweiss (Ed.), *Continuous measurement of blood oxygen saturation in the high risk patient* (p. 55). San Diego, CA: Beach International.

Kadota, L. T. (1986). Reproducibility of thermodilution cardiac output measurements. *Heart and Lung, 15,* 618–622.

Kersten, L. D. (1989). *Comprehensive respiratory nursing. A decision making approach.* Philadelphia: Saunders.

LeFort, S. M. (1993). The statistical versus clinical significance debate. *Image: The Journal of Nursing Scholarship, 25* (1), 57–62.

Liggett, S. B., St. John, R. E., & Lefrak, S. S. (1987). Determination of resting energy expenditure utilizing the thermodilution pulmonary artery catheter. *Chest, 91,* 562–566.

McCarthy, R. T. (1968). The metabolic cost of maintaining five fixed body positions. *Nursing Research, 17,* 539–544.

Nelson, L. D. (1986). Continuous venous oximetry in surgical patients. *Annals of Surgery, 203,* 329–333.

Peña, M. A. (1989). The effect of position change on mixed venous oxygen saturation measurements in open heart surgery patients during the immediate postoperative period. *Heart and Lung, 18,* 305.

Pomes Iparraguirre, H., Giniger, R., Garber, V. A., Quiroga, E., & Jorge, M. A. (1988). Comparison between measured and Fick-derived values of hemodynamic and oximetric values in patients with acute myocardial infarction. *American Journal of Medicine, 85,* 349–352.

Pond, C., Blessios, G., Bowlin, J., McCawley, C., & Lappas, D. G. (1992). Perioperative evaluation of a new mixed venous oxygen saturation catheter in cardiac surgical patients. *Journal of Cardiovascular and Vascular Anesthesia, 6,* 280–282.

Remolina, C., Khan, A. U., Santiago, T. V., & Edelma, N. H. (1981). Positional hypoxemia in unilateral lung disease. *New England Journal of Medicine, 304,* 523–525.

Rivara, D., Artucio, H., Arcos, J., & Hiriart, C. (1984). Positional hypoxemia during artificial ventilation. *Critical Care Medicine, 12,* 436–438.

Shively, M., & Clark, A. P. (1986). Continuous monitoring of mixed venous oxygen saturation: An instrument for research. *Nursing Research, 35,* 56–58.

Shively, M. (1988). Effect of position change on mixed venous oxygen saturation in coronary artery bypass surgery patients. *Heart and Lung, 17,* 51–59.

Stetz, C. W., Miller, R. G., Kelly, G. E., & Raffin, T. A. (1982). Reliability of the thermodilution method in the determination of cardiac output in clinical practice. *American Review of Respiratory Disease, 126,* 1001–1004.

Tidwell, S. L., Ryan, W. J., Osguthorpe, S. G., Paull, D. L., & Smith, T. L. (1990). Effects of position changes on mixed venous oxygen saturation in patients after coronary revascularization. *Heart and Lung, 19*(5), S574–S578.

Varon, J. (1994). *Practical guide to the care of the critically ill patient.* St. Louis, MO: Mosby Year Book.

Vierheller, A. I. (1993). The influence of hemoglobin on oxygen transport. In T. Aherns & K. Rutherford (Eds.), *Essentials of oxygenation* (pp. 33–39). Boston: Jones and Barlett Publishers.

Weissman, C., Kemper, B. A., Damask, M. C., Askanazi, J., Hyman, A. I., & Kinney, J. M. (1984). Effect of routine intensive care interactions on metabolic rate. *Chest, 86,* 815–818.

Winslow, E. H., Clark, A. P., White, K. M., & Tyler, D. O. (1990). Effects of lateral turn on mixed venous oxygen saturation and heart rate in critically ill adults. *Heart and Lung, 19,* S557–S561.

# Fictional Article: Demographic Characteristics as Predictors of Nursing Students' Choice of Type of Clinical Practice

*Abstract: This descriptive study examined predictors of nursing students' choice of field of clinical practice using a convenience sample of 30 baccalaureate students in a midwestern university. Students voluntarily completed a written questionnaire and responded to a subjective question about experiences influencing their choice of field. Students favored acute settings such as intensive care and emergency rooms over less acute settings and their age and self-rating of health were related to these choices. Three types of experiences were described as meaningful contributors to choice of field of practice.*

The nursing shortage is of grave concern to the public and to the profession of nursing itself, and nursing workforce planning is a priority. Nursing workforce planning needs to address numbers of nurses prepared and the level of nursing preparation at the national, as well as the international, level (Hegyvary, 2001; Peterson, 2001). In considering nursing workforce needs, not just the numbers of nurses, but also the choice of clinical practice of those nurses needs to be considered. While declining enrollments in schools of nursing affect the availability of nurses in all settings, settings that are less "popular" among new graduates will be even harder hit by this shortage. This includes long-term health care settings and primary care settings. The needs for nurses in these types of settings vary from country to country. For example, in South Africa the number of nursing positions in hospitals is much smaller than those in primary health clinics. In contrast, in the United States, the aging population makes needs in long-term care facilities greater than those in primary care.

## BACKGROUND

In the United States, the image of nursing to the general public continues to be the dedicated individual providing bedside nursing for acute health problems. Nurse Hathaway in the television show *ER* or the intensive care nurse responding to life-threatening crises are often the only images nursing students have of the field as they begin their education. Even nursing students who think they may be interested in primary care or public health nursing "someday," often plan to do "real nursing" in a hospital first. As long-term planning for the nursing workforce continues, it will be important to recognize which students are more likely to fill gaps in the different and varied fields of nursing practice. This will allow nursing programs to target student recruitment toward those students most likely to move into clinical practice in

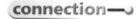

settings with the greatest need. Therefore, this study examined the relationships among nursing students' demographic characteristics and their choice for practice following graduation. Specifically the study addressed the following three questions.

1. Are age, gender, race and marital status associated with choice of clinical practice after graduation?
2. Do older students and those with higher levels of well-being select primary care settings for clinical practice after graduation more often than do younger students and those with lower levels of well-being?
3. What student experiences bring meaning to their choices of field of nursing practice?

## METHODS

### Sample

This study used a convenience sample of undergraduate baccalaureate nursing students in the second semester of the junior year of their program. The students were completing a required research course. The NLN accredited nursing program located in a large midwestern university enrolls 120 undergraduate students each year. The university draws students from throughout the Midwest and reports a generally diverse student body, including representative numbers of Latino and Black students. Programs to earn a bachelor's degree in nursing include a traditional four year program, an RN to BSN program and an LPN to BSN program. Students in all three of these programs take the research course that provided the sample for this study. Participation in the study was voluntary and completion of the questionnaire was anonymous. A total of 30 out of 33 students participated.

### Procedure

An independent faculty member who was not teaching the course administered the questionnaires. The subjects placed completed questionnaires in a sealed box. Subjects were told that the questionnaire was part of the nursing department's efforts to plan future programs. In order to avoid any overt breach of confidentiality, all students remained in the classroom while the questionnaires were being completed and all students placed questionnaires in the box, whether or not they had completed them.

### Measures

The entire questionnaire consisted of three sections. The first section asked about demographic characteristics, the second section asked about postsecondary education, perceived well-being, and planned choice of career, and the last section asked about subjects' preferences of automobiles. The last section was included to be used as a class exercise for the research course itself. Each section is described below.

Demographic characteristics included in this study were age, gender, and marital status. Each of these variables could reflect selected life experiences of students that might influence their choice of practice site after graduation.

The section asking about postsecondary education, well-being and planned career choice included items asking about completion of previous technical programs, or associate or undergraduate degrees. Subjects were asked if they were currently licensed to practice as either an LPN or RN, and to give the total number of years of postsecondary education they had completed. Well-being was measured on a four-point scale rating perceived health as excellent, good, fair, and poor (Kaplan & Camacho, 1983). This single self-report item has been used in a number of studies, including the Human Population Laboratory Studies in Alameda County (Kaplan & Camacho, 1983). The item has demonstrated reliability and validity. It has been shown to be strongly related to a persons' baseline physical health status, and to be significantly related to different mortality rates for both men and women of all ages who perceived their health as excellent versus poor (Kaplan & Camacho, 1983).

The last questions in the second section of the questionnaire asked subjects about their anticipated choice of field of nursing immediately postgraduation and long term. Responses were selected from a list of nursing career options, eliminating the need to code individual responses. Subjects also were asked a single open-ended qualitative question, "What experiences in your life have led to your anticipated choice for field of nursing practice?" Subjects were provided with a single page of lined paper for this response.

The third section of the questionnaire regarding automobile preferences included questions about ownership of an automobile, and a rating on a ten-point scale of the condition of that automobile or how much they want an automobile if they do not own one. Subjects were asked to rank their color preferences for automobiles, and to answer a series of dichotomous questions about their use of various forms of transportation.

The questionnaire was reviewed for face validity by three undergraduate faculty members of nursing. It was then pilot-tested with a sample of five graduate student nurses in their research course in order to assure clarity and relevance. Only very minor changes in language resulted from this pilot test.

### Analysis

Only the results from the first two sections of the questionnaire are reported here. Objective data from the questionnaires were analyzed using SPSS (Statistical Package for the Social Sciences) software program. Written subjective responses were directly transcribed and analyzed using common phenomenological methods (Munhall & Boyd, 1993). Analysis included data reduction, identification of common themes and conclusion drawing and was aided by use of QRS NUD.IST (Non Numerical Unstructured Data Indexing Searching and Theory building Multi-Functional) software program.

## RESULTS

The sample included 30 undergraduate baccalaureate nursing students, 25 female and 5 male. Ninety percent were single ($n = 27$) and the average age of subjects was 23 ($SD = 2$).

The majority of the subjects (60%) were traditional four-year baccalaureate students, however, subjects did represent all of the different programs offered. Many subjects had completed more than three years of postsecondary education ($M = 3.5$, $SD = 1$). Only 20% of subjects rated their own health as "fair or poor." Students' choices of field of nursing immediately postgraduation and for a long-term career are reported in Table B1–1. In both cases, the majority of students selected acute care settings, with an emphasis on intensive care and emergency department care as their anticipated field of nursing.

Choice of field or setting was dichotomized for acute setting versus nonacute setting for additional analysis. There was a significant difference in age of subjects who selected the two settings ($t = 2.4$, $p < .05$), with younger students selecting acute fields of practice. There also was a significant difference in rating of health ($t = 2.1$, $p < .05$), with subjects who rated their health higher choosing acute care fields of practice more than those with lower levels of self-rated health. Lastly, there was an association between type of nursing program and choice of field of study ($\chi^2_{[10, N = 30]}) = 23$, $p < .05$). There was no significant association between race or gender and choice of field of study, and no differences in number of years of postsecondary education and field of study. Logistic regression indicated that only age of subject and rating of health statistically contributed to the odds of selecting a nonacute care field of study

## TABLE **B1-1** Students' Choices of Field of Nursing

| Field of Choice | Number (Percent) Selecting Field Immediately Postgraduation | Number (Percent) Selecting Field as Long-Term Goal |
|---|---|---|
| Intensive Care (adult) | 18 (60%) | 9 (30%) |
| Neonatal or Pediatric Intensive Care | 3 (10%) | 6 (20%) |
| Emergency Department | 3 (10%) | 9 (30%) |
| Obstetrics | 1 (3%) | 0 |
| Medical/Surgical | 0 | 0 |
| Pediatrics | 2 (7%) | 2 (7%) |
| Health Department | 0 | 0 |
| Long-Term Care, Nursing Home | 2 (7%) | 0 |
| Primary Care Clinic or Health Care Provider Office | 1 (3%) | 4 (13%) |

when age, health rating and type of nursing program were entered. One-way analysis of variance indicated that students who were older were more likely to be in the LPN to BSN program or the RN to BSN program.

Analysis of subjective findings yielded three distinct themes that represent the meaning of life experiences related to choice of field of nursing. The themes and selected quotes from subjects are included in Table B1-2. The first theme was personal life experiences such as illness or death of a loved one, or their own acute illness. Subjects described experiences with nurses in the emergency room and the hospital and how these gave unique meaning to the health crisis being faced.

The second theme was direct experiences with family or close friends who provided nursing care in the field chosen by the subject. Subjects described love and respect and a desire to follow in the footsteps of these role models that had influenced their plans for field of nursing.

The last theme was experiences with fictional media including novels, movies and television shows. These subjects described being moved and excited by descriptions or scenes showing nurses providing care in the fields they expected to choose postgraduation.

**TABLE B1-2** Definitions of Themes and Examples That Represent Meaning of Experiences in Relation to Choice of Nursing Field

| Themes | Examples of Experiences |
| --- | --- |
| **Personal life experience:** Direct interactions with health care providers and the health care system surrounding student's own health or that of others | "Seeing how those nurses took care of my mother as she lay there unconscious with so many tubes and machines hooked to her made me decide right then and there that this was what I wanted to do." <br> "It was the nurse holding my hand as the doctor in the emergency room told me about my brother that made it possible for me to keep going. I want to be like that nurse and help others in such terrible times of life." <br> "After I got home from the hospital a nurse came to visit and change my dressing. She was so caring and kind and gentle. Taking nursing into people's homes is what I want to do." |
| **Experiences with nursing role models:** Direct interactions with significant others who are nurses | "My aunt was a nurse. She always was so strong and sure of herself—I wanted to be just like her and work in the emergency department." <br> "In our town Mrs. Timms was the person everyone went to with a question or for help. It seemed like her being a nurse just made her able to help everyone. Mrs. Timms worked in the Health Department Clinic so that seems to me to be a good place to practice nursing." |
| **Experiences with fictional media:** Vicarious experiences of providing nursing care in certain settings as described or depicted in books, television, and movies | "Watching the nurses in *ER*; they always knew what was going on and were really there for the patients—that is why I want to practice in the emergency room." |

## DISCUSSION

Overall, students in this study identified that their choice of nursing field was intensive care and emergency room care. Maternity care and care of children were the second most commonly identified fields, with public health, primary care and long-term care the least frequently chosen. Objectively, the major demographic characteristic that was associated with choice of acute care field of practice was age, with younger nursing students more frequently choosing acute fields compared to older students. Students who were older were more likely to be in the RN to BSN program or the LPN to BSN program, and therefore, type of baccalaureate program was also related to choice of field. Lastly, self-rating of health was related to choice of field of practice, with students who rated themselves in better health being more likely to choose acute care fields.

Subjectively, students described experiences in their personal lives, with role models and with fictional characters as meaningful in their decisions about choice of field. Age of students may very well relate to these types of experiences, since one would expect that older students would be more likely to have a range of personal life experiences with various fields of nursing. Younger students are more likely to have experienced health care primarily in the acute setting, if at all, and may depend on role models and fictional characters more than older students. Certainly, the fictional characters available to these students would create an emphasis on acute settings. The differences in self-rating of health further sup-

port this idea, since students who are in poor health are more likely to have personal experiences with a variety of health care fields, not just acute care. The subjective transcribed data was not connected to the objective demographic data, so it was not possible to explore these possibilities more completely.

Given the changes in health care in this country and throughout the world, and the increased emphasis on primary health care and early discharge from hospitals, it is clear that not all graduates who wish to practice in intensive care and emergency rooms will be able to do so. Nursing programs that are particularly concerned about shortages in nonacute settings may be able to expand this workforce by focusing their recruitment efforts on older students and by further developing or expanding RN to BSN and LPN to BSN programs. In addition, nursing needs to make fields of nursing other than acute care more visible to the public at large in order to widen the number of meaningful experiences nursing students might have that will affect their choice of field of practice.

## References

Hegyvary, S. T. (2001). Editorial: Roots of the shortage. *Journal of Nursing Scholarship, 33*(3), 204.

Kaplan, B. A. & Camacho, T. (1983). Perceived health and mortality: A nine-year follow-up of the Human Population Laboratory cohort. *American Journal of Epidemiology, 111,* 292–304.

Peterson, C. A. (2001). In short supply: Around the work, the need for nurses grows. *American Journal of Nursing, 101*(9), 61.

If the position is taken to implement recruitment strategies focused on older students will the schools of nursing get enough applicants. What of the health and physical abilities of older students. Would this be construed as somehow discriminatory? Logistic regression showed that age and health status affected the students choice of practice. Who is to say that only younger students can work in acute care settings?

Student age should not be used as a criteria for entrance into Nursing Programs. The study consisted of mostly single, young students. It does not significantly address the choices of nursing students after graduation as the sample for the study did not incorporate older students, male/female, married/single.

# APPENDIX C

# Historical Analysis of Siderail Use in American Hospitals

**Barbara L. Brush, Elizabeth Capezuti**

*Purpose:* To explore the social, economic, and legal influences on siderail use in 20th century American hospitals and how use of siderails became embedded in nursing practice.

*Design:* Social historical research.

*Methods:* Numerous primary and secondary sources were collected and interpreted to illustrate the pattern of siderail use, the value attached to siderails, and attitudes about using siderails.

*Findings:* The persistent use of siderails in American hospitals indicates a gradual consensus between law and medicine rather than an empirically driven nursing intervention. Use of siderails became embedded in nursing practice as nurses assumed increasing responsibility for their actions as institutional employees.

*Conclusions:* New federal guidelines, based on reports of adverse consequences associated with siderails, are limiting siderail use in hospitals and nursing homes across the United States. Lowering siderails and using alternatives will depend on new norms among health care providers, hospital administrators, bed manufacturers, insurers, attorneys, regulators, and patients and their families.

Throughout most of the 20th century, the use of siderails as safeguards against patients' falls from hospital beds has spurred debate. Although researchers and practitioners have argued the merits and pitfalls of siderail use, few have explored how use of siderails evolved and gradually became embedded in nursing practice. Raising bed siderails remains the most frequently used intervention to prevent bed-related falls and injuries among hospitalized patients and institutionalized older adults (Capezuti, 2000; Capezuti & Braun, 2001).

Examining the social, economic, and legal influences on siderail use in 20th century American hospitals, we explored the centrality of the hospital bed to the mission and purpose of nursing and the shifting focus of bedside care from patient comfort to patient safety. We argue that use of siderails has been based more on a gradual consensus between law and medicine than on empirical evidence for nursing practice. Nonetheless, nurses, as hospital employees, adopted siderail use as part of their standard of bedside care (Barbee, 1957).

Social historical research methods were used to collect and interpret data. Thus, the pattern of siderail use, the value attached to siderails as an example of benevolent care, and attitudes about raising siderails were examined as they evolved and shifted over time. Primary sources included medical trade catalogs, hospital procedure manuals, newsletters, photography, and other archival materials from the New York Academy of Medicine, the College of Physicians in

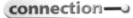
*Journal of Nursing Scholarship, 2001; 33:4, 381–385. © 2001 Sigma Theta Tau International.*

Philadelphia, and the Center for the Study of the History of Nursing at the University of Pennsylvania. Journal articles, government documents, published histories of hospital bed design, and nursing and medical texts provided additional sources of data.

## THE HOSPITAL BED AS CENTRAL TO NURSING'S MISSION

In 1893, Isabel Adams Hampton made clear, in a chapter devoted entirely to hospital beds, that nurses were the overseers of beds and their occupants. As she put it, "A nurse who works over [beds] daily ought to be a fair judge of what is required in the way of a bed for the sick" (Hampton, 1893, p. 75). Hampton charged nurses to coordinate bed type to patient condition, maintain a neat and uniform bed appearance at all times, and ensure patient comfort during the period of recuperation.

In Hampton's day, the ideal bed was 6 feet 6 inches long, 37 inches wide, and 24–26 inches from the floor (Hampton, 1893). Although similar in length and width to standard twin beds in homes, hospital beds were approximately 6–8 inches higher to facilitate patient care and prevent unnecessary strain on nurses. Because beds were a fixed "nursing" height, stools were often used to accommodate patients as they transferred from bed.

Bed height, more than any other bed dimension, has consistently influenced bedside nursing care in American hospitals and long-term care facilities. Bed height and the outcomes of bed-related falls in hospitals have been the basic issues underlying numerous legislative and practice initiatives in the 20th century. Despite changes meant to remedy injurious outcomes from bed-related falls, however, patients falling from high beds are deemed at risk for increased morbidity and mortality (O'Keeffe, Jack, & Lye, 1996). Bed siderails, initially used as a temporary means to prevent confused, sedated, or elderly patients from falling from bed, are now permanent fixtures on most institutional beds (Braun & Capezuti, 2000; Capezuti & Braun, 2001). Their increased use in the latter half of the 20th century reflects a shifting emphasis from patient comfort to patient safety as hospitals, evolving from charitable institutions to modern medical centers, became increasingly subject to litigation (Stevens, 1989).

### "Rendering the Obstinate Docile"

Bed siderails were rarely available on adult hospital beds until the 1930s. More common were cribs or children's beds equipped with full or partial crib sides, which, similar to siderails, were meant to protect infants and young children from falling from or leaving beds unattended. The primary intervention for agitated, confused, or other adults considered at risk of falling from bed was nurses' provision of "careful and continuous watchfulness" (*Merck Manual*, 1934, p. 36).

Haigh and Hayman's (1936) study of 116 "out of bed" incidents at the University Hospital of Cleveland, however, provided early evidence of siderail use to control adult patient behavior and prevent deleterious outcomes. The authors reported that in 31% of bed-related falls at the study institution, patients climbed over siderails, and an additional 7% removed a physical restraint and then proceeded over the rails before falling. Although siderails, as well as rails in combination with restraints, were ineffective in preventing falls or deterring patients from leaving beds unassisted, the nurse and physician authors concluded that siderails were a reasonable precautionary measure against falls from bed as well as necessary adjuncts in "rendering the obstinate docile" (Haigh & Hayman, 1936, p. 45).

When first used, siderails, also known as sideboards or side restraints, were not permanently fastened to hospital beds. Instead, they were accessories that nurses physically attached to beds when they deemed necessary or when prescribed by a physician (Tracy, 1942). Securing these devices was a time-consuming and cumbersome procedure that often required at least two people (Manley, 1944).

In the 1940s, siderail use on adult hospital beds gradually became the subject of legal action against personal injury and death. In 1941, for example, the parents of 21-year-old Edgar Pennington sued Morningside Hospital after their son fell from bed and sustained a fatal head injury (*Morningside Hospital v. Pennington et al.*, 1941). When Mr. Pennington was initially hospitalized, his bed siderails were raised because of his irrational behavior. A few days later and presumably calmer, his side rails were removed and his left leg was chained to the bed instead. The plaintiffs argues that the nurses' failure to maintain side rails on their son's bed caused him to sustain his fatal fall. Whether his leg was still chained to the bed when he was found "with his bloody head on the concrete floor" was unsubstantiated. Ultimately, the case was dismissed.

A year earlier, the surviving husband of Jennie Brown Potter sued the Dr. W.H. Groves Latter-Day Saints Hospital for his wife's fall-related death, claiming that the hospital's failure to attach side boards to her bed constituted negligence. As in *Morningside Hospital v. Pennington et al.* (1941), the court ruled for the defendant, citing lack of evidence that standard of due care required the hospital to place sideboards on patients' beds (*Potter et al. v. Dr. W.H. Groves*, 1940).

### The Nurse's Role in Hospital Safety

By the 1950s, siderail use became more visibly linked to institutional liability. Numerous factors contributed to this transition. First, many states adopted laws overturning charitable hospitals' immunity from the negligence of their employees, necessitating hospitals' purchase of expensive insurance policies (Hayt, Hayt, & Groeschel, 1952). Second, a severe post-war nursing shortage limited nurses' ability to provide previous levels of watchfulness over patients in their charge (Lynaugh & Brush, 1996). Finally, bed manufacturers expanded their focus in advertising to include patient safety along with patient comfort and rest. Consequently, institutional beds equipped with permanent full-length siderails became more readily available (Hospitals, 1954). Nurses raised siderails on patients' beds to reassure the public and hospital administrators that even if nurses were in short supply, at least patients were secure in their beds (Aberg, 1957; Barbee, 1957).

Ludham (1957) reinforced this notion in one of the first reported studies of hospital insurance claims involving bed incidents. In his study of 7,815 "out-of-bed" incidents in California hospitals, Ludham found that, although 63% (4,893) of reported incidents occurred when siderails were raised, claims paid by insurance companies increased ten fold when falls occurred in the absence of raised siderails. The imbalance in jury awards was largely attributed to the perception that raising siderails was a demonstrable effort, however unproved, to protect patients from falls and serious injury. With no supporting evidence, Ludham nonetheless echoed previous claims (Aston, 1955; Price, 1956) that out-of-bed incidents with raised siderails caused less severe injury because patients had something to grasp when falling. He recommended that hospitals establish standing orders or policies requiring siderail use with certain types of patients (e.g., sedated, confused, "older") as a national standard of hospital practice. Locally, the Council on Insurance of the California Hospital Association urged its hospitals to permanently attach siderails to every bed "as rapidly as possible" (Ludham, 1957, p. 47).

Professional journal articles and nursing texts also regularly encouraged nurses to use siderails as part of their therapeutic actions (Aberg, 1957; Harmer & Henderson, 1952; Price, 1954), especially because of the claim that "bedfalls, together with hot-water bottle burns account for more lawsuits involving nurses than all other risks combined" (Hayt, Hayt, Groeschel, & McMullan, 1958, p. 206). Although the standard hospital bed height was "not always comfortable to the patient (but) convenient for the nurse and the doctor" (Harmer & Henderson, 1952, p. 126), siderails, defined as restraints or restrictive devices, were advocated in the prevention of falls and injury from these high beds (Hayt, Hayt, & Groeschel, 1958; McCullough & Moffit, 1949; Price, 1954).

Meanwhile, bed manufacturers continued to sell to "safety-minded hospital administrators" (Hospitals, 1954, p. 197). The Hard Manufacturing Company's "Slida-Side" offered permanent siderails on every hospital bed, and the Inland Bed Company guaranteed portable siderails to "provide safety for your patients, protection for your hospital" (Hospitals, 1954, p. 194). Both the Hall Invalid Bed and the Simmons Vari-Hite bed could be manually lowered from the standard height of 27 inches to the "normal home bed height" of 18 inches (Hospitals, 1950). They were considered safer for two reasons: they eliminated the need for "slipping, tilting footstools" and they allowed patients to get up from a familiar bed height without calling for the nurse (Hospitals, 1950, pp. 87, 102). Thus, and most important, the Simmons Company reported, the Vari-Hite bed reduced "the likelihood of falling and serious injury" (Hospitals, 1950, p. 87).

The Hill-Rom Company also advertised its Hilow Beds as the pinnacle of modernization and fall prevention because the crank-operated bed could be lowered to 18 inches, making patients less likely to misjudge the distance to the floor, lose their balance, and fall (Hospitals, 1955). To make their point that lower beds eliminated the need for full siderails to prevent bed-related falls and injuries, advertisements depicted the Vari-Hite and Hall Invalid beds without siderails and the Hilow Bed with a half rail meant to assist patients to transfer independently.

Despite the availability of lower and variable height beds that eliminated the need for siderails, that were comfortable for patients, and increased nursing efficiency, fixed "nursing height" beds with permanent full-length siderails were used more regularly than were these new inventions (Smalley, 1956). The "common sense" notion that siderails were safety devices led to hospital-wide policies that standardized their use. Because nurses and hospital administrators failed to question siderail efficacy in preventing bedside falls, they also failed to use alternatives. Gradually, hospital-based nurses in the 1950s raised siderails to substitute for their physical presence at the bedside and to protect hospitals' legal interests.

### The Standard of Good Nursing Practice

An escalating nurse shortage in the 1960s and 1970s, coupled with changes in hospital architecture from multipatient wards to semiprivate and private patient rooms, prompted the continued use of siderails, as well as other physical restraints, as substitutes for nursing observation. By the 1980s, falls, especially from beds, were identified as a major hospital liability issue (Rubenstein, Miller, Postel, & Evans, 1983). In 1980 the National Association of Insurance Commissioners reported that falls represented 10% of all paid claims between 1975 and 1978; absence of siderails was identified as a principal justification. As a result, "routine use of bedrails" became "the standard of good nursing practice" (Rubenstein et al., 1983, p. 273).

As siderail use became common nursing practice, particularly to prevent falls among older patients, its scientific rationale was brought into question. Rubenstein and colleagues (1983) at Harvard Medical School labeled the continued use of siderails, in the absence of supporting data, an example of "defensive medicine" (p. 273). In other words, raising siderails was practice based on consensus rather than on scientific evidence. Based largely on legal action against hospitals and their personnel, siderail use became a means to promote patients' "right" to safety during hospitalization and nurses' "responsibility" to keep patients safe (Anonymous, 1984; Horty, 1973).

Shifting decisions about patient safety to nurses shifted liability from physicians to institutions. As a result, institutions took greater precautions to ensure that patients, especially the elderly, did not fall. Raising siderails for individuals deemed vulnerable to injury or death, in addition to using physical restraints for immobilization, reinforced the opinion that siderails and restraints were benevolent interventions (Cohen & Kruschwitz, 1997; Strumpf & Tomes, 1993). Although nurse attorney Jane Greenlaw found medication to be a major cause of negligence related to siderail use, she also noted the importance of a patient's mental state in determining liability. She noted, "Where it can be shown that a patient was senile, irrational, confused, or otherwise impaired, this can affect the hospital's duty to safeguard the patient" (Greenlaw, 1982, p. 125), and "Nursing responsibility to evaluate each person's safety and to act accordingly, regardless of whether the attending physician has done so" (Greenlaw, 1982, p. 127).

The nurse's duty to render independent judgment about siderail use was evident in the 1977 fall and injury case of John Wooten. Eighty-three-year-old Wooten suffered a severe head injury after falling at the Memphis, Tennessee Veterans Administration Hospital. During the evening, Wooten had risen from his bed unattended and walked a short distance before falling. Before the fall, Wooten's physician deemed him "stable" and gave an order for "bedrest with bedside commode and up in chair three times per day" (Anonymous, 1984, p. 4). Despite the physician's medical opinion, the U.S. District Court of Tennessee ruled that hospital personnel were negligent in caring for Wooten because his condition "mandated the use of siderails" (Anonymous, 1984, p. 4). The Court held that raised siderails was a reminder for patients to call nurses when they needed assistance to transfer from bed. Moreover, because

Wooten was "older", he was at greater risk for confusion and disorientation. The Court awarded $80,000 in damages.

In 1981, 80-year-old Esther Polonsky was injured during her stay at Union Hospital in Lynn, Massachusetts, upon attempting to use the bathroom during the night. Several hours before the incident, the nurse had administered 15 milligrams of Dalmane to Polonsky to aid sleep. The Appeals Court of Massachusetts found that because the nurse failed to raise her bed siderails, a confused and disoriented Polonsky fell and fractured her right hip. She recovered $20,000 in damages (Regan, 1981).

While Polonsky's fall was directly linked to her medication, the case of Catherine Kadyszeski, like that of Wooten, illustrated the ageism often associated with siderail use (Tammelleo, 1995). Kadyszeski was 67 years old in 1985 when she fractured her left hip in a bathroom-related fall at New York's Ellis Hospital. Although heavily sedated with Demerol, Vistaril, and Phenobarbital, Kadyszeski did not win her claim on the basis of oversedation. Rather, the hospital was found negligent for failing to comply with its own rule that siderails be raised for all patients over age 65.

The continued use of siderails and restraints in the 1980s and 1990s sharply contrasted with new ideas about the importance of mobility during recuperation from acute illness or surgery (Allen, Glasziou, & Del Mar, 1999). The trend toward decreasing bedrest and increasing ambulation in hospitalized patients did not translate to the care of frail elders (Creditor, 1993; Sager et al., 1996). While younger patients' beds were equipped with half instead of full-length siderails to facilitate transfers, older patients continued to be immobilized in bed, in large part because nurses equated full siderail use with greater patient protection (Rubenstein et al., 1983). Even as negative consequences of immobilizing hospital elders, such as deconditioning, pressure ulcers, and pneumonia, were reported in the literature (Creditor, 1993; Hoenig & Rubenstein, 1991; Inouye et al., 1993; Sager et al., 1996), the use of siderails in this population did not abate.

### Implications for Current Practice

Reports of siderail-related entrapment injuries and deaths over the past decade (Food and Drug Administration, 1995; Parker & Miles, 1997; Todd, Ruhl, & Gross, 1997) continue to challenge perceptions of siderails as safety devices. Many legal claims are not being won against hospitals for siderail misuse (Braun & Capezuti, 2000; Capezuti & Braun, 2001). The Health Care Finance Administration (HCFA) has issued surveyor guidelines redefining siderails as restraints when they impede the patient's desired movement or activity, such as getting out of bed (U.S. Department of Health & Human Services, 2000). The fundamental goal of these guidelines is to deter health care providers from routinely using siderails. Instead, they encourage a thorough assessment of patients' individualized needs and consideration of alternative interventions to siderail use (Capezuti et al., 1999; Capezuti, Talerico, Strumpf, & Evans, 1998). More broadly, the HCFA guidelines will likely influence siderail use by hospitals accredited through the Joint Commission on Accreditation of Healthcare Organizations (JCAHO). Because JCAHO must, at a minimum, meet applicable federal law and regulation, new standards, consistent with HCFA regulations, likely will be promulgated in the near future (Capezuti & Braun, 2001).

The acceptance and use of alternatives to siderails, however, will depend on a new consensus among health care providers, hospital administrators, bed manufacturers, insurers, attorneys, regulators, and patients and their families. To reach consensus, all parties need to understand how and why siderails became common practice in the first place and why, despite evidence to the contrary, they remain firmly entrenched as acceptable bedside care. Rethinking siderail use, especially with the elderly, will require new incentives for their discontinuation. The new guidelines by HCFA (U.S. Department of Health & Human Services, 2000) are a beginning step in this direction.

Bed manufacturers have also reintroduced adjustable low-height beds, similar to the models first proposed in the 1950s. These "new" beds, as well as siderails with narrower rail gaps, will be on the market over the next few years. Financing the purchase of this equipment and retrofitting outdated bed systems will likely raise new concerns about siderail-related liability (Braun & Capezuti, 2000; Capezuti & Braun, 2001). Nurse researchers are in key positions to evaluate how legislative and manufacturing trends affect clinical outcomes.

Given the gradual evolution of siderail use in American hospitals, nurses can anticipate that attitudes and practices about use of siderails will not change quickly or easily. Changing views and practices of siderail use will require reinterpretation of nursing care standards and benevolent care. Given the evidence of these shifting ideas and practices now (Braun & Capezuti, 2000; Capezuti & Braun, 2001; Capezuti, 2000; Donius & Rader, 1994), new perceptions and habits will develop. Those changes should be based on empirical outcomes rather than on untested consensus.

## References

Aberg, H.L. (1957). The nurse's role in hospital safety. *Nursing Outlook, 5,* 160–162.

Allen, C., Glasziou, P., & Del Mar, C. (1999). Bed rest: a potentially harmful treatment needing more careful evaluation. *Lancet, 354,* 1229–1233.

Anonymous. (1984, February). Hospital policy re: "siderails" nurses' responsibility [Journal article]. *Regan Report on Nursing Law, 24,* 4.

Aston, C.S., Jr. (1955). Grasping bars means added safety. *Hospitals, 29,* 102–104.

Barbee, G.C. (1957). More about bedrails and the nurse. *American Journal of Nursing, 57,* 1441–1442.

Braun, J.A., & Capezuti, E. (2000). The legal and medical aspects of physical restraints and bed siderails and their relationship to falls and fall-related injuries in nursing homes. *DePaul Journal of Healthcare Law, 3,* 1–72.

Capezuti, E. (2000). Preventing falls and injuries while reducing siderail use. *Annals of Long-Term Care, 8*(6), 57–63.

Capezuti, E., Bourbonniere, M., Strumpf, N., & Maislin, G. (2000). Siderail use in a large urban medical center (Abstract). *The Gerontologist, 40* (Special Issue, 1), 117.

Capezuti, E., & Braun, J.A. (2001). Medicolegal aspects of hospital siderail use. *Ethics, Law, and Aging Review, 7,* 25–57.

Capezuti, E., Talerico, K.A., Cochran, I., Becker, H., Strumpf, N., & Evans, L. (1999). Individualized interventions to prevent bed-related falls and reduce siderail use. *Journal of Gerontological Nursing, 25,* 26–34.

Capezuti, E., Talerico, K.A., Strumpf, N., & Evans, L. (1998). Individualized assessment and intervention in bilateral siderail use. *Geriatric Nursing, 19*(6), 322–330.

Cohen, E.S., & Kruschwitz, A.L. (1997). Restraint reduction: Lessons from the asylum. *Journal of Ethics, Law, and Aging, 3,* 25–43.

Creditor, M.C. (1993). Hazards of hospitalization of the elderly. *Annals of Internal Medicine, 118,* 219–223.

Donius, M., & Rader, J. (1994). Use of siderails: Rethinking a standard of practice. *Journal of Gerontological Nursing, 20,* 23–27.

Food and Drug Administration. (1995, August 23). *FDA Safety Alert: Entrapment hazards with hospital bed side rails.* Rockville, MD: U.S. Dept. of Health and Human Services, Public Health Service, Center for Devices and Radiological Health.

Greenlaw, J. (1982, June). Failure to use siderails: When is it negligence? *Law, Medicine & Health Care, 10*(3), 125–128.

Haigh, C., & Hayman, J.M., Jr. (1936). Why they fell out of bed. *The Modern Hospital, 47,* 45–46.

Hampton, I.A. (1893). *Nursing: Its principles and practice.* Philadelphia: W.B. Saunders.

Harmer, M., & Henderson, V. (1952). *Textbook of the principles and practice of nursing.* New York: Macmillan.

Hayt, E., Hayt, L.R., & Groeschel, A.H. (1952). *Law of hospital and nurse.* New York: Hospital Textbook Co.

Hayt, E., Hayt, L.R., Groeschel, A.H., & McMullan, D. (1958). *Law of hospital and nurse.* New York: Hospital Textbook Co.

Hoenig, H.M., & Rubenstein, L.Z. (1991). Hospital-associated deconditioning and dysfunction. *Journal of the American Geriatrics Society, 39,* 220–222.

*Hospitals.* (1950). Hall Invalid Bed; Simmons Vari-Hite [Advertisements]. *Hospitals, 24,* 86–87, 102.

*Hospitals.* (1954). Inland Bed Company; Hard Slida-Side [Advertisements]. *Hospitals, 28,* 19, 197.

*Hospitals.* (1955). Hill-Rom Hilow Beds [Advertisement]. *Hospitals, 29,* 161.

Horty, J.F. (1973). Hospital has duty to maintain premises, but employees have duty to be cautious. *Modern Hospital, 120,* 50.

Inouye, S.K., Wagner, D.R., Acampora, D., Horwitz, R.I., Cooney, L.M., Hurst, L.D., et al. (1993). A predictive index for functional decline in hospitalized elderly medical patients. *Journal of General Internal Medicine, 8,* 645–652.

Joint Commission on Accreditation of Healthcare Organizations (JCAHO). (1996). Comprehensive accreditation manual for hospitals (restraint and seclusion standards plus scoring: Standards TX7.1–TX7.1.3.3, 191–193j). Oakbrook Terrace, IL: Author.

Ludham, J.E. (1957). Bedrails: Up or down? *Hospitals, 31,* 46–47.

Lynaugh, J.E., & Brush, B.L. (1996). *American nursing: From hospitals to health systems.* Cambridge, MA: Blackwell.

Manley, M.E., & The Committee on Nursing Standards, Division of Nursing, Department of Hospitals. (1944). Chapter VI: Preparation and care of beds. In *Standard Nursing Procedures of the Department of Hospitals, City of New York* (109–125). New York: Macmillan.

Merck & Company. (1934). *The Merck manual of therapeutics and materia medica* (6th edition). Rahway, NJ: Author.

McCullough, W., & Moffit, M. (1949). *Illustrated handbook of simple nursing.* New York: McGraw-Hill.

*Morningside Hospital & Training School for Nurses v. Pennington et al.,* 189 Okla. 170, 114P.2d 943 (1941).

National Association of Insurance Commissioners. (1980). *Medical claims: Medical malpractice closed claims, July 1, 1975 through June 30, 1978* (Vol. 2) Brookfield, WI: Author.

O'Keeffe, S., Jack, C.I., & Lye, M. (1996). Use of restraints and bedrails in a British hospital. *Journal of the American Geriatrics Society, 44,* 1086–1088.

Parker, K., & Miles, S.H. (1997). Deaths caused by bedrails. *Journal of the American Geriatrics Society, 45,* 797–802.

*Potter et al. v. Dr. W.H. Groves Latter-Day Saints Hospital,* 99 Utah 71, 103 P.2d 280 (1940).

Price, A.L. (1954). *The art, science and spirit of nursing.* Philadelphia: W.B. Saunders.

Price, A.L. (1956). Short side guards are safer. *Hospital Management, 82,* 86–89.

Regan, W.A. (1981). Legal case briefs for nurses. *Regan Report on Nursing Law, 21,* 3.

Rubenstein, H.S., Miller, F.H., Postel, S., & Evans, H.B. (1983). Standards of medical care based on consensus rather than evidence: The case of routine bedrail use for the elderly. *Law, Medicine & Health Care, 11,* 271–276.

Sager, M.A., Franke, T., Inouye, S.K., Landefeld, C.S., Morgan, T.M., Rudbert, M.A., et al. (1996). Functional outcomes of acute medical illness and hospitalization in older persons. *Archives of Internal Medicine, 156,* 645–652.

Smalley, H.E. (1956). Variable height bed: A study in patient comfort and efficiency in care. *Hospital Management, 82,* 42–43.

Stevens, R. (1989). *In sickness and in wealth: American hospitals in the twentieth century.* New York: Basic Books.

Strumpf, N.E., & Tomes, N. (1993). Restraining the troublesome patient: A historical perspective on a contemporary debate. *Nursing History Review, 1,* 3–24.

Tammelleo, A.D. (1995). Siderails left down—patient falls from bed: "Ordinary negligence" or "malpractice"? *Regan Report on Nursing Law, 36,* 3.

Todd, J.F., Ruhl, C.E., & Gross, T.P. (1997). Injury and death associated with hospital bed side-rails: Reports to the U.S. Food and Drug Administration from 1985–1995. *American Journal of Public Health, 87,* 1675–1677.

Tracy, M.A. (1942). *Nursing: An art and a science.* St. Louis, MO: CV Mosby.

U.S. Department of Health & Human Services. (2000, June). Health Care Financing Administration, guidance to surveyors. Hospital conditions of participation for patients' rights (Rev. 17). Retrieved from http://www.hcfa.gov/quality/4b.htm.

# Sample In-Class Data Collection Tool

This questionnaire is for use in this research class only. Completing the questionnaire is entirely voluntary. If you choose to fill out the questionnaire please answer each question thoughtfully.

### DO NOT PUT YOUR NAME ON THIS FORM

**Section One**
What is your AGE in years? _____

Are you—          MALE   FEMALE (circle one)

What is your MARITAL STATUS? (check one)          ____ Single
                                                  ____ Married
                                                  ____ Divorced or Widowed

**Section Two**
*How many YEARS of school have you *completed* since finishing high school? _____

*In general how would you rate your OVERALL HEALTH? (circle one)
          Excellent          Good          Fair          Poor

*Below you will find a list of possible fields for nursing practice. Please check your ONE FIRST CHOICE for area of practice when you first graduate from this nursing program.

___ Emergency Department
___ Health Department
___ Intensive care of adults
___ Long-Term Care, Nursing Home
___ Medical/Surgical Unit
___ Neonatal or Pediatric Intensive Care
___ Obstetrics
___ Pediatric Unit
___ Primary Care Clinic or Health Care Provider Office

**connection**

\*Below you will find the same list of fields of nursing. This time please check your ONE FIRST CHOICE for practice as a **long-term goal**.

___ Emergency Department
___ Health Department
___ Intensive care of adults
___ Long-Term Care, Nursing Home
___ Medical/Surgical Unit
___ Neonatal or Pediatric Intensive Care
___ Obstetrics
___ Pediatric Unit
___ Primary Care Clinic or Health Care Provider Office

**\*On the blank piece of paper attached to this questionnaire please describe the one major experience in your life that you believe has led you to your first choice of a field of practice in nursing.**

*Section Three*
Do you currently own a car? (check one)     ___ YES     ___ NO

- If "YES" please answer the following questions for the car you own.
- If "NO" please answer the following questions for the car you expect to own in the *immediate* future.

Is the car (check one)     ____NEW     ____ USED

Please **rate** the overall condition of the car you own or expect to own in the immediate future by circling ONE rating from the scale below.

| 1 | 2 | 3 | 4 | 5 | 6 | 7 | 8 | 9 | 10 |
|---|---|---|---|---|---|---|---|---|----|
| Terrible | | | | OK | | | | | Excellent |

Please select below your preferences for the CAR OF YOUR DREAMS.

Color (please write in primary color choice) _____

Type (such as SUV, sedan, convertible) _____

Transmission type (check one)     _____ Automatic     _____ Standard 5 speed

Engine cylinders (check one)     _____ 4 cylinder     _____ 6 cylinder     _____ 8 cylinder

From a range of 0% to 100%, how often do you wear seatbelts while riding or driving in a vehicle? _____ % of the time.


**Thank you for completing this questionnaire that we will use for practice in this class only.**

# In-Class Study Data for Practice Exercise in Chapter 5

| Case Number | Marital Status | Health Rating |
|---|---|---|
| 1 | Single | 4 |
| 2 | Married | 3 |
| 3 | Divorced/widowed | 3 |
| 4 | Married | 2 |
| 5 | Married | 1 |
| 6 | Single | 3 |
| 7 | Single | 1 |
| 8 | Single | 4 |
| 9 | Single | 4 |
| 10 | Divorced/widowed | 3 |
| 11 | Married | 2 |
| 12 | Single | 3 |
| 13 | Single | 3 |
| 14 | Single | 2 |
| 15 | Married | 2 |
| 16 | Married | 3 |
| 17 | Single | 4 |
| 18 | Single | 3 |
| 19 | Divorced/widowed | 3 |
| 20 | Single | 4 |

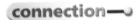

For additional activities go to
http://connection.lww.com/go/macnee.

| Case Number | Marital Status | Health Rating |
|---|---|---|
| 21 | Married | 3 |
| 22 | Married | 2 |
| 23 | Single | 3 |
| 24 | Single | 2 |
| 25 | Single | 3 |
| 26 | Divorced/widowed | 4 |
| 27 | Single | 3 |
| 28 | Single | 3 |
| 29 | Married | 2 |
| 30 | Married | 3 |

# Glossary

**A**

**Abstract:** a summary or condensed version of the research report. Chapter 1, p. 11.

**Aggregated data:** data that are reported for an entire group rather than for individuals in the group. Chapter 11, p. 244.

**Analysis of variance (ANOVA):** a statistical test for differences in the means in three or more groups. Chapter 5, p. 90.

**Anonymous:** a participant in research is anonymous when no one, including the researcher, can link the study data from a particular individual to that individual. Chapter 7, p. 129.

**Assent:** to agree or concur; in the case of research assent reflects a lower level of understanding about the meaning of participation in a study than consent. Assent is often sought in studies that involve older children, or individuals that have a level of impairment that limits their ability but does not preclude their understanding some aspects of the study. Chapter 7, p. 135.

**Assumptions:** ideas that are taken for granted or viewed as truth without conscious or explicit testing. Chapter 11, p. 236.

**Audit trail:** written and/or computer notes used in qualitative research that describe the researcher's decisions regarding both the data analysis process and collection process. Chapter 8, p. 164.

**B**

**Beta (β):** a statistic derived from regression analysis that tells us the relative contribution or connection of each factor to the dependent variable. Chapter 5, p. 93.

**Bias:** some unintended factor that confuses or changes the results of the study in a manner that can lead to incorrect conclusions; bias distorts or confounds the findings in a study, making it difficult to impossible to interpret the results. Chapter 6, p. 107; Chapter 7, p. 135.

**Bivariate:** statistical analysis involving only two variables. Chapter 4, p. 60.

**C**

**Categorization scheme:** an orderly combination of carefully defined groups where there is no overlap amongst the categories. Chapter 4, p. 69.

**Central tendency:** a measure or statistic that indicates the center of a distribution or the center of the spread of the values for the variable. Chapter 4, p. 66.

**Clinical trial:** a study that tests the effectiveness of a clinical treatment; some researchers would say that a clinical trial must be a true experiment. Chapter 9, p. 207.

**Cluster sampling:** a process of sampling in stages, starting with a larger element that relates to the population and moving downward into smaller and smaller elements that identify the population. Chapter 6, p. 111.

**Code book:** a record of the categorization, labeling, and manipulation of data for the variables in a quantitative study. Chapter 11, p. 242.

**Coding:** reducing a large amount of data to numbers or conceptual groups (see data reduction) in qualitative research; giving individual datum numerical values in quantitative research. Chapter 4, p. 70.

# GLOSSARY

**Coercion:** involves some element of controlling or forcing someone to do something. In the case of research, coercion would occur if a patient were forced to participate in a study to receive a particular test or service, or to receive the best quality of care. Chapter 7, p. 130.

**Cohort:** a selected subgroup that reflects a certain characteristic, often age-related. Chapter 6, p. 103.

**Comparison group:** a group of subjects that differs on a major independent variable from the study group, allowing comparison of the subjects in the two groups in terms of a dependent variable. Chapter 9, p. 198.

**Conceptual framework:** an underlying structure for building and testing knowledge that is made up of concepts and the relationships among the concepts. Chapter 10, p. 216.

**Conceptualization:** a process of creating a verbal picture of an abstract idea. Chapter 3, p. 45.

**Conclusions:** the end of a research report that identifies the final decisions or determinations regarding the research problem. Chapter 2, p. 18.

**Confidentiality:** assurance that the identities of participants in the research will not be revealed to anyone else, nor will the information that participants provide individually be publicly divulged. Chapter 7, p. 129.

**Confidence intervals:** the range of values for a variable, which would be found in 95 out of 100 samples; confidence intervals set the boundaries for a variable or test statistic. Chapter 5, p. 82.

**Confirmation:** the verification of results from other studies. Chapter 3, p. 44.

**Confirmability:** the ability to consistently repeat decision-making about the data collection and analysis in qualitative research. Chapter 8, p. 163.

**Construct validity:** the extent to which a scale or instrument measures what it is supposed to measure; the broadest type of validity that can encompass both content- and criterion-related validity. Chapter 8, p. 171.

**Content analysis:** the process of understanding, interpreting, and conceptualizing the meanings imbedded in qualitative data. Chapter 4, p. 69.

**Content validity:** validity that establishes that the items or questions on a scale are comprehensive and appropriately reflect the concept they are supposed to measure. Chapter 8, p. 170.

**Control group:** a randomly assigned group of subjects that is not exposed to the independent variable of interest to be able to compare that group to a group that is exposed to the independent variable; inclusion of a control group is a hallmark of an experimental design. Chapter 9, p. 198.

**Convenience sample:** a sample that includes members of the population who can be readily found and recruited. Chapter 6, p. 106.

**Correlation:** the statistical test used to examine how much two variables covary; a measure of the relationship between two variables. Chapter 5, p. 87.

**Correlational studies:** studies that describe interrelationships among variables as accurately as possible. Chapter 9, p. 198.

**Covary:** when changes in one variable lead to consistent changes in an-

# GLOSSARY

other variable; if two variables covary then they are connected to each other in some way. Chapter 5, p. 87.

**Credibility:** the confidence that the researcher and user of the research can have in the truth of the findings of the study. Chapter 8, p. 165.

**Criteria for participation:** identify how individuals were selected for the study and what were the criteria for participation in the study; describe the common characteristics that define the target population for the study. Chapter 6, p. 103.

**Criterion-related validity:** the extent to which the results of one measure match those of another measure that is also supposed to reflect the variable under study. Chapter 8, p. 170.

**Cross-sectional:** a research design that includes the collection of all data at one point in time. Chapter 9, p. 196.

## D

**Data:** the information collected in a study that is specifically related to the research problem. Chapter 2, p. 21.

**Data analysis:** a process that pulls information together or examines connections between pieces of information to make a clearer picture of all of the information collected. Chapter 2, p. 21.

**Data reduction:** organizing large amounts of data, usually in the form of words, so that it is broken down (or reduced) and labeled (or coded) to identify to which category it belongs. Chapter 4, p. 70.

**Deductive knowledge:** a process of taking a general theory and seeking specific observations or facts to support that theory. Chapter 10, p. 214.

**Demographics:** descriptive information about the characteristics of the people studied. Chapter 4, p. 72.

**Dependent variable:** the outcome variable of interest; it is the variable that depends on other variables in the study. Chapter 4, p. 58.

**Descriptive designs:** research designs that function to portray as accurately as possible some phenomenon of interest. Chapter 9, p. 198.

**Descriptive results:** a summary of results from a study without comparing the results to other information. Chapter 2, p. 21.

**Directional hypothesis:** a research hypothesis that predicts both a connection between two or more variables and the nature of that connection. Chapter 10, p. 225.

**Discussion:** the section of a research report that summarizes, compares, and speculates about the results of the study. Chapter 3, p. 42.

**Design:** the overall plan or organization of a study. Chapter 9, p. 181.

**Distribution:** the spread among the values for a variable. Chapter 4, p. 64.

**Dissemination:** the spreading or sharing of knowledge; communication of new knowledge from research so that it is adopted in practice. Chapter 11, p. 243.

## E

**Electronic databases:** categorized lists of articles from a wide range of journals, organized by topic, author, and journal source available on CDs or online. Chapter 1, p. 10.

**Error:** the difference between what is true and the results from the data collection. Chapter 8, p. 153.

**Ethnographic method:** a set of qualitative research methods used to

# GLOSSARY

participate or immerse oneself in a culture in order to describe it. Chapter 9, p. 192.

**Evidence-based practice:** the conscious and intentful use of research and theory-based information to make decisions about delivery of care to patients. Chapter 1, p. 5.

**Experimental design:** a quantitative research design that includes manipulation of an independent variable, a control group, and random assignment to groups. Chapter 9, p. 200.

**Experimenter effects:** a threat to external validity that occurs when some characteristic of the researchers or data collectors themselves influences the results of the study. Chapter 8, p. 189.

**External validity:** the extent to which the results of a study can be applied to other groups or situations; how accurate the study is in providing knowledge that can be applied outside of or external to the study itself. Chapter 9, p. 184.

## F

**Factor analysis:** a statistical procedure to help identify underlying structures or factors in a measure; it identifies discrete groups of statements that are more closely connected to each other than to all the other statements. Chapter 5, p. 94.

**Field notes:** notes about the participant's tone, expressions, and associated actions, and what is going on in the setting at the same time; they are a record of the researcher's observations about the overall setting and experience of the data collection process while in that setting or field itself; field notes are used to enrich and build a set of data that is thick and dense. Chapter 8, p. 155.

**Frequency distribution:** a presentation of data that indicates the spread of how often values for a variable occurred. Chapter 4, p. 64.

## G

**Generalization:** the ability to say that the findings from a particular study can be interpreted to apply to a more general population. Chapter 3, p. 46.

**Generalizability:** the ability to say that the findings from a particular sample can be applied to a more general population; see generalization. Chapter 6, p. 105.

**Grounded theory:** a qualitative research method that is used to study interactions to understand and recognize linkages between ideas and concepts, or to put in different words, to develop theory; the term "grounded" refers to the idea that the theory that is developed is based upon or grounded in participants' reality. Chapter 9, p. 193.

**Group interviews:** the collection of data by interviewing more than one participant at a time. Chapter 8, p. 156.

## H

**Hawthorne effect:** a threat to external validity that occurs when subjects in a study change simply because they are being studied, no matter what intervention is applied; reactivity and the Hawthorne effect are the same concept. Chapter 9, p. 188.

**History:** a threat to internal validity that occurs because of some factor outside those examined in a study that affects the study outcome or dependent variable. Chapter 9, p. 186.

# GLOSSARY

**Historical research method:** a qualitative research method used to answer questions about linkages in the past to understand the present or plan the future. Chapter 9, p. 193.

**Hypothesis:** a prediction regarding the relationships or effects of selected factors on other factors under study. Chapter 2, p. 30.

## I

**Independent variable:** those factors in a study that are used to explain or predict the outcome of interest; independent variables also are sometimes called predictor variables, because they are used to predict the dependent variable. Chapter 4, p. 58.

**Inductive knowledge:** a process of taking specific facts or observations together to create general theory. Chapter 10, p. 214.

**Inference:** the process of concluding something based on evidence. Chapter 4, p. 56.

**Informed consent:** the legal principle that an individual or his or her authorized representative is given all the relevant information needed to make a decision about participation in a research study and is given a reasonable amount of time to consider that decision. Chapter 7, p. 127.

**Instrument:** a term used in research to refer to a device that specifies and objectifies the process of collecting data. Chapter 8, p. 158.

**Instrumentation:** a threat to internal validity that refers to the changing of the measures used in a study from one time point to another. Chapter 8, p. 186.

**IRB:** Institutional Review Board (IRB) is a board created for the explicit purpose of reviewing any proposed research study to be implemented within an institution or by employees of an institution to ensure that the research project includes procedures to protect the rights of its subjects; the IRB is also charged to decide whether or not the research is basically sound in order to ensure potential participants' rights to protection from discomfort or harm. Chapter 7, p. 127.

**Internal consistency reliability:** the extent to which responses to a scale are similar and related. Chapter 8, p. 168.

**Internal validity:** the extent to which we can be sure of the accuracy or correctness of the findings of the study; how accurate the results are within the study itself or internally. Chapter 9, p. 184.

**Internet:** the network that connects computers throughout the world. Chapter 1, p. 8.

**Interrater reliability:** consistency in measurement that is present when two or more independent data collectors agree in the results of their data collection process. Chapter 8, p. 167.

**Items:** the questions or statements included on a scale used to measure a variable of interest. Chapter 8, p. 159.

## K

**Key words:** terms that describe the topic or nature of the information sought when searching a database or the Internet. Chapter 1, p. 10.

**Knowledge:** information that furthers our understanding of a phenomenon or question. Chapter 1, p. 7.

## L

**Likert-type scale:** a response scale that asks for a rating of the item on a continuum that is anchored at either end by opposite responses. Chapter 8, p. 160.

# GLOSSARY

**Limitations:** the aspects of a study that create uncertainty as to the meaning or decisions that can be made from the study; the aspects may refer to the design, sample, or procedures. Chapter 2, p. 20.

**Literature Review:** a synthesis of existing published writings that describes what is known or has been studied regarding the particular research question or purpose. Chapter 2, p. 29; Chapter 10, p. 219.

**Longitudinal research design:** a research design that includes the collection of data over time. Chapter 9, p. 196.

## M

**Matched sample:** the intentful selection of pairs of subjects so that they share certain important characteristics to prevent those characteristics from confusing what is being explained or understood within the study. Chapter 6, p. 109.

**Maturation:** a threat to internal validity that refers to changes that occur in the dependent variable simply because of the passage of time, rather than because of some independent variable. Chapter 8, p. 186.

**Mean:** the arithmetic average for a set of values. Chapter 4, p. 66.

**Measures:** the specific method(s) used to assign a number or numbers to an aspect or factor being studied. Chapter 2, p. 27.

**Measurement effects:** a threat to external validity because various procedures used to collect data in the study changed the results of that study. Chapter 9, p. 188.

**Measure of central tendency:** a measure that shows the common or typical values within a set of values; central tendency measures reflect the "center" of a distribution, or the center of the spread; the mean, the mode and the median are the three most commonly used. Chapter 4, p. 61.

**Median:** a measure of central tendency that is the value in a set of numbers that falls in the exact middle of the distribution when the numbers are in order. Chapter 4, p. 66.

**Member checks:** a process in qualitative research where the data and the findings from analysis of the data are brought back to the original participants to seek their input as to the accuracy and completeness of the data and the interpretation of the data. Chapter 8, p. 165.

**Meta-analysis:** a quantitative approach to knowledge by taking the numbers from different studies that addressed the same research problem and using statistics to summarize those numbers looking for combined results that would not happen by chance alone. Chapter 2, p. 35.

**Methods:** the methods section of a research report describes the overall process of implementing the research study, including who was included in the study, how information was collected, and what interventions, if any, were tested. Chapter 2, p. 23.

**Mixed methods:** some combination of research methods that differ in relation to the function of the design, the use of time in the design, or the control included in the design. Chapter 9, p. 205.

**Mode:** the value for a variable that occurs most frequently. Chapter 4, p. 66.

**Model:** the symbolic framework for a theory or a part of a theory. Chapter 9, p. 199.

**Mortality:** a threat to internal validity that refers to the loss of subjects from a study due to a consistent factor that is related to the dependent variable. Chapter 9, p. 186.

# GLOSSARY

**Multifactorial:** a study that has a number of independent variables that are manipulated. Chapter 9, p. 201.

**Multivariate:** more than two variables; multivariate studies examine three or more factors and the relationships among the different factors. Chapter 2, p. 23.

### N

**Nondirectional hypothesis:** a research hypothesis that predicts a connection between two or more variables but does not predict the nature of that connection. Chapter 10, p. 225.

**Nonparametric:** a group of inferential statistical procedures that are used with numbers that do not have the bell-shaped distribution or that are categorical or ordinal variables. Chapter 5, p. 84.

**Nonprobability sampling:** a sampling approach that does not necessarily assure that everyone in the population has an equal chance of being included in the study. Chapter 6, p. 107.

**Normal curve:** a type of distribution for a variable that is shaped like a bell and that is symmetrical. Chapter 4, p. 65.

**Novelty effects:** a threat to external validity that occurs when the knowledge that what is being done is new and under study somehow affects the outcome, either favorably or unfavorably. Chapter 9, p. 188.

**Null hypothesis:** a statistical hypothesis that predicts that there will be no relationship or difference in selected variables in a study. Chapter 5, p. 95.

### O

**Operational definition:** a variable that is defined in specific, concrete terms of measurement. Chapter 8, p. 151.

### P

**P-value:** a numerical statement of the percentage of the time the results reported would have happened by chance alone. For example, a p-value of .05 means that in only 5 out of 100 times would one expect to get the results by chance alone. Chapter 2, p. 22.

**Parametric:** a group of inferential statistical procedures that can be applied to variables that are: 1) normally distributed and 2) interval or ratio numbers such as age or intelligence score. Chapter 5, p. 84.

**Participant observation:** a qualitative method where the researcher intentionally imbeds himself or herself into the environment from which data will be collected; the researcher becomes a participant himself or herself. Chapter 8, p. 156.

**Peer review:** the critique of scholarly work by two or more individuals who have at least equivalent knowledge regarding the topic of the scholarly work as the author of that work. Chapter 10, p. 221.

**Phenomenology:** a qualitative method used to increase understanding of experiences as perceived by those living the experience; assumes that lived experience can be interpreted or understood by distilling the essence of that experience. Chapter 9, p. 190.

**Pilot study:** a small research study that is implemented for the purpose of developing and demonstrating the effectiveness of selected measures and methods. Chapter 11, p. 248.

**Population:** the entire group of individuals about whom we are interested in gaining knowledge. Chapter 6, p. 102.

**Power analysis:** a statistical procedure that allows the researcher to

# GLOSSARY

compute the size of a sample needed to detect a real relationship or difference if it exists. Chapter 6, p. 119.

**Predictor variable:** a factor or factors in a study that are expected to affect the dependent variable in a specified manner; predictor variables are also called independent variables. Chapter 4, p. 58.

**Pre–post testing:** a research design that includes an observation both before and after the intervention. Chapter 9, p. 200.

**Primary source:** use of a source of information as it was originally written or communicated. Chapter 10, p. 220.

**Printed indexes:** written lists of professional articles that are organized and categorized by topic and author, covering the time period from 1956 forward. Chapter 1, p. 8.

**Probability:** the percent of the time the results found would have happened by chance alone. Chapter 5, p. 82.

**Probability sampling:** strategies to assure that every member of a population has an equal opportunity to be in the study. Chapter 6, p. 109.

**Problem:** section of a research report that describes the gap in knowledge that will be addressed by the research study, or a statement of the general gap in knowledge that will be addressed in a study. Chapter 2, p. 29.

**Procedures:** specific actions taken by researchers to gather information about the problem or phenomenon being studied. Chapter 2, p. 26.

**Prospective:** a research design that collects data about events or variables moving forward in time. Chapter 9, p. 196.

**Purpose:** a section of a research report that describes the specific factors that will be examined in the research study. Chapter 10, p. 216.

**Purposive sample:** inclusion in a study of participants who are intentionally selected because they have certain characteristics that are related to the purpose of the research. Chapter 6, p. 107.

## Q

**Qualitative methods:** approaches to research that focus on understanding the complexity of humans within the context of their lives and tend to focus on building a whole or complete picture of a phenomenon of interest; qualitative methods involve the collection of information as it is expressed naturally by people within the normal context of their lives. Chapter 2, p. 24.

**Quality improvement:** a process of evaluation of health care services to see if they meet specified standards or outcomes of care. Chapter 12, p. 260.

**Quantitative methods:** approaches to research that focus on understanding and breaking down the different parts of a picture to see how they do or do not connect; quantitative methods involve the collection of information that is very specific and limited to the particular pieces of information being studied. Chapter 2, p. 24.

**Quasi-experimental design:** a research design that includes manipulation of an independent variable but will lack either a control group or random assignment. Chapter 9, p. 201.

**Questionnaire:** a written measure that is used to collect specific data, usually offering closed or forced choices for answers to the questions. Chapter 8, p. 159.

**Quota sampling:** selection of individuals from the population who have one or more characteristics that are important to the purpose of the

# GLOSSARY

study, and these characteristics are used to establish limits or quotas on the number of subjects who will be included in the study. Chapter 6, p. 108.

**R**

**Random assignment:** ensures that subjects in a study all have an equal chance of being in any particular group within the study. The sample itself may be one of convenience or purposive, so there may be some bias influencing the results. But, since that bias is evenly distributed among the different groups to be studied, it will not unduly affect the outcomes of the study. Chapter 6, p. 115.

**Random sample:** a sample in which every member of the population had an equal probability of being included; considered the best type of sample because the only factors that should bias the sample would be present by chance alone, making it highly likely that the sample will be similar to the population of interest. Chapter 6, p. 109.

**Random selection:** the process of creating a random sample; selection of a subset of the population where all the members of the population are identified, listed, and assigned a number and then some device, such as a random number table or a computer program, is used to select who actually will be in the study. Chapter 6, p. 110.

**Reactivity:** a threat in external validity that refers to subjects' responses to being studied. Chapter 9, p. 188.

**Regression:** a statistical procedure that measures how much one or more independent variables explain the variation in a dependent variable. Chapter 5, p. 91.

**Reliability:** the consistency with which a measure can be counted on to give the same result if the aspect being measured has not changed. Chapter 8, p. 167.

**Repeated measures:** a design that repeats the same measurements at several points in time. Chapter 9, p. 196.

**Replication:** a study that is an exact duplication of an earlier study; the major purpose of a replication study will be confirmation. Chapter 3, p. 44.

**Research design:** the overall plan for acquiring new knowledge or confirming existing knowledge; the plan for systematic collection of information in a manner that assures the answer(s) found will be as meaningful and accurate as possible. Chapter 9, p. 181.

**Research hypothesis:** a prediction of the relationships or differences that will be found for selected variables in a study. Chapter 5, p. 94.

**Research objectives:** clear statements of factors that will be measured in order to gain knowledge regarding a research problem; similar to the research purpose, specific aims or research question. Chapter 10, p. 218.

**Research problem:** a gap in existing knowledge that warrants filling and can be addressed through systematic study. Chapter 10, p. 212.

**Research purpose:** a clear statement of factors that are going to be studied in order to shed knowledge on the research problem. Chapter 10, p. 216.

**Research questions:** statements in the form of questions that identify the specific factors that will be measured in a study and the types of relationships that will be examined to gain knowledge regarding a research problem; similar to the research objectives, purposes, and specific aims. Chapter 10, p. 218.

# GLOSSARY

**Research utilization:** the use of research in practice. Chapter 12, p. 258.

**Response rate:** the proportion of individuals who actually participate in a study divided by the number who agreed to be in a study but did not end up participating in it. Chapter 7, p. 139.

**Results:** a summary of the actual findings or information collected in the research study. Chapter 2, p. 21.

**Retrospective:** a quantitative design that collects data about events or factors going back in time. Chapter 9, p. 196.

**Rigor:** both a strict process of data collection and analysis, and a term that reflects the overall quality of that process in qualitative research; rigor is reflected in the consistency of data analysis and interpretation, the trustworthiness of the data collected, the transferability of the themes, and the credibility of the data. Chapter 8, p. 163.

**Rights of human subjects:** five human rights that have been identified by the ANA guidelines for nurses working with patient information that may require interpretation; they include: the right to self-determination, the right to privacy and dignity, the right to anonymity and confidentiality, the right to fair treatment, and the right to protection from discomfort and harm (ANA, 1985). Chapter 7, p. 126.

**Risk/benefit ratio:** a comparison of how much risk is present for human subjects compared to how much benefit there is to the study. Chapter 7, p. 128.

## S

**Sample:** a subset of the total group of interest in a research study; the individuals in the sample are actually studied to learn about the total group. Chapter 2, p. 24; Chapter 6, p. 103.

**Sampling frame:** the pool of all potential subjects for a study; that is, the pool of all individuals who meet the criteria for the study and, therefore, could be included in the sample. Chapter 6, p. 108.

**Sampling unit:** the element of the population that will be selected for study; the unit depends on the population of interest and could be individuals, families, communities, or outpatient prenatal care programs. Chapter 6, p. 116.

**Saturation:** a point in qualitative research where all new information collected is redundant of information already collected. Chapter 4, p. 71; Chapter 6, p. 113.

**Scale:** a set of written questions or statements that in combination are intended to measure a specified variable. Chapter 8, p. 159.

**Secondary source:** use of someone else's description or interpretation of a primary source. Chapter 10, p. 220.

**Selection bias:** refers to subjects having unique characteristics that in some manner relate to the dependent variable, raising a question as to whether the findings from the study were due to the independent variable or to the unique characteristics of the sample. Chapter 9, p. 187.

**Selectivity:** the tendency of certain segments of a population agreed to be in studies. Chapter 7, p. 139.

**Significance:** a statistical term indicating a low likelihood that any differences or relationships found in a study happened by chance alone. Chapter 2, p. 22.

**Skew:** a distribution where the middle of the distribution is not in the

# GLOSSARY

exact center; the middle or peak of the distribution is to the left or right of center. Chapter 4, p. 67.

**Snowball sample:** a strategy to get individuals in a study that starts with one participant or member of the population and uses that member's contacts to identify other potential participants in the study. Chapter 6, p. 106.

**Specific aims:** clear statements of the factors to be measured and the relationships to be examined in a study to gain new knowledge about a research problem; similar to research purpose, objectives, or questions. Chapter 10, p. 218.

**Speculation:** a process of reflecting on the results of a study and putting forward some explanation for them. Chapter 3, p. 44.

**Standard deviation:** a statistic that is the square root of the variance; it is computed as the average differences in values for a variable from the mean value; a big standard deviation means there was a wide range of values for the variable; a small standard deviation means there was a narrow range of values for the variable. Chapter 4, p. 63.

**Stratified random sampling:** an approach to selecting individuals from the population by dividing the population into two or more groups based on characteristics that are considered important to the purpose of the study and then randomly selecting members within each group. Chapter 6, p. 110.

**Systematic:** a planned, organized set of actions. Chapter 1, p. 6.

**Systematic reviews:** the product of a process that includes asking clinical questions, doing a structured and organized search for theory-based information and research related to the question, reviewing and synthesizing the results from that search, and reaching conclusions about the implications for practice. Chapter 1, p. 6.

**Systematic sample:** an approach to selection of individuals for a study where the members of the population are identified and listed and then members are selected at a fixed interval (such as every fifth or tenth individual) from the list. Chapter 6, p. 111.

## T

**Testing:** a threat to internal validity where there is a change in a dependent variable simply because it is being measured or due to the measure itself. Chapter 9, p. 186.

**Test–retest reliability:** consistency in the results from a test when individuals fill out the questionnaire or scale at two or more time points that are close enough together that we would not expect the "real" answers to have changed. Chapter 8, p. 168.

**Theory:** an abstract explanation describing how different factors or phenomena relate. Chapter 2, p. 29; Chapter 10, p. 213.

**Theoretical framework:** an underlying structure that describes how abstract aspects of a research problem interrelate based on developed theories. Chapter 10, p. 216.

**Themes:** results in qualitative research that are ideas or concepts that are implicit in the data and are recurrent throughout the data; abstractions that reflect phrases, words, or ideas that appear repeatedly as a researcher analyzes what people have said about a particular experience, feeling, or situation. A theme summarizes and synthesizes discrete ideas or phrases to create a picture out of the words that were collected in the research study. Chapter 2, p. 21; Chapter 4, p. 70.

# GLOSSARY

**Theoretical definition:** a conceptual description of a variable. Chapter 8, p. 151.

**Transferability:** the extent to which the findings of a qualitative study are confirmed or seem applicable for a different group or in a different setting from where the data was collected. Chapter 8, p. 164.

**Triangulation:** a process of using more than one source of data to include different views, or literally to look at the phenomenon from different angles. Chapter 8, p. 165.

**Trustworthiness:** the honesty of the data collected from or about the participants. Chapter 8, p. 163.

**t-test:** a statistic that tests for differences in means on a variable between two groups. Chapter 5, p. 86.

## U

**Univariate:** information about only one variable. Chapter 4, p. 59.

**Unstructured interviews:** questions asked in an informal open fashion without a previously established set of categories or assumed answers, used to gain understanding about a phenomenon or variable of interest. Chapter 8, p. 155.

## V

**Validity:** how accurately a measure actually yields information about the true or real variable being studied. Chapter 8, p. 169.

**Variable:** some aspect of interest that differs among different people or situations; something that varies: it is not the same for everyone in every situation. Chapter 4, p. 58.

**Variance:** the diversity in data for a single variable; a statistic that is the squared deviations of values from the mean value and reflects the distribution of values for the variable. Chapter 4, p. 61.

**Visual analog:** a response scale that consists of a straight line of a specific length that has extremes of responses at either end but does not have any other responses noted at points along the line. Subjects are asked to mark the line to indicate where they fall between the two extreme points. Chapter 8, p. 161.

## W

**Withdrawal:** a right of human subjects to stop participating in a study at any time without penalty until the study is completed. Chapter 7, p. 130.

# INDEX

Note: Page numbers followed by f indicate figures; those followed by t indicate tables, and those followed by b indicate boxed material.